An Inner Approach to Cranial Osteopathy

of related interest

**Cranial Osteopathy: Principles
and Practice – Volume 1**
TMJ and Mouth Disorders, and Cranial
Techniques, Fourth Edition
Torsten Liem
Forewords by Jean Pierre Barral,
Fred L. Mitchell Jnr. and Richard A. Feely
ISBN 978 1 91342 671 2
eISBN 978 1 83997 612 4

**Cranial Osteopathy: Principles
and Practice – Volume 2**
Special Sense Organs, Orofacial Pain,
Headache, and Cranial Nerves, Fourth Edition
Torsten Liem
Forewords by Jean Pierre Barral,
Fred L. Mitchell Jnr. and Richard A. Feely
ISBN 978 1 91342 669 9
eISBN 978 1 83997 615 5

Cranio-Sacral Integration
Foundation, Second Edition
Thomas Attlee, D.O., R.C.S.T.
ISBN 978 1 84819 361 1
eISBN 978 0 85701 320 0

The Fascial Distortion Model
Philosophy, Principles and Clinical Applications
Todd Capistrant, Georg Harrer and Thomas Pentzer
Foreword by Ole Saether
ISBN 978 1 91208 556 9
eISBN 978 1 91208 557 6

Osteopathy and Obstetrics, Second Edition
Stephen Sandler
Foreword by Eric Jauniaux
ISBN 978 1 91342 623 1
eISBN 978 1 91342 624 8

The Five Osteopathic Models
Rationale, Application, Integration: From an
Evidence-Based to a Person-Centered Osteopathy
*Ray Hruby, Paolo Tozzi, Christian
Lunghi and Giampiero Fusco*
ISBN 978 1 90914 168 1
eISBN 978 1 90914 169 8

An **INNER APPROACH** to **CRANIAL OSTEOPATHY**

Timothy Marris

Forewords by Hollis H. King and Liz Hayden

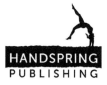
HANDSPRING PUBLISHING

First published in Great Britain in 2023 by Handspring Publishing,
an imprint of Jessica Kingsley Publishers
Part of John Murray Press

Copyright © Timothy Marris 2023

Foreword copyright © Hollis H. King 2023
Foreword copyright © Liz Hayden 2023

Disclaimer: This book is intended to convey inspiration and information to the reader. It is not intended
for medical diagnosis or treatment. The reader should seek appropriate professional care and attention
for any specific healthcare needs. The exercises in this book are for qualified practitioners only, who
have a current and valid professional indemnity insurance. Neither the author nor the publisher has any
responsibility for your work with your model at the treatment table in respect of the practical exercises
accessed via the QR codes in this book. The author has taken great care when creating these audio files, to
make them as useful and beneficial to you as possible but cannot be held responsible for your use of them.

A CIP catalogue record for this title is available from the British Library and the Library of Congress

ISBN 978 1 91342 637 8
eISBN 978 1 91342 638 5

Printed and bound in Great Britain by CPI Group Ltd

Jessica Kingsley Publishers' policy is to use papers that are natural, renewable and recyclable
products and made from wood grown in sustainable forests. The logging and manufacturing
processes are expected to conform to the environmental regulations of the country of origin.

Jessica Kingsley Publishers
Carmelite House
50 Victoria Embankment
London EC4Y 0DZ

www.handspringpublishing.com

John Murray Press
Part of Hodder & Stoughton Limited
An Hachette UK Company

Contents

Foreword by Hollis H. King

Handspring has published several books in the last few years by British osteopaths that have elucidated osteopathic philosophy and practice with greater insight and explication of principles than any before, except for those by A.T. Still himself. This book by Tim Marris is one such. It is likely that the cranial concept opens more doors for philosophical discourse than most other modalities of osteopathic clinical application because of the need to be centred and focussed on subtle, not-easily palpated structures and somatic dysfunction.

This is both a 'why' and a 'how' book. The why is most illuminating and to me, a seldom presented perspective in teachings on the cranial concept. The how is certainly an intermediate to very advanced set of teachings with something for the osteopath with only one or two cranial courses under their belt, to those with 40-plus years of studying and practising based on the cranial concept, referred to by Tim Marris as Osteopathy in the Cranial Field (OCF). We American osteopathic physicians call it Osteopathic Cranial Manipulative Medicine, a phrase coined to appeal to 'mainstream medicine', but which I think diverts our attention from its true meaning and potential.

Among the 'why' or conceptual discussions are those in Chapter 2. First, we explore the attitude the cranial osteopath would most productively bring to the treatment encounter which is 'Being non-judgemental and without preconceptions' and to think, 'I have no idea what I will feel nor find.' Second, the concept of Centring is described, accompanied by an audio exercise on how to enhance one's clinical focus in practice. Third, drawing on his training and experience with Rollin Becker, DO, we explore the use of 'the third hand', or the 'one between our ears', which is our consciousness. This concept is illustrated by examples throughout the chapter and in the audio exercises. In the mid-1980s, at about the same time as Tim Marris, I had the privilege of training with Rollin Becker, and I can say that Tim has stayed very true to Becker's teaching.

It has been an honour to teach in dozens of basic courses in Osteopathy in the Cranial Field over the last 40 years, and the level of instruction and practice presented in this book are most rare indeed. It may be Tim Marris's psychological training that provides the insights that seamlessly flow from biomechanical aspects of OCF to the point in a treatment where 'You can only be conscious of stillness', '[N]ot a still point but a stillness that *is* [my italics] that individual [patient].' These concepts, so well articulated, are the quintessence of 'an inner approach', and are just a few of the examples of treatment insights offered in this book.

This book truly could be a basic reference for any level of training course on OCF as it covers, in state-of-the-art form, all the necessary anatomy and physiology which are part and parcel of the cranial concept. There are chapters on embryology, bone, fascia and cellular structure, meninges, cerebrospinal fluid, and cranial nerves, comprising both 'why' and 'how' aspects. That is, why the anatomy and physiology are essential to health and healing, and how the practitioner facilitates the recovery of health by application of OCF, amplified and informed by 'the inner approach'.

In contrast to some biodynamic cranial courses, Tim states, 'Where possible use as full a hand contact to the patient as you can.' This contrasts with a propensity in some circles to teach fingertip or distal phalangeal contact. I agree with the author that while it is not always possible when working on the face, there is a fuller palpatory experience and treatment effect by using the whole hand.

The ability to understand and apply the treatment principles described in Chapters 15–18 – Back to the time, The inner relationship of mind, body and emotions, The inner relationship of inter-tissue relationships, and Working at the intracellular level – requires substantial mastery of the preceding lessons to achieve meaningful therapeutic outcomes. Throughout the book there is emphasis on proceeding sequentially, as the principles build on one another and important concepts would be missed if the order of presentation were not followed. In following the order of chapters, the reader is rewarded with a very advanced set of OCF teachings; the dialogue between osteopath and patient transcends verbal discourse, as, by 'asking the right questions', one allows the patient's body to tell its story.

Having also trained and practised as a clinical psychologist before attending osteopathic medical school, I appreciate the very great contribution Chapters 15–18 represent for advanced training in OCF. The discussion in these final chapters, enhanced by the audio exercises, is alone worth the price of the book.

Hollis H. King, DO, PhD
San Diego, California
October 2022

Foreword by Liz Hayden

The practice of osteopathy is both a science and an art, and it takes an osteopath many years of experience to develop and perfect their skills. Every osteopath is different and unique, developing their own individual skills and style of working whilst remaining grounded within the fundamental principles of osteopathy, anatomy and physiology. The aim of a good osteopathic teacher is to inspire the student to continue to learn, to challenge them to refine their knowledge of the body and its internal and external relationships and thus enhance their palpatory skills. This can only help to deepen the efficacy of their osteopathic treatments, to the lasting benefit of their patients.

Tim Marris has a wealth of skill and experience developed over his long career as an osteopath and teacher, and in this book, he takes the reader on an experiential journey deep inside the body. Tim guides the reader in the philosophy and principles of an osteopathic approach to supporting health in the whole body. As a teacher, Tim is able to help other osteopaths develop clarity and specificity in their palpation and stimulate them to continue to question and explore the full potential of osteopathy.

Osteopathy is best known for the treatment of musculoskeletal conditions, but it can be so much more than this. Tim demonstrates in this book that osteopathy is a system of healthcare that engages and facilitates the body's own self-healing ability throughout the whole body, and osteopathic treatment can help a much wider range of symptoms and problems.

Palpation, or our sense of touch, is perhaps the special sense that is least well considered – sight, hearing, balance, smell and taste are more widely recognised. Palpation goes far deeper than tactile sensation through our skin. It also includes proprioception, a whole-body awareness of where we are in space and the relationship of the body and individual structures to their surroundings. In this book Tim helps us to understand and develop our sense of touch and proprioception in relation to the anatomy under our hands.

In developing and perfecting highly skilled palpation, one of the greatest challenges for an osteopath is being able to communicate the fine detail of their practice. Language always seems inadequate when describing the finest of changes in tissue quality or the expression of function that we are privileged to witness with our palpation. We help to assist the body on its journey to improved health by utilising the innate responses and self-correcting ability of the tissues in the body. Tim has the remarkable ability to explain with incredible detail his experiences of palpation and treatment, and is able to pass these on to osteopaths who are still developing those skills.

The inclusion of audio-guided practical exercises is unique in an osteopathic text. Osteopaths learn best from having their hands on the body, and every osteopath needs to develop his or her own palpatory library of experiences, and learn to recognise the unique quality or function of different structures deep inside the body. The guided exercises allow the reader to learn with their hands, following the concepts taught in the text, and to directly embed these concepts in their own experience and practice. This is an invaluable resource and one that can be returned to time and time again.

This book will benefit an osteopath who has some basic skills in the palpation of involuntary motion as taught in Osteopathy in the Cranial Field courses. By far the best way to develop palpatory skills and broaden osteopathic thinking is through attending courses and working with an individual tutor. However, our experiences gained by working with and treating patients who present with innumerable conditions also contribute a huge amount to the development of our palpatory senses. This book is an invaluable resource for self-study that I am sure many osteopaths will value.

Liz Hayden D.O. F.S.C.C.O
Churchdown, Gloucestershire
February 2023

About the Author

Tim Marris has been practising cranial osteopathy since 1978, and lecturing in this approach since 1982. He currently lectures internationally in six countries in Europe and South America. He has spent his whole professional life researching and seeking more profound cranial osteopathic ways to help his patients. He was taught by, and had hands on tutoring, from several of William Sutherland's key students: Drs Rollin Becker, Anne Wales, Robert Fulford, Alan Becker, and Herb Miller. Tim was one of the original faculty members of the Sutherland Cranial College of Osteopathy, which is one of the largest postgraduate osteopathic teaching organisations in the world.

Acknowledgements

I would like to acknowledge the understanding from my loving wife Yanwen, who accepted that I had to spend many hours sitting at a computer keyboard for much of these past two years.

I also am indebted to Alyson Groom, who has read and corrected all my grammatical mistakes in the chapters, of which each chapter had many.

I also thank Nicholas Gosset, with whom I have spent many days regularly over the past six years, to explore osteopathy without conventional boundaries, and to explore my technique ideas which were outside the box of normal cranial osteopathic approaches.

There are many osteopathic teachers, sadly most of whom have passed on to new pastures. Many of these have been quoted in this book in the various chapters.

Lastly, I wish to thank my osteopathic teaching colleagues who have enriched my osteopathic journey, and my osteopathic students who inspired me to write this book.

Part 1

INTRODUCTION AND DIAGNOSTIC PALPATION SKILLS

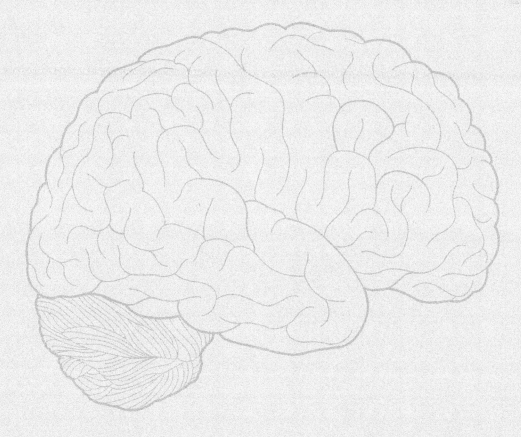

CHAPTER 1

Introduction and How Best to Use This Book

William Garner Sutherland developed an osteopathic approach, which within the profession is called Osteopathy in the Cranial Field (The Osteopathic Cranial Academy 2021), but is more commonly referred to as 'cranial osteopathy'. This term implies that it is just about the head. This could not be further from the truth, yet it has become an established term in the public domain. Sutherland studied the anatomy of the skull, and the more he looked at the specificity of the sutures, concluded that they must be expressing motion, and that this motion varied in differing parts of the skull. He termed this motion, one that had been mentioned in neither osteopathic teaching nor medical textbooks, the involuntary motion, or the primary respiratory mechanism.

THE PRIMARY RESPIRATORY MECHANISM

Sutherland discussed five very important aspects of his way of working. Please note that these five aspects all have equal significance and one is not more important than others.

These subsequently became called Sutherland's Five Phenomena.

1. The mobilty of the cranial bones.
2. The involuntary mobility of the sacrum between the iliac bones.
3. The mobility of the bones of the skull.
4. The inherent motility of the brain and spinal cord.
5. The fluctuation of the cerebrospinal fluid.

In this book, it is not my intention to cover the teachings required to gain an initial therapeutic skill in Osteopathy in the Cranial Field. I leave the teaching of the principles and basic techniques to the undergraduate schools and postgraduate courses. This book is aimed at the existing keen student of the cranial approach, who wishes to take their knowledge, and hence experience and therapeutic success, to a significantly higher level.

THE FIVE PHENOMENA

The Osteopathic Cranial Academy (2021) outlines the underlying phenomena which Sutherland observed and taught as his Cranial Concept below – some call these components Sutherland's five phenomena. The primary respiratory mechanism has five basic components: please note, these are *not* listed in order of importance – all are equally important!

The inherent motility of the brain and spinal cord

The fluctuation of the cerebrospinal fluid (CSF) – Potency in the Tide

The mobility of the intracranial and intraspinal membranes

The mobility of the cranial bones

The involuntary mobility of the sacrum… between the ilia… (The Osteopathic Cranial Academy 2021)

In this book I will take the reader on a journey which will not only explore these five phenomena, but will also look at the whole body including the cellular level, the mind and emotions, and timelines from an osteopathic perspective.

HOW TO USE THIS BOOK AND GAIN THE MOST BENEFIT TO HELP YOUR PATIENTS

I kindly ask you to read each chapter and participate in the practical exercises in sequence, reading this book from the beginning and progressing through each chapter in turn. Even if one topic seems dull or presents an aspect of the physiology with which you are remarkably familiar, you may still discover new insights and deeper perceptions from reading the chapter and following the practical sessions. I have placed the chapters in order of experience required for the associated practical exercises. Each chapter will increase your experience in readiness for the subsequent chapters.

Exercises in this book

In most chapters, you will find QR codes to access practical exercises. These are not open to the public and only accessible via the QR codes in this book. By scanning the QR codes with your phone or tablet (or entering the web links into your browser), you will then be able to hear the audio files I have created of the practical sessions relevant to that section of the chapter, or the whole chapter. The image associated with the audio simply allows the audio to be turned into a video which has then been posted on YouTube for safekeeping and access by you the reader. As they are just audios, you can simply listen to me at your treatment table, as I take you on a journey within the physiology, without visual distractions.

I ask you to respect that these tracks are for you the reader and not for other practitioners who have not read the book and have not engaged with all the practical sessions. In some of the later chapters, the practical sessions are very profound, and non-readers of the book may not have the required skill level to safely perform the exercises on a model.

In these audios, I will take you through practical exercises where you will require a colleague, friend or family member lying down on your treatment couch. In each audio exercise I will indicate places to investigate and assess on each journey, and at the same time, give guidance, knowledge and osteopathic therapeutic tips at different locations within the physiology.

I strongly advise the use of headphones/earphones, if you have them, to listen to the audio files.

This will override any outside noises which could otherwise distract your awareness. If necessary, pause the track if you need more palpation time at any stage.

> Please note that these exercises are for qualified practitioners only, who have a current and valid professional indemnity insurance. Neither the author nor the publisher has any responsibility for your work with your model at the treatment table in respect of the practical exercises accessed via the QR codes in this book. The author has taken great care when creating these audio files, to make them as useful and beneficial to you as possible but cannot be held responsible for your use of them.

If you do not currently have a friend/partner/colleague with whom you can kindly palpate their physiology and have to wait for such an opportunity, I recommend that you read the text for about 20–30 minutes, then take a break for mental digestion time before returning to the book.

I was fortunate in the 1990s to have had educationalist training from the late Eric Sotto (author of *When Teaching Becomes Learning*, 1994). When teaching me he would often say:

> Educationally it is considered that a 20-to 30-minute lecture on a new or complex topic gives the student as much learning as a 60-to 90 minute (or longer) lecture. Sadly, but truly, we mentally switch off and/or lose our focus and concentration after about 20–30 minutes. (Sotto 1994)

I have applied this wise principle in my osteopathic teaching since that time and recommend it to you, especially with the reading of this book and the practical sessions in each chapter. Most chapters have more than one practical session, and again I recommend that you take your time to work through them, and not spend excessive amounts of time on one session, to avoid fatigue and tiredness. Do not rush your learning: it is learning quality, not speed that is important. Reading this book and going through the practical sessions is not a race, it is about increasing your understanding and palpation/therapeutic skills.

Part 1: Introduction and diagnostic palpation skills
Chapter 2: The inner perception and the osteopathic toolbox

Part 1 asks who we are as practitioners, and how we relate to diagnostic palpation and working with fluids, diagnostic skills, the inner perception and the 'osteopathic toolbox'.

These are the essentials of what we bring into the consultation room. The patient brings their complaint and their physiology expressing those symptoms. But what do we bring to this interaction between patient and practitioner? Which part of ourselves do we bring and how well is that part working? These are fundamental questions for us all!

In my experience very little is discussed in osteopathic circles about who we are as practitioners. Yes, in the modern day, many teaching schools do teach 'Centring' (see Chapter 2), but there are still many that may not. In my opinion, being centred is essential to becoming a good osteopath, irrespective of which methods of treatment you choose to employ.

Here we will also discuss the contents of the osteopathic toolbox, which is full of the tools and approaches we can select when working with our patients.

Chapter 3: Diagnostic palpation and working with fluids

This will be an overview and revision of osteopathic diagnostic skills, which you should have learned at college, and a discussion of added questions and considerations you will need to contemplate as you further your skills in Osteopathy in the Cranial Field.

Part 2: Embryology and differing anatomical areas of the physiology
Chapter 4: Embryology and its inner relevance to osteopaths

In this chapter we will discuss how the knowledge of embryology is of therapeutic value to us as practitioners. It is not intended to be a lengthy discourse on the topic, but will explain how this knowledge enriches what we feel at the treatment table. I also include a table showing a timeline of embryological development for the cranial base and vault, which is very necessary to working on the skull.

Chapters 5 to 13: The inner approach

In these chapters, we will take an inner journey, to explore many aspects of the whole physiology as we deepen our awareness and perception. These chapters are to introduce some concepts and treatment approaches with which you may or may not be familiar, and provide practical exercises on different parts of the body. I will aim to take your palpatory skills to new levels and to explore more subtle areas of the physiology.

Each chapter takes on a different part of the anatomy or a different theme. As the chapters progress, so the skill level requirement will generally be higher, building on your experiences from previous chapters. Initially I do not expect all readers to be able to feel and work at some of the skill levels required – each reader will have their own unique skill level before commencing with this book. However, with repeated practice and increasing experience, everyone will acquire increasing skills.

Time is an important aspect of our learning process. Attending training courses is also essential to developing our skills. So, if you find a suggested approach or a practical session initially too difficult or not possible, *do not try* to achieve the task, as 'trying' may put your model at risk. Instead, it is imperative to acknowledge that you are finding an aspect tricky. I then recommend that you make a note of your difficulty in the margin of the book and date it. At a future time, come back and re-read the section of the book to see if your skills have now progressed to a sufficiently good level for the exercise.

Going back and re-reading and re-practising the exercises taken before you came to a tricky point will also be highly beneficial, and as such I recommend this to all readers. By repeating and seeing how long it takes you to achieve (without any trying or striving) some of these exercises, you will reveal your professional progress. To perceive your skillset progressing is highly satisfying and deeply rewarding! As I have said above, do not rush your learning, it is learning quality, not speed that is important.

Part 3: Advanced osteopathic considerations

In the remaining chapters we will look at the physiology in ways that perhaps you may have never considered before.

Chapter 14: An overview of working with babies and children

This chapter is not intended to make you a competent paediatric practitioner but is included here to stimulate your interest in this rewarding work, for exploring further reading and courses in paediatric osteopathy.

Chapter 15: Back to the time: an inner approach

In this chapter we will explore how time, as the fourth dimension, needs to be included in our diagnostic awareness. Time not only determines how long a condition or tissue state has been present, but time also has a strong psychological influence on the physiology. In this chapter we explore how to use timelines diagnostically and to understand how the mind and body are influenced by time.

Chapter 16: The inner relationship of mind, body and emotions

Following the previous chapter on time and its relationship to the psychophysiology, here we will look at other tissues and organs which are strongly influenced by the state of the mind, and how we can help the psyche with osteopathic treatment to the tissues of the physiology.

Chapter 17: The inner relationship of inter-tissue relationships

In this chapter we will explore how many organs and tissues influence other aspects of the physiology in a manner not always expected, or perhaps we thought impossible!

Chapter 18: Working at the intracellular level along with tissue and cellular consciousness

This chapter will explore the other side of the cell membrane, looking inside the cell wall. We will be noting the differences in fluid quality between the extracellular matrix and the intracellular fluid. We will then proceed to explore the cell contents: the organelles. In this chapter we will also explore tissue and cellular consciousness and how such parts of the body can express their own emotional state, separate from that of the personal psyche.

Chapter 19: Experiences of refined perception

Here we will not only discuss working with the body potency as a therapeutic tool, but will also discuss the nature of practitioners' perceptual experiences whist working, including topics such as liquid light.

Chapter 20: Conclusion

Summary and final discussion.

REFERENCES

The Osteopathic Cranial Academy, 2021. Osteopathy in the Cranial Field. Available from: https://cranialacademy.org/students/principles-of-ocf/

Sotto, E., 1994. Conversation with Timothy Marris. October.

CHAPTER 2

The Inner Perception and the Osteopathic Toolbox

WHO AM I?

Who am I? This is the first 'inner' question a practitioner needs to ask! Who am I, that I bring into the clinical relationship with my patients? What is my state of consciousness? How accurate is my perception and hence my palpation and understanding?

Although you may have considered these aspects before, it is worth exploring them in some detail, as our understanding of who we bring to the treatment table is integral to our inner work as osteopaths. What we see, what we feel and what we hear from our surroundings reflects our perception and our consciousness as a practitioner.

As human beings, unless we are graced with being fully enlightened (I will assume the reader has not achieved this supremely esteemed state of consciousness), we are all wearing sunglasses. These sunglasses are all different levels of opacity and colour and there are millions of different grades of each, such that we are all wearing a unique pair, different to everyone else on the planet. Consequently, we all see the world differently from each other: different colours, shades, or tones from other people.

We also are all wearing earmuffs. These earmuffs distort or delete certain sounds, words, or inflections in the spoken words of people talking to us. These distortions and deletions result in our not comprehending the words with the exact

same meaning as that given to the words by the speaker.

When we palpate the body, what we feel is again distorted – we are all wearing varying types of gloves distorting the truth of the palpation. Therefore, our proprioception will be limited and over simplified or over complicated to varying degrees, compared with reality. Our interpretation of our palpatory findings will also express an amount of distortion, and perhaps also be narrowed by our lack of anatomical awareness – none of us are perfect (even though we live in hope).

So, *who am I?* Do you ask your inner self, before you see each patient? In their book *The Structure of Magic,* on communication and how we interpret what we see, hear and feel, Grinder and Bandler, the founders of Neurolinguistic Programming (NLP), give a clear understanding that how we act in response to an event will very much depend on our 'meta programmes' (unconscious programmes within our unconscious mind which filter our experiences) (Grinder and Bandler 1975). In their 2003 paper 'Neuro-linguistic Programming: its potential for learning and teaching in formal education', Tosey and Mathison discuss the significant educational benefit of an understanding of this psychological insight. I do not intend in this book to delve deeply into the benefits of understanding the NLP perspective when in the consulting room, however I do recommend further reading on the topic. To whet your appetite on this topic, I will discuss taking case histories and palpation with your patients.

When taking a case history, the responses you will receive from your patient, or especially from the parent if treating a child, will be their current version of reality, a reflection of today's 'sunglasses' that they are now wearing. Not only will their clinical symptoms differ day to day, but their interpretation of what they feel within their body will be distorted by other factors such as who they have spoken to and what they have read (in books or more likely, online). These 'expert opinions' on their condition may be from genuine authorities which should be valued, or from a friend, neighbour or social media, with little authoritarian knowledge, and which should therefore be questioned. When your patient is a child, do talk to them when taking the case history in addition to the parent, as the parent is only interpreting what the child is feeling. This also makes the child feel included in the discussion about their condition.

We should also consider what colour of sunglasses and type of earmuffs and gloves we practitioners may be wearing. This is especially true if the condition the patient presents with is one that you or someone you know has had in the past, or may currently have. It could be extremely easy to mishear a patient's description and dwell on your own experience instead.

STATE OF THE PHYSIOLOGY

As osteopaths we know from our training and experience, that almost all aspects of the physiology are affected by the state of our mind. The autonomic nervous system, the state of our musculoskeletal system, our organs, our circulation, all change with the state of our consciousness. If we have recently been experiencing negativity or distress within ourselves from any reason or cause, it is vital that we put those feelings to one side (see discussion on 'Centring' below). If we do not do this or are unable to do so, we distort our understanding of the patient and their physiology.

In a clinical setting, our patients will express not only their complaint, and, with our questioning, their case history, but possibly also they will express their fears, concerns and apprehensions about being in our consulting rooms, especially if they are a new patient. Consequently, we have to bear in mind that there will be distortions at play when we listen to the case history. Listen out for how patients describe events. Are they filtering or distorting the reality? When we listen to our patients, this is also an event for us as practitioners. Therefore, we should be aware of how we interpret the case history and be mindful of any distortions from within us in addition to those within the patient.

ASPECTS TO CONSIDER WHEN AT THE TREATMENT TABLE

When, as practitioners, we are in a state of tension (physical or mental), this will reflect on our state of awareness. Physical tensions in our physiology may cause blocking or distortion of our afferent neural pathways, making it more difficult to feel the physiological truth about the tissue state within our patients. If we are not mindful at such moments, we may then *try harder* to feel the tissues. This process of trying to feel then further blocks our receptive ability. Hence *trying to feel* creates the opposite of what we want to achieve. It is therefore vital to eliminate our ego and all our pre-expectations in our work. Being non-judgemental and without preconceptions is one of the most important aspects I attempt to instil in my students when teaching osteopathic courses.

As osteopaths, we must palpate our patients with an attitude of: 'I have no idea what I will feel nor find.' Only with this attitude can any true state of the tissues be expressed in our awareness. If we do have a preconception, it is possible that this will influence what we will feel and diagnose. Therefore, we need to be without ego – that aspect of who we are, the ego which thinks and assumes we are right in what we do. We need to be very mindful to eliminate our ego when working with the involuntary mechanism (IVM), otherwise we could impose ourselves on the patient's mechanism, even if only subtly. This has ethical issues as well as distorting the accuracy of our diagnosis, and can create tissue tensions and treatment reactions within the physiology of the patient.

If we feel rushed, perhaps when a patient arrives late in our practice and we are pushed for time, it is still important to take time to centre ourselves (see below). In such a situation, reduce your expectation as to what you will achieve during that appointment. When there's not enough time for a full treatment session, consider mentally asking the physiology what to treat. Surprisingly, the patient's physiology (because it is aware of our consciousness too) will come up with the correct answer for that shortened session.

When we get ourselves into a neutral receptive state in order to palpate, it enables our own IVM to receive what it needs to gain better balance. If we are fatigued, we commonly find that tiredness kicks in when we work with the IVM, and our perception of what we can feel becomes cloudy and foggy. In these circumstances, the usual process of *trying* happens, to compensate for the dullness we perceive in our ability. As already mentioned, trying only makes matters worse.

Many practitioners (who are honest enough to admit it) have had some very drowsy (or even short sleepy moments) when treating patients. Drowsiness may be associated with feeling tired yourself, but can also be caused by states within the patient. In a lecture I attended by Dr Anne Wales, a key student of William Garner Sutherland (and co-editor of the book *Contributions of Thought*), she described an experience she had with a patient:

> I was treating a patient's head, sitting at the head of the table. I then became very sleepy. My neck relaxed and whilst asleep my head dropped forwards and my forehead made contact with the patient's frontal bone! This immediately woke me up and then straight away I said to the patient 'Did you feel that?' (to give the impression I had done it on purpose!). (Wales 1980)

So, if you have ever fallen asleep when treating, usually just momentarily, remember it has happened to one of our osteopathic greats, the late Dr Anne Wales. If it ever happens to you again, remember her comment to the patient!

CENTRING AND REDUCING THE DISTORTIONS OF OUR SUNGLASSES, EARMUFFS AND GLOVES

Centring is an integral component of the inner approach to osteopathy. Centring can improve our sensory accuracy of what we see, hear, feel and mentally interpret. This enhances our assessment, deepens our diagnosis, makes our treatment plan more relevant, and thus increases success when treating our patients.

What is centring?
There are many methods for centring ourselves. It is a method or technique for reducing the external and internal sensory input so that we experience more of our true inner self. Cultures all over the world use different names and a variety of ways for achieving the same goal.

Mindfulness is a relatively new buzzword in the West, and is used as a more acceptable term for meditation, which some consider too much of a 'New Age' or Eastern activity.

Meditation has been around for many millennia in the East, and for 100 or more years in the West. Larkin (n.d.) discusses in his article how 'contemplative or centring prayer' are aspects of the Christian faith with similar psychological goals, exploring the spiritual benefits of being still and quiet within oneself. Sutherland himself used the phrase, 'Be still and know' (Sutherland 1967). All these approaches have a common theme, to find that profound inner stillness within the core of oneself. By doing so, the ego is reduced or eliminated, thereby allowing the sensory awareness or consciousness to be heightened and more accurate.

Much scientific research has been done on the benefits of meditation, such as the Transcendental, Buddhist and Zen Meditation techniques. This research indicates a range of physiological and psychological benefits: for example, in the study by Nidich *et al.* (2009) on the effects of Transcendental Meditation on blood pressure, psychological distress and coping in young adults. Whilst I have no wish to advocate one centring approach over another, I do want to demonstrate that centring has a known benefit to mankind in cultures worldwide, including scientifically demonstrated benefits. Consequently, our osteopathic community will certainly benefit too!

BODY LANGUAGE

In his article 'Cognition: The Science of Body Language & The Debates' (2012), Jeff Thompson discusses an understanding of body language. Developing higher skills in body language perceptions can be highly beneficial in osteopathic case history taking and treatment. It is not uncommon for patients to say something with a specific meaning; the meaning they want us to understand and take as the truth. Being aware of the body language may allow to us to pick up on the unconsciously expressed truth. Our body language expresses the 'felt sense' about what we are thinking. Most of the time, our conscious mind is not aware of our body language expression (there are some exceptions, such as a skilled actor when consciously choosing to act a part).

Taking time to study and notice the body language of our patients will give you a greater degree of understanding about your patient. If the body language corresponds with the spoken meaning, then it is true for this person.

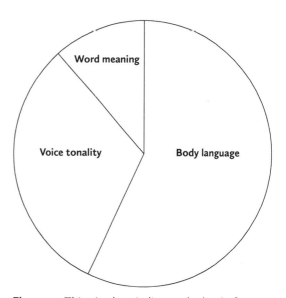

Figure 2.1 This pie chart indicates the level of importance that we should give to the communication from our patients, both the spoken (conscious) words and the unconscious body language and voice tonality. These ratios apply to general conversations and differ to when someone is giving a speech or a lecture.

If the body language and spoken meaning are at variance and not congruent, then as osteopathic diagnosticians, we should consider why this should be so. Why is the patient not happy to tell you the whole story?

Imagine a second-hand car salesperson selling you a choice of cars. You are most likely to consider buying the car where the body language and voice tonality of the salesperson mimics the meaning of their words. What will affect your choice when both cars look good at the garage, and sound/feel OK on a test drive? The salesperson's words may be the same in both cases, but their mannerisms or body language may differ.

> Do remember that the patient will not be aware that their body language is telling you information other than what their spoken words convey. Therefore, you must be tactful in how you proceed with the incompatibility of body language and voice tonality information with that of the spoken words.

To help further your perception of body language, you need to exercise your peripheral vision skills. When looking straight ahead we notice the details of our focal vision and are less aware of our peripheral vision. When we take a case history from our patients we should, out of courtesy and to show we are interested in them and their condition, give gentle (not over focussed) eye contact during their consultation. However, much information may be missed if we only look at their face region. We need to culture our skills for noticing detail with our peripheral vision *whilst* maintaining eye to eye contact. This peripheral vision, which involves looking out of the corner of your eyes, can pick up on highly beneficial visual clues as to the body language of your patient. Equally, it is important to note the quality of the vocal tone when they speak.

Aspects you may want to notice about your patient when taking the case history:

- How are they sitting? Are they facing you or facing slightly to the left or right by rotating the shoulder girdle or hips? You should do your best to face them if your consulting room furniture placement allows it.
- Are their shoulders hunched, up and around the neck, braced back, etc.?
- Do they fidget and fiddle with their fingers, hair, etc., or keep reasonably still?
- Do they cross/uncross their legs or ankles several times?
- Are there any facial movements around the mouth, cheeks, eyes, or forehead that occur during the case history?
- Are there any changes in skin colour?
- What is the tone and intonation of their voice like? Is it gentle, stern, confident, hesitant, concerned, harsh, forceful, fearful, etc.?

(See Seppälä 2017 for further reading on body language.) If a parent and a child (or more than one child) is in the room at the same time, our peripheral vision can give hidden clues as to the family dynamic. You will naturally be asking the parent most of the questions depending on the child's age, but do remember that if the child is the patient, to give the child that important recognition. However, when talking to the parent, notice the facial expression or body language of the child/children present. They may or may not be agreeing with the parent's comments (if old enough to comprehend them). If more than one child is present, notice the interactions going on between siblings whilst talking to the parent. The children will not realise you are noticing, and hidden truths may be expressed about their interrelationships with the parent or with each other, which the parent may not mention.

From time to time, you may have a patient whose relationship partner attends the initial consultation (if the patient gives their permission). Body language in these circumstances can be very revealing. Whenever a partner is present in my waiting room in addition to the patient, I always ask the patient if they are happy for their partner to come in. Only once or twice in my career have they said: 'I think it might be easier if I come on my own.' In which case I acknowledge that and give the partner some reassurance as to why they must wait outside the consultation room.

I once treated a patient who had sustained a very serious head injury nine months before coming to see me. The injury was so significant that it was a miracle he did not die. After recovering from a loss of consciousness, he had a severe headache with numbness to his face and left arm. He certainly should have gone to hospital immediately, but he drove a couple of hours home. He did not tell his wife about the injury, nor did he go to the hospital. He only went to his doctor and hospital as his headaches persisted five months later. An X-ray was taken of his head and neck which revealed that he had fractured his C1 vertebra! He did not tell his wife anything about the incident for those five months. When he related this story to me, his wife was sitting just behind his left shoulder. I could see both of them, but he could not see his wife. Both their body languages as he related his story were an absolute picture, but each in their own different manner.

THE OSTEOPATHIC TOOLBOX

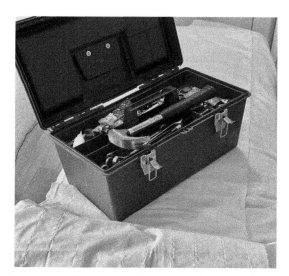

Figure 2.2 The osteopathic toolbox that we take to each consultation – however, it should not be full of spanners, screwdrivers and hammers like this one! It contains our posture, our degree of centring, the matching of our elbow fulcrum and our hand contact, and our 'third hand' matching.

One of my personal teachers, and Sutherland's 'right hand man', Dr Rollin Becker DO, instilled in me the importance of a number of factors which we should all bring to the treatment table. I call these factors 'the osteopathic toolbox'. Let us examine the contents of this toolbox.

Personal comfort

The first item in the toolbox to consider when sitting at the treatment table is evaluating our own personal comfort. Of course, we all should ensure our patients are comfortable lying or sitting on our treatment couches, but do we pay as much attention to our own comfort? Have we consciously chosen our seat position or are we just using it as it was for the last patient? Have we chosen to adjust the height of the chair/treatment table (if adjustable)? If not adjustable, I recommend soon acquiring such a chair and table. Is the chair in the best position at the table for your elbows to be well supported (see below)? Will you have a good position to access those parts of the patient's anatomy you wish to contact with your hands?

If your body comfort is not as good as *you consciously* (not just accepting the status quo) decide it to be, then your sensory apparatus will not be in the best state for receiving information via your fingers to your conscious awareness. If, as many of us do, you have a full list of patients to see in a day, then your personal comfort levels will determine how you will feel at the end of the day. If fatigued from a poor working posture, then it is likely that you will be tired, and your thinking then becomes less clear. With fatigue, the danger point kicks in and you start *trying* to feel, resulting in poor perceptiveness, misdiagnosis and less beneficial treatment, which put the patient at risk of treatment reactions.

Tensegrity

Donald Ingber discussed the principles of tensegrity in the physiology (Ingber 1998). Via the principle of tensegrity I have developed a simple method of enhancing our postural efficiency. Do share with your patients.

Tensegrity exercise

- Sit on a chair with your eyes closed.
- Do not have your spine touching the back of the chair.
- Take 4–5 minutes or more and allow any tension you experience anywhere in your body to dissipate to adjacent tissues.
- Imagine all tensions being spread across your cell membranes, across the extracellular matrix and to the cell neighbours in all three dimensions, and then continuing to move farther and farther away. Allow any tension to spread and be dissipated or shared throughout the whole body.
- As you do this, allow your posture to be led into a better position, without your intellect interfering.

- Keep doing this until you feel a sense of lightness and spaciousness throughout your whole body.
- You may notice how this has made your mind feel lighter and calmer, yet more alert.
- Adjust your treatment table/chair to the height which allows you to work from this tensegrity position.
- Remember your posture is king and everything else which is adjustable should be adjusted to this position.
- You can do the same exercise for your car seat and any adjustable seats at home.

Hand contact

This is another important feature of our toolbox. Our hand contact should be light and delicate yet still purposeful. Sutherland in his teaching, often used the phrase:

> Let your hands be like the bird lighting on the branch of a tree, quietly touching and then settling down on the area. While your fingers are there feeling, seeing, and knowing, they can tell you more in one minute than a firm grasp can gain in an hour's observation. (Sutherland and Wales 1990)

Remember to use both hands. This should be obvious, however at times I have observed students on courses with one hand under the sacrum and the other on their own thigh. Whilst their own thigh might be interesting, the patient's tissues are more interesting!

Where possible use as full a hand contact to the patient as you can. Some practitioners like to just put fingertip contact on the patient, especially if working on the face. However, in my experience, using a fuller hand, whilst making sure your hands are not obtrusive over the eyes, allows a greater surface area contact. A greater surface area of your hand means that any one specific part of your hand has less pressure from the weight of your hand. A full soled shoe causes less pressure than a stiletto heeled shoe! When I advise this to my students, the model lying down then acknowledges that a fuller contact is more comfortable. It should go without saying but just for completeness, beware the length of fingernails!

Forearm muscles

We need to be conscious of the degree of forearm tone required, which will alter our palpatory pressure of our fingertips. If you have some experience in working with the IVM, you will probably be doing this automatically. Even if this is the case, occasionally go back to basics and *consciously* alter and change the degree of forearm flexor tone and notice how this changes your perception. Dr Rollin Becker advises:

> ...just let your hands make contact somewhere on the body. Then, don't do anything except barely contract your flexor digitorum profundus (FDP) muscles. Do you feel something which you didn't before? Now, go back to not feeling with the proprioceptors. There is a difference in the quality of the feel because with the proprioceptive contact, you are reaching through to a body of fluid and a set of ligaments and muscles, and they are all in motion. With superficial contact you are not feeling motion; all you have is a hold of the body. When you use the proprioceptors, you are mechanically listening to the function that's going on in that particular area. (Becker, quoted in Brooks 1997a)

Elbow fulcrum

The elbow is the main fulcrum of the lever between the shoulder and the hand/fingers. Rollin Becker was very keen to instil in me, as a student on courses, that I should have my elbows fully supported by the treatment table whenever physically possible (i.e., most of the time). An example of when this may not be possible would

be standing to work in the mouth, or some other such situation when standing is required. By having the elbow of the palpating hand(s) supported, it allows the practitioner to vary the degree of lean onto the elbow, thus changing the fulcrum pressure. This change in fulcrum pressure will change your perception of what you feel, generally taking your perception deeper and further into the physiology.

By consciously adjusting both the forearm tone and your elbow fulcrum tone, you will find a whole range of palpatory experiences come to your awareness without making any other changes. Consciously choose which degree of forearm and elbow tone gives you the maximum useful information about the tissues from which you are seeking more knowledge.

The third hand

The third hand is the one between our ears! Our third hand is our consciousness. This is by far our most powerful tool and as such needs to be used extremely carefully. Because it is our most powerful tool it can give us amazing insights, however it can also lead us up the garden path with misinformation!

Becker gives us a brilliant understanding of why we should use our third hand when palpating for the stillness within the tissues, as long as it is done with due care and consideration. I consider this to be a key aspect of the advanced practitioner's skill:

> I get my hands under the given area of problem and I try to be aware of stillness. Not a still point, but a stillness that is that individual. You can only be conscious of stillness; you cannot palpate stillness with your hands. The stillness is that which centres every molecule of being of that living body. The body physiology is the outward expression of that stillness. They are in total unity, in balance interchange. In health, it is a free-flowing interchange. In disease and trauma, patterns of disability are set up that

have stillness within them. So, the energy of that motive power is built into these patterns of disability as it is into the health. (Becker, quoted in Brooks 2000)

However, if the use of our mind, our third hand, is done *without* due care there can be negative consequences. Imagine you are meeting someone you do not know for the first time. You go to greet them, but you stand under 10 cm away from their nose. What will be their immediate body response? They will instantly back away! They will be thinking: 'I don't know you. I didn't invite you to stand that close, go away and if you don't, I'm moving back away from you!'

We all know as adults that there are only certain people in our life whom we allow to come inside our personal space – generally speaking, our loved ones. Other people must stay outside that area. In many cultures we shake hands on greeting someone that we don't know that well. The handshake keeps the other person at arm's length, outside of our personal space. Only when you know that person much, much better might you allow them into your personal space, when you trust them.

If you focus with too much intention on your patient's tissues, then they feel, usually at an unconscious level, intruded upon and uncomfortable. If this happens then their tissues will start to go into a defensive process, tighten up and become compressed. This clearly is not good. However, what can make matters worse, is when the practitioner then considers the compressed state as part of the patient's condition that needs diagnosing, not realising that they have caused it to occur. This is then added to the treatment plan, with the subsequent treatment rapidly going downhill and treatment reactions highly likely to occur.

When we come into palpatory contact with our patients, we need to introduce our palpatory awareness to our patient's tissues in the same manner that we would if we were meeting an important person for the first time. We would meet them with respect. As the patient's tissues gradually come to accept our presence, they become further relaxed and then start to open up to us and can more fully 'tell us their story'.

Listening

Dr Rollin Becker describes how listening is a key aspect of our work:

> Feeling motion is not enough. One needs to 'listen' to what the motion means: listen with the mind, reason with the mind, interpret with the mind, read with the mind. Develop a mental picture of what, when, and why the patient's physiological mechanism wants this type of motion. (Becker, quoted in Brooks 1997b)

In addition, I would suggest feeling the tissues with your whole body, not just the hands and upper limbs. By absorbing the tissue state quality with your whole-body awareness, you gain a much deeper connection to the tissues and a deeper consciousness of how those tissues experience being in the state they are. We will discuss this tissue consciousness in Chapter 18.

Do not get 'drawn in'

Keep being conscious and not overshadowed by the experience of what you find when palpating. Sometimes it can be quite easy to get 'drawn in', or as I like to describe it, seduced by the patient's problem or condition.

Perhaps if we feel a strong pulling occurring between two areas of the patient's body as part of a strain pattern, or they present with a condition we have not seen before, we are at risk of losing our objective consciousness and allowing ego to creep in. Or we may start to over focus on the problem and stop 'being polite' to the tissues, as discussed above. We should be able to acknowledge these findings but not let them overshadow us. Practise looking at the patient's tissue state with your peripheral vision, keeping part of your awareness on your own still centredness plus the health and potency within the patient.

Anatomy, anatomy, anatomy!

Where are we treating? This may seem a strange question to ask. The reality is that for over 95 per cent of the time we just have our hand contact on skin, hair, or clothing, but are we treating where we have our hand contact? Perhaps if we are doing intraoral work to treat the facial mechanics, this may be one of the exceptions when we touch somewhere away from skin, hair, or clothing, but this is only a small percentage of our therapeutic time in practice.

However, how often have you ever treated skin, hair, or clothing? Only very occasionally have I chosen to treat the skin, less than that for hair follicles, but never clothing! So, we must acknowledge that we do not treat where we place our hands. We treat where our *attention* goes. Now, our attention is an amazing thing. We can take it anywhere. We can consider the planet Jupiter, we can think of a lovely holiday destination. We can take our awareness to times in the past and to events coming up. Our attention is incredibly elastic, not fixed.

Osteopathy is anatomy, anatomy, anatomy. If we know our anatomy extremely thoroughly, then we can take our awareness to any part of the physiology. The possibilities are limitless, depending on our knowledge of the road map. Our anatomy knowledge is our road map (or in modern terms our sat nav). As osteopaths we are highly familiar with feeling bones, joints and muscles. By working with the involuntary mechanism, we become familiar with the physiology of the meninges, the bony cranium and the central nervous system. We do this by taking our awareness to these tissues, and can do so by knowing where they are and what the *tissue quality* feels like.

Each tissue type has its own unique tissue quality. As a simple example, bone is firm and hard compared with muscle, which is pliant and soft. Fascia and membranes have more of a fabric-like quality with varying degrees of strength dependent on the amount of collagen and whether the collagen is laid down in bundles or is random.

As will be explored in later chapters, if we know our road map and start at a place with which we are highly familiar, we can journey into new anatomical regions and tissues of the body, previously unexplored by us. Generally speaking, if we can feel a tissue, we can engage diagnostically and therapeutically with it. When palpating, do not just feel the bone, but take your awareness within the bone so that your experience is of *being* the bone. Then the bone can reveal its whole life story, as and when you become perceptive enough and without ego to 'listen' to the story.

Tissue matching

This is something I learned from Dr Rollin Becker – not from his words, but once when I was under his tutelage and he treated me at the end of the day, simply saying (in a very firm tone), 'Lie down!' Not knowing what he was about to do and not wanting to argue with Sutherland's 'right hand man', I did.

When I was 10 years old, I had dived into a swimming pool that was not my local pool (which I knew intimately as a member of my local swimming club). This was a much older pool, that unknown to me was much shallower at a point two-thirds along its length. I dived in, thinking it was 2.5 metres (a little over 8 feet) deep, when in fact it was only about 1.55m (5 feet) deep. The next experience I had was a state of 'pure consciousness'. I was not aware of my body, just a blissful state of 'at oneness'. After a while, which could in reality have been just fractions of a second, but seemed to me timeless, I became conscious of thinking and thought: 'I'm under the water, if I stay here, I'll drown (pause), if I drown, my parents will get upset (pause, without emotion), I don't want my parents to get upset.'

I then became aware of my body and swam to the surface, climbed out and had a strange, rather clear, nosebleed. Many years later I realised this clear nosebleed was probably from raised intracranial pressure and it was probably cerebrospinal fluid (CSF) which was diluting the blood. I did not tell anyone (not even my parents) nor seek any medical examination. It was 13 years later when, on that cranial course with Rollin Becker, I palpated a crater on my frontal bone where I had fractured my skull in the swimming pool and realised why the nosebleed was not very red!

On my lying down, Rollin quickly assessed my cranial base and then took a contact with my temporal bones. The next thing I became aware of was his hands having a very gentle but at the same time quite firm contact. His two hands plus his third hand contact, his consciousness, were at the exact level of matching as the compressive state of my right petrous temporal bone, which I then could feel had been compressed since the swimming pool accident.

It felt as if Rollin's whole being was my temporal bone, matching it in every way. He was not compressing it, nor was he undermatching it. As he did so, all the tension in my temporal bone melted and seemingly disappeared. This near death experience under the water, when I felt I made a conscious choice to live, changed my life, permanently removing in me any fear of death! Thirteen years later under the hands of Rollin, that life-changing event changed the way I work. Matching became a key element of my osteopathic toolbox, one which I bring to every patient.

When we match tissue tone in the area we are working with (perhaps an area that already feels compressed and has varying degrees of tightness), and we get closer to matching the tissue tension to 100 per cent accuracy, the compression state within the tissues automatically reduces and the tissues become more comfortable. We achieve this by adjusting our forearm muscle tone, our elbow fulcrum, and our level of attention focus with our third hand. All three need to be neither too great nor insufficient (your accuracy will increase with practice). By monitoring the tissue response to these subtle adjustments, we can perceive the tissues becoming softer, more open, and amenable to treatment. In fact, when the matching of the tissue tone is extremely close to 100 per cent accuracy, it feels like the treatment is already more than half done without us having even started to treat.

Fist matching

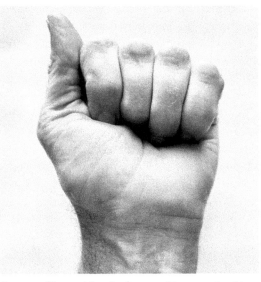

Figure 2.3 Fist position for fist matching exercise. Note that the thumb is on the outside, not tucked under the fingers. Both the owner of the fist and the practitioner need to have their elbows supported.

This is a useful exercise which helps you to practise matching the patient's tissues to an extremely high degree. You need a partner to assist you in the exercise. They do not need to do anything except make a fist with their hand.

Fist matching exercise

- The fist of your partner needs to have the thumb on the outside of the fingers, with their hand, forearm and elbow on a firm surface with palm facing upwards, as in Figure 2.3.

- Instruct your partner to make their fist as tight as possible and to keep it tight throughout the exercise.
- Place one of your hands gently under their fist.
- Next:
  - Very gradually increase the tone of your forearm muscles until you feel some matching of the tone in the fist.
  - Then adjust the lean on your elbow fulcrum of the palpating arm again until you feel some matching and a degree of fist relaxation.
  - Finally adjust the tone of your third hand – the level of your mental intention – into the fist until you feel further relaxation of the fist.
- Make further subtle adjustments of the forearm, elbow fulcrum and third hand until the softening is as best as it can be.

As you match, you will feel gradual changes within the tension of the person's fist. When you get close to matching the tension, by adjusting these above three factors, to about 95 per cent accuracy or better, you will suddenly feel a significant shift in the feel of the tissues and a relaxation of the fingers of the hand. You will find that you are now able to gently move their fingers more open with your other hand, whereas before it would have been exceedingly difficult to go against the power of them keeping a tight fist.

If you do not match the tone of the fist sufficiently (less than 95 per cent accuracy), the fist will stay strong and tight. If you go past the 100 per cent accurate level, then the tightness very quickly reasserts itself and the person can keep a strong hand as long as they want. When you get within 95–100 per cent accuracy, the person knows they cannot keep a tight fist and if honest will tell you. You will also see their fingers and thumb soften.

This exercise demonstrates exactly what happens when treating. We should match the tissue tone of the area we wish to treat to the same 95–100 per cent accuracy. This results in the tissues softening, even before we start treating, making the actual treating process more successful. If we over match (going beyond the 100 per cent level and thus compressing, not matching the tissues), then the tissues stay tight!

Therefore, it is incredibly important to generate matching the tones of your forearm, elbow fulcrum and third hand *very gradually* so that you do not miss the magical 95–100 per cent point where tissues soften. If you match too quickly, then you will soon go to 110 per cent or more and tissues will stay tight. When feeling tightness in this circumstance, it is easy to assume you have not matched enough and add even more – causing a total locking up of the tissues!

If at any time you cannot understand why tissues have not softened, take your hands away, recentre yourself and start the matching process again. The recentring will remove any ego which may have led you to think you had been doing it right before. Clearly you had not, because otherwise the tissues would have softened. Just put it down to experience and a good learning process.

We should remember that we match the tissues in any therapeutic situation. However, different tissues and tissue types will require differing levels of matching. If I am working on the lung tissue or the eyes, for example, it requires a *very* delicate level of tissue matching compared with working on an arthritic hip joint! Both should still be matched but each to their *own* tissue level. Matching the lung tissue or eyes needs to be very, very delicate, whereas an arthritic hip will require much more matching. So, you need to initially acknowledge the true tissue state and then match *that specific* level.

Time

As Einstein taught us, space and time are intimately intertwined, and he referred to it as space-time (Mann 2021). This is as true in osteopathy as it is in physics. We need to give the tissues space by accurately and not over matching as mentioned above, but we also need to give them time. They need time, to get used to our presence, time to inform us of their story, time to experience a therapeutic process and time to settle back to a new and improved state of function. As with space, if we do not give the tissues time, they get irritable and react negatively to our work.

Divided awareness

If you have a hand on one aspect of the anatomy and the other hand palpating a related area, you may wish to place your third hand, your awareness, somewhere else. Doing this is what we call 'divided awareness'. Part of your awareness, your consciousness, is on the sensory input from your hands and another part is feeling or sensing, somewhere else in the physiology at the same time. Divided awareness is a skill which develops over a period of time, sometimes several years, so do not expect it to happen quickly.

Again, for the reasons stated above, we must be very aware of the results of our actions and ensure we are not creating a false diagnosis by adding problems to the patient's tissues, which we then feel need treating! The ego can say: 'I must be doing this right, so anything I feel is the patient's problem.' I have observed this egoist type of thinking when teaching students. Beware, the ego *must* be removed when using the 'third hand' in our work!

Repetition of centring

Another feature of the toolbox is repetition of centring. It is often a good idea to recentre yourself one or more times during a single treatment, particularly with a trickier patient. We all have some patients whose condition requires a higher level of skill and awareness than others. In such

situations I may centre myself two or three times during a single appointment to ensure my perception stays clear and without ego, without sunglasses, earmuffs and gloves interacting on what I palpate. You will find a set of instructions on centring at the end of this chapter.

Intuition: A sense of knowing or gut feeling

Many practitioners, when they have been working with the involuntary mechanism for several years, tend to start getting intuitive insights about the psychophysiology. Intuition is a sense of gaining data through our senses (yes, the input is still through our senses, it is not magic) but at a rate and volume of input not yet able to be comprehended by the conscious mind. The answer seems to jump out at us.

Commonly these experiences *may* be a sudden sense of knowledge about:

- treatment
  - 'I need to do some work at (x) area of the physiology.'
  - 'I need to treat them in this manner.'
  - 'The treatment is finished.'
  - 'I should leave (y) amount of time before the next treatment.'
- something to do with the patient's current or past psychological state
  - He/she has a problem at work/financial issues.
  - He/she has a problem with their relationship.
  - He/she has a problem with other family members, friends, boss, etc.
  - Or any other issue.

These intuitive insights can arise without any spoken information from the patient. It is as if the tissues are telling you directly, not the conscious person.

If you gain such an insight, do not ignore it, but give it some serious consideration. If you have an insight about treatment to an area of the body (even if it is an area you might not think is involved with their problem), once the current area being treated has settled down, go to that area indicated by your intuition. You will probably surprise yourself by how accurate, informative and therapeutically valuable that insight becomes. If your insight is more about the patient's life/psychological state, again be prepared to accept that this *may* be a true situation. The patient has chosen not to provide this information, so you do not know for certain. Here great tact must be engaged. That patient will not know that you may have gained this insight. It may be highly inappropriate to speak about it to them, in which case keep it to yourself and let that 'possibly true' knowledge give you greater wisdom on your further treatment of their condition. However, you can ask non-obtrusive questions which do not give away any clues as to your reason for the questions, which may reveal more useful information.

My question of choice in these situations is to ask: 'Do you sleep well?' If they indicate 'No', by words *or* body language, then *tactfully* ask more questions such as: 'How long has this poor sleep pattern been going on for?' *Always* make sure that you are looking at the body language at the same time as asking these types of questions. The body language will tell you when to stop asking about this topic and change the subject of your conversation.

On the surface these are perfectly innocent questions. However, if the patient is going through a difficult emotional time for any reason, they probably are not sleeping well. They may open up a little more about the issue or may choose to keep quiet. If this occurs, then *do not ask about it.* Remember, unless you have extra qualifications in the psychological field, we are osteopaths. We have every right to ask questions which are tissue based, but *not* purely psychological questions, even though we all know that the state of the psyche affects the tissue state.

As your osteopathic skills, anatomical knowledge and palpatory experience grow on an intellectual level, so your intuitive skills will also grow and develop. However, always remember to back up your intuitive insights with your reasoned intellect: we need both aspects of knowledge.

A final quotation on intuition is from Einstein:

I believe in intuition and inspiration. Imagination is more important than knowledge. For knowledge is limited, whereas imagination embraces the entire world, stimulating progress, giving birth to evolution. It is, strictly speaking, a real factor in scientific research. (Einstein, quoted in Samples n.d.)

Knowing when to finish

This is another incredibly important aspect of the osteopathic toolbox. Over treatment is a common issue with less experienced practitioners. Over treatment can result in creating irritation and mild inflammation in the tissues from spending too much time in one area or on the whole body. This can occur just locally, within a specific region or tissue, or it may be expressed by a larger area or even the whole body, depending on the nature of the condition and treatment.

This usually happens from our old adversary, the ego, coming too much into play. Our ego becomes too keen to get the patient better: 'I am going to/want to get this person better.' The 'I' in this sentence is the ego talking! The reality is that the patient gets themselves better, the osteopath is merely the assistant.

In any treatment, there is a process:

- We feel a negative tissue state.
- We engage with the tissues and match that state to a high level, close to 95 per cent-plus accuracy.
- We add our osteopathic thinking, the tissues respond by softening and we

feel activity or change happening to our sensory awareness.

- The tissues start settling down towards a still point.
- The still point occurs and within the still point, a sense of the potency expression increasing within the tissues occurs.
- The patient may take a deep breath – very common but not always.
- The tissues then express a flexion and extension, external/internal rotation motion, with a different healthier quality than before the treatment. It is as if the tissues take a deep breath and feel more relaxed afterwards.
- So, when you feel a sense of the tissues going into a state of ease and a healthier flexion and extension, the treatment to that area of the body is finished. If you only worked on a specific area, you may find the body calling to your awareness saying: 'Come and treat this area now.'
- Or you may get the impression the body is saying: 'Thanks for what you have done but that's enough for today.'

It is particularly important to listen to these messages, and with time and repeated experience you will learn to trust these truths from the patient's body.

Centring and the osteopath

Here are two methods to centre yourself. As osteopaths we have a good knowledge of anatomy and physiology. We can use this anatomical and physiological awareness to help our centring ability.

Centring exercise

Scan these QR codes (or enter the web links into your browser) to listen to the author taking you through this centring exercise.

https://youtu.be/oOoT_rYOcCo

Then after 10–15 minutes scan these codes and centre yourself even deeper.

https://youtu.be/mqePHZ9dwfQ

https://youtu.be/4dpxHeZKknk

https://youtu.be/dJKrLCIgtWM

You will probably now feel more settled and calmer. It is a good idea to practise centring (such as the longer version as described above) daily at a time when not seeing patients, when you have plenty of time and are not rushed. Doing so will deepen your centring skills when you are in clinic and have less time. This inner calmness will enable your sensory systems to give you truer and less distorted information about your patient. You will be more aware of the manner in which your patient is giving you the information, the body language which they express when talking. You will hear inflections in the sound of their voice which may or may not be the same or congruent with the meaning of their words. Your awareness will be more settled, allowing your tactile and proprioceptive skills to be more accurate as there will be less distortion for the reasons already described.

The next centring exercise takes about 30 minutes. It is not designed to be done just before you see a patient, but perhaps at the start of your day in the morning, or at the end of your work day. It is also a method which would be good for your patients too. It was developed based on osteopathic principles to become centred and to clear the mind of unwanted thoughts. When we work, we should be focussing on the health not symptoms, not lesions, and this principle is used in this centring approach.

If you ask anyone where they feel uncomfortable anywhere in their body, they will immediately say something such as: 'My left shoulder or my lower back.' It is usually a quick response. If, however you ask the opposite question: 'Where specifically in your body do you feel *most comfortable?*', their thinking pauses and has a 'double take'. It is probably something they have never thought of before, and also is not something that the mind consciously registers.

Centring exercise, based on the osteopathic principles of vitality and potency being the forces behind therapeutic change

This is a much longer centring exercise (33 minutes), so you will need to do it when not seeing patients. It also includes a powerful self-healing exercise.

https://youtu.be/hx6YwW3Vfpl

Here is the same long centring exercise as above that includes the self-healing exercise which you can give to your patients. Just photograph the QR code and web link below and pass it on to patients and those whom you think may value it. This version is better for your patients as does not include the specific message for you the practitioner, which is at the end of the version above.

https://youtu.be/OWo_dXH3f4I

Trust the involuntary mechanism!

This is perhaps the most important feature of our osteopathic toolbox. Rollin Becker once told me, when personally teaching me on a course, that there are three opinions in any consultation. First, the opinion of the patient, or worse, the patient's next-door neighbour (or social media, though this was not around at the time of Rollin Becker) – this is what the patient thinks their condition is about and will be limited by their understanding of medical sciences; second, the opinion of the practitioner – this is what the osteopath (or a medical colleague) has decided is the diagnosis; and third, the involuntary mechanism within the patient's physiology which *knows* what the diagnosis is! 'This third opinion is the only true one, which we as osteopaths should seek to understand' (Becker 1975).

I often say to my patients: 'You have more ability to get yourself better than anyone else on the planet! Your doctor, your medicines, the medical specialist, even me as your osteopath: we can only be the assistants to your body treating itself.' In addition to this being a true statement, it helps to put the practitioner – patient relationship on the right footing – instead of patients putting all the responsibility for their healing onto the practitioner, it helps to own it themselves.

REFERENCES

Becker, R.E., 1975. Conversation with Timothy Marris during Sutherland Cranial Teaching Foundation training course. 15–19 September.

Brooks, R.E., 1997a. Developing palpatory skills. Sutherland Cranial Teaching Foundation lecture 1986. In: Brooks, R.E., ed. *Life in Motion, The Osteopathic Vision of Rollin E Becker DO.* Portland, OR: Rudra Press, pp. 141–147.

Brooks, R.E., 1997b. Learning to listen. Excerpts from various lectures by Dr Becker. In: Brooks, R.E., ed. *Life in Motion, The Osteopathic Vision of Rollin E Becker DO.* Portland, OR: Rudra Press, p. 149.

Brooks, R.E., 2000. Using the stillness. A transcription of a tape-recorded message from Dr Becker to his close colleague Dr Anne L Wales in the early 1970s. In: Brooks, R.E., ed. *The Stillness of Life, The Philosophy of Rollin E Becker, DO.* Portland, OR: Stillness Press, p. 68.

Grinder, J., & Bandler, R., 1975. *The Structure of Magic.* Palo Alto, CA: Science and Behaviour Books.

Ingber, D.E., 1998. The architecture of life. *Scientific American.* Available from: http://time.arts.ucla.edu/Talks/Barcelona/Arch_Life.htm.

Larkin, E.E., n.d. Carmelite tradition and centring prayer Christian meditation. Available from: https://ocarm.org/en/item/2201.

Mann, A., 2021. What is space-time? Available from: https://www.livescience.com/space-time.html.

Nidich, S.I., Rainforth, M.V., Haaga, D.A.F., Hagelin, J., *et al.,* 2009. Randomized controlled trial on effects of the transcendental meditation program on blood pressure, psychological distress, and coping in young adults. Available from: https://academic.oup.com/ajh/article/22/12/1326/182024?login=true.

Samples, B., n.d. The intuitive mind is a sacred gift and the rational mind is a faithful servant. Quote Investigator. Available from: https://quoteinvestigator.com/2013/09/18/intuitive-mind/

Seppälä, E., 2017. 8 ways your body speaks louder than your words. *Psychology Today.* Available from: https://www.psychologytoday.com/gb/blog/feeling-it/201704/8-ways-your-body-speaks-way-louder-your-words.

Sutherland, W.G., 1967. Final lecture seminar in cranial osteopathy. Des Moines. Iowa, 1948. In: Wales, A.L., ed. *Contributions of Thought: Collected Writings of William Garner Sutherland 1914–1954.* Kansas City, MO: Sutherland Cranial Teaching Foundation, p. 146.

Sutherland, W.G., & Wales, A.L., eds., 1990. *Teachings in the Science of Osteopathy.* Portland, OR: Rudra Press, p. 151.

Thompson, J., 2012. Cognition: the science of body language & the debates. *Psychology Today.* Available from: https://www.psychologytoday.com/us/blog/beyond-words/201210/the-science-body-language-the-debates.

Tosey, P., & Mathison, J., 2003. Neuro-linguistic Programming: its potential for learning and teaching in formal education. Available from: https://www.researchgate.net/publication/228789398_Neuro-linguistic_programming_Its_potential_for_learning_and_teaching_in_formal_education.

Wales, A., 1980. Conversation with Timothy Marris during Sutherland Cranial Teaching Foundation Training course, London. 20 September.

CHAPTER 3

Diagnostic Palpation and Working with Fluids

Andrew Taylor Still did not just palpate his patients – he 'became' his patients' tissues! This is a powerful statement which I believe can transform the way we work. John Lewis, in his biography on Still, relates Ernest Tucker's words about this aspect of Still when palpating and teaching: 'When Still was investigating a particular topic, he would say he was "living in the liver" or "being the bone." He made himself *en rapport* with the body he studied, he tried to be that bone' (Lewis 2012).

Note that Still used the words 'being the bone' not 'thinking the bone', 'living in the liver' not 'feeling the liver'. The use of the words 'being the bone' or 'living in the liver' implies that Still sought to experience what it was like to be that tissue, to experience what that tissue was feeling as it lived its life. By taking our palpation to this level of perception, we then start to gain an inner insight into its function on both gross and more subtle levels.

Rollin Becker describes palpation in another manner: 'Feeling motion is not enough. One needs to listen to what the motion means, listen with the mind, reason with the mind. Develop a "mental picture" of what, when and why the patient's physiological mechanism wants this type of motion' (Brooks 1997).

To palpate in the manners described by both Still and Becker, we need to engage more than just our thinking, our intellect. To be the bone, or any other tissue, we have to engage our whole self, our being. This also means we have to engage our 'heart felt' senses too. This does not mean we allow our emotions to get caught up in the consultation, as that would be highly unprofessional. However, incorporating an egoless sense of universal love for our fellow man/woman or a deep level of compassion, is probably the level at which Still was working with patients, which helped him to open the door and work on the level of 'being'.

We could call this being in a professional, heart-felt state towards our patients alongside our being mindful and engaging our physical touch. As described in the previous chapter, my experience of Becker treating me was experiential evidence that he also certainly worked by 'being the tissue'. In Chapter 18 we will be discussing some of these inner aspects when looking at tissue and cellular consciousness, but please do not jump ahead to that chapter. Do just work your way through each and every chapter in sequence.

HOW DO YOU CHOOSE WHERE TO TREAT?

When we put our hands on a patient (or a model at the treatment table in a practical session), when we begin, we can have a specific area or tissue in mind that we wish to evaluate or explore. This is likely to occur with a patient after having made your evaluation and osteopathic diagnosis. During a practical session, e.g., doing the exercises in this book, again you will consciously choose to look at a specific area of the anatomy.

However, particularly as your experience level increases, you will find there are times when, for no apparent reason, you get a 'hunch', 'get called', or 'get a feeling', that you should move your contact point and your attention to a different anatomical area. Sometimes this can be some distance away. When this happens, and there will be times when it happens to you, you have no logical reason as to why you should do so. At such times, please ignore the 'Why, this doesn't make logical sense?' question – follow the intuitive, gut feeling and move your attention and hand contact to that place. Very often the 'why' becomes much more obvious after you have moved to that area and perceive this area's role in the diagnosis.

We must acknowledge that our physiology receives sensory input at a phenomenal rate, usually faster than the conscious mind can handle. Think of the mind like a computer. Your computer has both hard drive memory and RAM memory. The hard drive on a modern computer may be 500 GB or even 1 TB in capacity and have a RAM of 8 or 16 GB at the time of writing (though will probably have increased by the time you read this). In other words, the hard drive is phenomenally larger than the RAM memory. The RAM is what is actively being used at any one moment, the rest is storage. Our minds are similar: the conscious activity of our brain (our RAM) is only a small proportion of the total activity (hard drive).

Our senses are receiving a phenomenal amount of input, way beyond that which our conscious mind can handle. In the brain stem (see Chapter 12) there is the filtering area which makes us only conscious of that which is immediately necessary. When for example we watch the TV, our attention is on the programme we want to see. Our eyes are still seeing other things in our living room, bedroom or wherever the TV is

located. But at that moment our brain is saying: 'The cleanliness of the window is not important now; I am watching the news.' If, however, someone throws a stone against the window, then suddenly the window hit by the stone becomes vitally important and our attention shifts there instead of the TV.

When you get the hunch, gut feeling, or intuitive thought to look elsewhere in the physiology, that information is not coming by magic. It is coming from the brain processing the sensory data at a rate faster than the conscious mind can achieve, at the unconscious level. Such events are probably carrying much more sensory input than when you consciously choose to look at a specific tissue or area of the physiology. Therefore, learn to trust your gut feelings, intuition and hunches as you will find they are frequently correct. This, however, *does not* mean we just work intuitively. If an intuitive insight occurs, follow that intuition, but *back up that thought with rational thinking*, to verify the correctness of your intuition afterwards. We do need to intellectually understand what we are doing and why, to the best of our ability and current knowledge.

A clinical example which stands out in my career to demonstrate this occurred some years ago when treating someone who had a poorly functioning immune and lymphatic system. I was working on the sacrum and pelvis of the patient, and a colleague and close friend was working on the cranial base at the same time. After working on the sacrum and pelvis for a little while, the thought occurred to 'jump into the back of the head, go to the thymus'. I had not been thinking about that area of the physiology as my awareness had been on the lumbar region, sacrum and pelvic tissues, leaving my colleague to pay attention to the upper body. However, I listened to this intuitive thought, and felt I must follow it.

To be honest, at that time I had never considered the thymus in my therapeutic work and certainly not treated it, and so this was a step into the unknown. When I put my hands there, my colleague (still working on the head), was surprised (as was I) at my contacting the thymus. What I then felt was significant heat in the thymus gland. After my being with the gland and staying centred, and then inviting it to treat itself (if it wanted to), it became cooler and a more normal temperature. My rational mind kicked in as the cooling occurred, giving me the understanding that the thymus had been overworking (hence the heat), due to the patient's poorly functioning immune system, linked to his condition.

I acknowledged that my intellect was not sharp enough when at the sacrum to have considered working with the thymus, as it was not an aspect of the physiology I had ever fully appreciated before in a clinical situation. I would have never gone there if the sudden thought in my head had not told me to do so. I had never had a patient where I had been called to look at the thymus before. This specific experience reinforced the importance of my intuition, and equally important, that I needed to study more about the thymus gland! Our patients teach us where we need to increase our study of the anatomy and physiology.

WHAT ARE YOU LOOKING FOR?

When you take your hands to an area of the physiology, what are you initially looking for? Let us explore some possibilities.

What is the vitality/health level of the tissues/fluid?

This I consider to be a key question. If a tissue has good vitality in or around it, or a fluid has a high level of potency, then it can handle the consequences of a negative disturbance more effectively or more efficiently. Any attempt to describe what a high level of vitality or potency feels like is extremely difficult, and it soon becomes difficult to find the right adjectives. The *Cambridge Dictionary* gives 'energy and strength' as a definition of vitality (Cambridge University Press 2021).

Although this is a reasonable definition, it does not help so much when looking at a tissue state. In simple terms, a good healthy vitality of a tissue is one of having 'good energy'. Ouch, I just fell into the trap of a poor description as the next question then becomes: 'What does good energy feel like?' OK, I will make another attempt: a tissue with high vitality has a bright vibrancy, it feels as if the battery in the system and specifically the tissue being evaluated has good charge, allowing it very easily to cope calmly with the current physiological demands.

If the tissue quality has low vitality, it feels as if the battery has low charge, is depleted or drained. Here the tissues feel dull or exhausted. They will easily become over stressed and lead to degrees of dysfunction and pre-pathology, which if allowed to continue become symptomatic. If the battery is over charged beyond the natural capacity for those tissues, then they feel irritated, buzzy, over-active, or moving in the direction of inflammation. This over charged state is where the tissues are in a state of over demand, and they are not responding *calmly* to the current demand. This is very different from high vitality, where the energy is coherent and coordinated.

Such information is extremely useful. It reveals how the tissue is currently expressing its life quality, and from this, we can extrapolate how we need to work with the tissues. It also tells us how the tissues are likely to respond to osteopathic help, and hence give us prognostic information. This is also important as our patients frequently ask: 'How long before I will feel better?' or 'How many treatments will I need?' We should remember that the unhealthier the tissue state, the less treatment it can handle, without making strong treatment reactions.

I like to use a vitality scale to rate my patient's vitality. I ask the patient to rate their own score, as well as making my own private estimate. It is a score out of 10. Level 1 is what I call 'death warmed up' (though I do not say this explanation to patients), and level 10 is phenomenal health and vitality, a level way beyond feeling 'OK' or 'no discomfort'. These two vitality scores (your own and the patient's) can be especially useful to relate back to after a few treatments to give perspective on your patient's progress.

Suppose you had a patient whose vitality you assessed as 'death warmed up', a level 1 out of 10 on my vitality scale. If you then gave that person an hour of osteopathic treatment, because you were so keen to help them, it is extremely likely that the person could, over the next few days become quite nauseous, achy and/or painful, along with other symptoms depending on their pre-existing pathological state. These symptoms would be occurring because of the significant tissue changes arising from the treatment, and the consequent level of toxicity released into the circulation.

I have treated a significant number of terminal cancer patients in my career, ensuring that the patient fully understood that I was not treating the tumour(s) but giving osteopathic care to enable them to cope better with the condition. In each case I had to be extremely careful and knowingly under treat to make sure I did not over treat them. Think back to a time when you had a bad dose of influenza, or some other disabling condition. One day you can be feeling awful on many levels, due to the fever, perhaps a bad sore throat, cough etc. However, the next day you still have the same level of symptoms, but somehow they do not bother you as much. The fever, the sore throat and cough are all still there, but it is as if there is part of you which can rise above the condition. When we refer to treating the whole person, not just the condition, this is what we mean. We look to treat and hence help the person to cope better with their condition, even if that condition may be terminal.

One lady I treated had breast cancer with secondary tumours in her omentum in the upper abdomen. She had been having chemotherapy once per week. She found that the effects of the 'chemo' made her feel dreadful for about five days afterwards. After her first visit to me she said that she felt much better and the negative side effects of the chemo were far less. When I carefully questioned her about it, she said that it was because she, as a person, could cope better with the side effects. I used to treat her the day following the chemotherapy, which allowed her to have a 'good week' between her weekly osteopathy sessions. She was so incredibly grateful as she was able to have more quality time with her family right up to the last week of her life. I felt the osteopathic help enabled her to live out the last months and weeks of her life, and to say her goodbyes in a manner that she wanted.

Conversely, the healthier the person, and the tissues, the greater the ability to accept change without the risk of treatment reactions. When treating babies (see Chapter 14) they generally have such high vitality that they can tolerate greater levels of tissue change compared with adults, though one should still be very mindful not to over treat them.

Generally speaking, you never see 'level 10's in practice as they have no symptoms, have good coordination so do not have accidents, and so are highly unlikely to come to your practice. I have only once seen a 10 in my whole career. She was a lady who must have been in her late 40s but who looked in her mid-20s. She had been on a continuous residential meditation course for over 20 years, and at that time I was on a short course at the same venue, a beautiful place in Switzerland. She had heard about me from a mutual acquaintance who was an ex-patient of mine and asked me for a treatment. She had no symptoms!

Her physiology felt quite extraordinary. There was only an extremely vague cranial rhythmic impulse, virtually no mechanism. Her membranes and fasciae felt like silk. There was only the mildest of patterns in her cranial base and sacrum. Quite simply there was nothing to treat! Her vitality levels were outstanding and smooth. She obviously only wanted me to give her a treatment out of curiosity, but I was delighted to have the opportunity to experience her subtle physiology!

Before we leave the topic of vitality, I would like to discuss patients' comments on their own perceived progress under a course of treatment. When a patient comes to see us for a follow-up appointment, we naturally ask: 'How have you been since your last treatment?', or words of a similar nature. Sometimes the patient may answer: 'Oh, yesterday and today it has been feeling quite painful.' They may then even follow up this sentence with: 'I'm not sure if we are getting anywhere.'

I always make sure that they are making correct comparisons. It is extremely easy to compare a good day with a bad day. However, this is not a correct comparison. A good day will always be better than a bad day, that is why it is a good day! I then ask them to compare a good day now, with a good day one, two, or three weeks ago, depending on when they started their course of treatment. Then, I also ask them to compare a bad day this week with a bad day, one, two, or three weeks ago. This way it will make the patient realise the degree of their progress by making true comparisons, not by comparing a good day with a bad day.

Is the area expressing involuntary motion?

As osteopaths we all know that tissue and fluid involuntary motion is key to our health. Do we want our fluids to be like a mountain stream or a dirty pond? Our osteopathic founder Andrew Taylor Still wrote about the importance of our body fluids, seeing them as a key to maintaining health, and poor fluid physiology as a reason behind ill health: 'Sickness is an effect caused by the stoppage of some supply of fluid or quality of life' (Still 1908).

Without healthy motion, stasis occurs and that leads to congestion and sluggishness. Congestion and stagnancy lead to degrees of biochemical shock and distress to the tissues, which then respond by going into varying degrees of tension which we feel as compressive states under our fingers. Healthy motion, on the other hand, helps to facilitate cellular nutrition and excretion to and from the capillaries.

If an area is expressing a lack of involuntary motion, it could be an expression of supreme health (a '10' patient) as described in the patient above. However, in over 99.9999 per cent of patients, it will be an expression of the tissues being locked down and/or compressed. In the case of the central nervous system (see Chapter 12), this shock may well be from psychological distress in addition to, or instead of, those from physical trauma.

William Garner Sutherland sometimes used the phrase 'to irrigate the withering fields in order to grow healthy plants' when discussing the benefits of his fluid techniques. Here Sutherland was actually quoting his own teacher A.T. Still:

Another period of observation appears to the philosopher. We find partial or universal discord from the lowest to the highest in action and death... We continue our investigation, but the results obtained are not satisfactory, and another leaf is opened, and the question appears, why and where is the mystery, what quality and element of force and vitality has been withheld? A thought strikes him that the cerebrospinal fluid is one of the highest known elements that are contained in the body, and unless the brain furnishes this fluid in abundance, a disabled condition of the body will remain. He who is able to reason will see that this great river of life must be tapped, and the withering field irrigated at once, or the harvest of health be forever lost. (Still 1902)

William Sutherland (1873–1954) was born in

Wisconsin, USA, and initially worked in the American Midwest as a newspaper reporter. He, like Still before him, came from a farming community, and liked to use farming analogies.

PATTERN OF HEALTH

It should always be remembered that the body is always working perfectly! You may now be wondering how that can be. Surely when we get illnesses, aches and pains, that is not perfect! What this statement really means is that the body is working perfectly, the best it can, for the current state in which it finds itself at that moment in time.

My definition of the pattern of health, the patterns of involuntary motion happening when we palpate our patients, is: the pattern of health is the expression of the body at the time when palpating, expressing how it is best coping with all the historical events it has experienced in the past. Most of these events will have been very mild in terms of their consequences, and the body, always self-treating, has dealt with them. As you palpate, there may be areas where you can feel the body is currently working to resolve its tensions.

The body adapts the motion of the sphenobasilar symphysis and the Sutherland Fulcrum, the latter being the relative still point of the meninges and fascial system, and through these, the whole body. In this manner, the physiology finds the best way to adapt to life events, and in doing so it minimises the consequences of such events on the whole body. In other words, it is always finding the perfect solution, the best it can do, in its current state of the physiology, in the circumstances it now finds itself in, at this moment in time.

The pattern of health is actually a combination of patterns which have been named by Sutherland to enable us to gain a clear picture of what is occurring. He called these patterns 'strains and shears'. He named these individual patterns by the relationship of how they affect the sphenoid and occiput bones at the sphenobasilar symphysis (see below). We should always remember that these named patterns of health are expressed throughout the whole body, to differing degrees, even though they are named by the relationship of the sphenoid to the occiput bone.

An understanding of the patterns may give us an explanation of why the various tissues of the body are behaving in their own specific manner, when looking at the body as a whole. Consequently, knowing the patterns being expressed is *part* of the diagnostic information we have so far gained, as any osteopathic diagnosis can only be our current working diagnosis. The next time you see the patient, some other verbal information or tissue knowledge will add further depth and development to your developing diagnosis.

The pattern types

For the following images, the darker grey box represents the basisphenoid, and the lighter grey box represents the basiocciput at the sphenobasilar symphysis. The notochordal axis is represented by the dotted line. What happens to the notochordal axis will determine how well the physiology can accommodate the pattern.

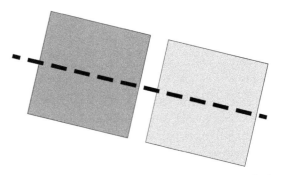

Figure 3.1 This is a neutral state. However, a so-called neutral state of the sphenobasilar symphysis in reality does not exist.

In Figure 3.1, the sphenoid and occiput are shown in their relative anatomical relationships indicating the diagonal positioning of the sphenobasilar symphysis when viewed laterally, the notochordal axis being in a straight line. It should be acknowledged that this 'normal' relationship does not exist in nature as we have had 'events' which result in patterns of health.

With the extension pattern (Figure 3.3), the opposite motion is expressed compared with the flexion pattern, resulting in an easier, more full extension phase of motion compared with flexion. For both the flexion and extension patterns there is a slight angulation of the notochordal axis. The pattern is named by the amplified phase of flexion or extension.

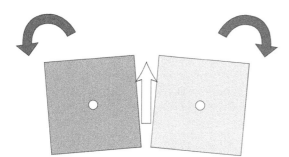

Figure 3.2 Flexion pattern. Here the flexed state is slightly exaggerated and the sphenobasilar symphysis both flexes and extends from this starting point.

From this position (Figure 3.2) the person's physiology would then further flex in the flexion phase and extend towards 'normal' or slightly into true extension (depending on the degree of the flexion pattern). Here (on palpation), the flexion phase feels easier, more comfortable, or moves further than the extension phase of movement.

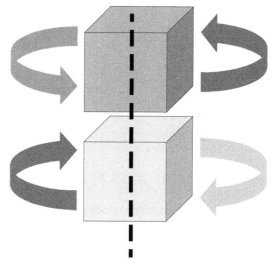

Figure 3.4 A left torsion pattern. This pattern is named by the high greater wing of the sphenoid. The flexion and extension motions occur within this pre-existing state. As the notochordal axis is intact, the body accommodates easily to this pattern.

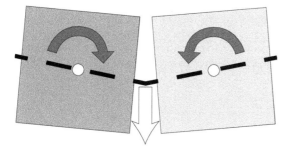

Figure 3.3 Extension pattern. Here the sphenobasilar symphysis is already in a slightly greater extension position, and so it then flexes and extends from this starting point.

In a torsion, we have a twisting occurring around the notochordal axis. Here as shown in a left torsion (Figure 3.4), the greater wing of the sphenoid bone on the left side is rotated high, and low on the right side. Conversely, the left side of the occiput has rotated low, and the right side of the occiput has rotated higher. Because the axis of both rotations is through the notochordal axis, it keeps the notochordal axis intact. For a right torsion, the rotations would be in the opposite direction. It is named (whether left or right), by the position of the high greater wing of the sphenoid bone.

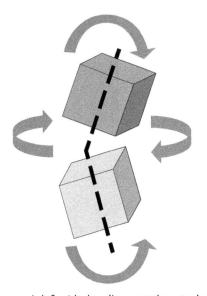

Figure 3.5 A left side-bending rotation strain. The pattern is named after the side of the pattern which 'bulges' and rotates inferiorly towards the feet. The body can accommodate easily to this pattern as the notochordal axis remains intact.

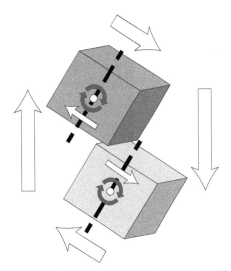

Figure 3.6 A left lateral shear. Here the notochordal axis is interrupted and the body does not find this pattern so easy to accommodate. It is named by the direction that the body of the sphenoid travels towards (left or right).

In Figure 3.5, the sphenoid and the occiput side-bend towards each other creating a concavity on the right side, and away from each other on the left side creating a convexity. At the same time,

the convex side moves in an inferior direction towards the feet. For a right side-bending rotation pattern, the movements would be reversed. The notochordal axis remains intact. The pattern is named by the side of the convexity.

In Figure 3.6, the basisphenoid moves to the left and the basiocciput to the right. Both bones are rotating clockwise (or anticlockwise for a right lateral pattern). The motion occurs around a superior/inferior axis through each bone. This creates a parallelogram type shaped head. The notochordal axis is now no longer intact. The pattern is named by the side to which the basisphenoid moves relative to the basiocciput.

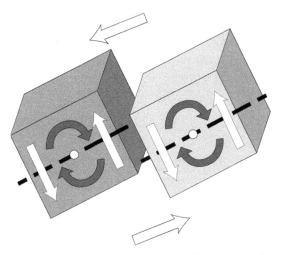

Figure 3.7 A vertical shear sphenoid high. Here the notochordal axis is again disrupted and so the body does not accommodate very easily to this pattern. It is named by the direction to which the body of the sphenoid moves (high or low).

In Figure 3.7, both the sphenoid and the occiput are rotating anticlockwise *when viewed from the left side*. For a vertical shear sphenoid low, it would be a clockwise motion when also viewed from the left side. These motions occur around a lateral axis passing through the middle of the basisphenoid and basiocciput respectively. Here the notochordal axis is no longer intact. The pattern is named by the direction to which the basisphenoid moves relative to the basiocciput.

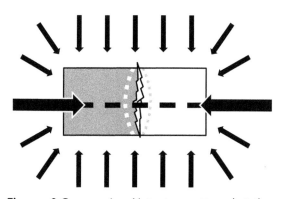

Figure 3.8 Compression. Not a true pattern, but the consequences of compression result in a reduced quality of any pattern within the body.

In Figure 3.8, the basisphenoid and basiocciput are compressed towards each other. This could be from physical trauma, psychological trauma, or any other significantly distressing event to the mind or body. The palpatory quality of the compression would vary depending on the causation. With psychological trauma, there is no force vector, unless the psychological event occurred at the same time as a physical trauma. There is, however, a palpatory feeling of 'implosion', as if the head is retreating back into itself – a fear response. In Figure 3.8, the small arrows coming from all directions express the palpatory felt sense of psychological trauma. In a compression pattern, the notochordal axis becomes 'crumpled' and consequently the quality of all involuntary motion is compromised. When the compression is occurring alongside a physical event, then there usually will be compression alongside one or more of the above patterns.

Flexion pattern, extension pattern, torsion strain (left or right), side-bending/rotation strain (left or right): these four types are called the physiological patterns. Here the notochordal axis remains intact. The notochord is the energetic line which develops early during the embryological phase and gives the body reference of its internal positions, lying between the coccyx and the junction of the pre- and post-sphenoid, the two halves of the body of the sphenoid bone. When the notochordal axis remains intact, involuntary motion at the sphenobasilar symphysis, and elsewhere in the body, is more easily expressed.

Lateral shear left or right, and vertical shear sphenoid high or sphenoid low, are called shears, not strains. They are called the unphysiological patterns. In these situations, the notochordal axis loses a degree of its continuity, and hence involuntary motions becomes less easy.

Compression is not technically a strain or a shear, but it also results in a poor quality of involuntary motion. The palpatory quality is that of the sphenoid body and the basiocciput being closer together than is comfortable. As mentioned above, this may result from both physical trauma and from psychological trauma, or both at the same time, although the palpatory quality is different between the two types.

It should be borne in mind that virtually all patients have two, three, or more patterns occurring simultaneously, to greater or lesser degrees of severity. When it comes to our diagnostic interpretation of these patterns, it is the degree of severity or mildness and the consequent quality of motion which we need to assess. Then we should be asking ourselves: 'How well is this person's physiology coping, living within their patterns of health?'

A pattern assessment is not a diagnosis!

Whilst teaching courses, I have come across students who when asked what their diagnosis is, give a reply such as: 'They have a left side-bending rotation pattern with a sphenoid high vertical shear.' This is often expressed in a proud manner for having accurately assessed the cranial base pattern of the model at the treatment table. Even if the pattern testing is accurately evaluated, it is not a diagnosis, it is a 'finding'. Such patterns are not wrong, they just make it less easy for the body to cope, but they are still *the perfect solution* for those events (usually traumatic) that the physiology is having to resolve within itself.

Does the tissue feel compressed?

Physics tells us you cannot compress fluids (as they can flow out of the way of the compressive force). So, this question should not be relevant for body fluids, however some fluid states can be quite viscous and less easily able to flow away from the compressive forces.

As has been discussed in the section above on patterns of health, frequently we find areas of the body in a relative state of compression, where the patterns are being expressed quite strongly either in the body as a whole or in a local area. Fortunately for our patients, we less frequently see strong whole-body compressions, though we do see them from time to time. The patterns arise out of the body needing to compensate for the traumas, physical and/or mental, to the body and consequent compressive states. We all take note of significant findings of compression in patients, both the degree and location, as they are a part of our diagnosis and become part of our treatment rationale.

POSSIBLE CAUSES OF COMPRESSED, TIGHT AND REDUCED, OR LOCALLY ABSENT INVOLUNTARY MOTION

First, we need to look at what is a compressed tissue state. A compression is a response by the body to an event which can be from a variety of aetiologies. Listed below are the more common ones.

Physical trauma

As osteopaths, the most common type of compression in tissue that we see in our practices is caused by physical trauma. This can be sudden in onset and include birth injury, a fall, or an accident – either that only affects the patient or involves other people too, such as a car accident. However, we must not forget that postural stresses and strains, or work-related repetitive strain injuries are slow onset traumas. These, as we know, manifest in a different palpatory quality from the sudden onset variety, as there is no felt sense of a sudden shock in the tissue.

Chemical trauma

Here there has been an insult to the body without physical trauma, but it is certainly in a manner which is damaging, causing shock and distress. Various examples include:

- Eating food that has 'gone off'. Do remember that food is chemical.
- Food or drink excesses, for instance general overeating, poor diet, excesses of tea or coffee.
- Recreational toxicity such as alcohol (toxic if taken to excess), nicotine, recreational drugs, etc.
- Environmental pollution, for example if the patient lives near a polluting factory, near high powered electricity cables, in a crowded industrial city, etc.
- Toxic liquids which can be either accidently ingested or in contact with the skin, such as farmers exposed to sheep dip, workers in a chemical factory with poor ventilation, etc.
- Pharmaceutical prescriptions.

Please note, that I am not against prescribed medications, but we all know that some can and do cause side effects with some patients. We must remember that the medications are taken because the benefit outweighs possible side effects. Any side effects are the body responses to chemical input.

Each of these differing types of chemical stress will create its own unique palpatory quality to the patient's mechanism. Chemical trauma in general creates a qualitative change such as being more irritable (if acute), or dull (if chronic). The chemical input is not physically traumatic so there will not be any force vectors present unless the patient also has a history of mechanical trauma. Depending on where your practice is located, so you will be exposed to some examples more than others. For example, I used to live and work in a sheep farming area where sheep dipping was an annual event in the farming calendar. Sheep dip poisoning was not uncommon in farmers there, but on a positive note there was little environmental pollution. Wherever you live and work, you will gain expertise in assessing your type of patients.

Psychological trauma

Many of our patients are suffering with degrees of psychological or emotional traumas (I will be discussing this in much greater detail in Chapter 16: The inner relationship of mind, body and emotions). In the pattern illustrations and descriptions above, I have mentioned how psychological trauma expresses quite differently from physical trauma in its palpatory quality due to there being no directional force vectors involved, and it feels more like an implosion happening from within.

There can be certain incredibly sad situations where a physical and psychological trauma occur at the same time. Such situations could be from a history of violence, or from a car accident where a person was severely injured, or even worse, died. In these examples the physical effect becomes amplified within the tissues, due to the added psychological trauma. Fortunately, such cases are uncommon, but you will see such cases from time to time.

Infectious traumas

If someone receives a microbial or viral input into their physiology, that becomes a trauma to the system. When the infectious and symptomatic phase has passed, their tissues may still be suffering from the consequences of the infectious trauma. At the time of writing, Covid-19 and its potential sequela long Covid are very much in the news.

If you are asked to treat such a patient, do wisely assess the risk to your own health before agreeing to see them, and where necessary take the required personal protective measures. If you then decide to proceed, then the tissue quality when palpating such a patient will depend on the aetiological onset, plus the type and severity of the condition. The pathological processes in responding to the infection will vary as the condition progresses, and so the palpatory quality of the tissue will reflect these changes. However, a patient with an illness can still complain about a musculoskeletal issue. Consequently, we may be asked to treat an infected patient's other symptoms such as back or hip issues. Do remember in such circumstances that you would have to 'under treat' them, as their physiology will already be under demand from the illness and thus more reactive.

N.B. We should *never* claim that osteopathy can and will successfully treat infectious conditions, neither to the public nor to individual patients. Such proclamations would not sit well with our medical colleagues. However, it is ethically professional, to say: 'In my opinion, osteopathy *may* help your body to fight the illness more effectively.' We know from his writings that Still often used to treat illnesses: 'To cure disease the abnormal parts must be admitted to the normal' (Still 1910).

In my professional career, I have knowingly treated a number of patients (including members of my own family) when they were suffering from an illness or disease. My experience is that generally they either felt a positive benefit within 24–48 hours of having had osteopathic treatment, or they felt worse for 24 hours, then afterwards significantly better. In the latter scenario I think that the osteopathic treatment initiates a strong immunological response which results in the immediate symptomatic aggravation, with a subsequent strong decline in the fever and symptoms.

Depending on the long-term vitality of the patient, follow-up treatments may need to be more frequent than in non-infectious conditions. In general, I would advise 'under treating'

patients with an active infection. Their physiology is having to cope with the infection, and we should not create an excessive added demand for change. Remember that osteopathic treatment requires tissue adaptation and change, and we must keep the change to within the tissue's ability at that time.

WHY DOES THE BODY RESPOND TO AN EVENT WITH COMPRESSION, EITHER LOCALLY OR GLOBALLY?

If we look at what is behind the compression, we see a trauma, as outlined above. Any type of trauma is a shock, a distress to the psychophysiology. My *current* understanding of why tissues enter a state of compression is as follows: the traumatic input creates a 'fear' in the affected cells and tissues of the body. If they could speak, they would be saying something like: 'Help, what has just happened to me?' Just before the event happened, they were living happily and calmly, behaving as they are supposed to do, carrying out their individual role for the good of the whole physiology. Suddenly, now they are not! That fear reaction at the cellular or tissue level is to shut down to a greater or lesser extent and tighten up as a protective response. As osteopaths we call this response compression. (See more on cellular consciousness in Chapter 18.)

I like to use an analogy of how a young child responds to an unknown threat. Imagine, or perhaps you can remember this from your own childhood, a young child experiencing their first powerful and very loud lightning and thunderstorm. Because they have never experienced anything like this before they have no reference to give support to their feelings. They experience very bright flashes of light, which their closed eyelids will not keep out, followed by very loud bangs and possible house vibrations from the thunderclaps. This, to them, is a very frightening experience. Quite often the child may then go

to somewhere safe, a small place, under the bedclothes, behind a settee, in the cupboard under the stairs, etc., to an enclosed place. Then they tend to sit in a hunched posture, often with their knees up to their chest, with arms fully crossed around their body, as protective posture. The small surroundings give or provide an added feeling of security.

Compressed tissues

In a state of fear and shock from trauma of any type, the tissues are doing the same as the frightened child. However, unlike the child they cannot move to somewhere safe, but they do tighten up to become a bit smaller and 'feel safer' in response to the outside threat. That tightening process creates a sense of being partially cut off from the rest of the body and its vitality, its potency, and cut off from the wholeness to varying degrees. When we palpate a compressed tissue state, it does feel as if it is a bit separate from the full health of the patient, and consequently behaves differently. It needs treatment!

So now we have a compressed tissue, which is feeling partially separated from the wholeness, the health of the rest of the physiology. Because it is now compromised, lacking the full resources of the health of the body, it is unable to treat itself like it would do under normal circumstances. Areas which were initially compressed due to a response from a type of trauma, but to one of a lesser degree, will retain or have greater communication with the health of the body. Consequently, they are able to treat themselves and, quickly or slowly, resolve their compressive state. From this self-treatment, they become improved, and hence asymptomatic.

Going back to the frightened child analogy, how do parents respond to the frightened child hiding under the stairs, under the duvet or behind the settee, etc.? A parent lacking sympathy for the child's fear might just say in a stern voice: 'Don't be so silly, come out of there!' In such a situation, this statement and harsh tone of the parent only adds to the child's fear and makes them want to stay where they are, and to stay safe even more. The child's refusal would anger the parent who will say it again with an even stronger voice tonality and a vicious circle will arise between them, perhaps resulting in the child being physically pulled out of their safe place by the parent.

By contrast, the wise parent responds *very* differently. They gently go and sit with the child in their safe place and give the child a warm and supportive cuddle, holding the child just right, not too tightly, but also not too loosely like a wet fish, and say in a tender, sympathetic voice: 'Yes, it is a bit frightening isn't it.' This *immediately* makes the child feel *acknowledged, understood and protected* by the parent. The wise parent, instead of telling the child to get out, stays with the child in their safe place, keeping the reassuring cuddle, gently saying reassuring things, until they feel the tension in the child release. Only after having felt the child relax, the wise parent would then encourage the child to leave that space, by saying something such as: 'Would you like to come and have a glass of juice and a biscuit in the kitchen?' The child, now feeling understood, reassured and relaxed, would naturally agree and go with the parent, leaving that safe place behind to have a treat in the kitchen, ready to continue their day.

When we treat a compressed tissue with the involuntary mechanism, we should act like the wise parent. Here is a suggested checklist:

- Acknowledge the tissue state of the compression, to develop an understanding that it has lost a sense of connectivity to the wholeness of the body due to the trauma, which is a relatively frightening state for that tissue to experience. This is what we do when we are centred and put our hands on such a tissue.

- Match the tissue tone of the compression, not too much (which would exacerbate the compression), nor too little, but just right, like the parent giving the perfect cuddle (see fist matching exercise in Chapter 2). The more centred we are, the more accurately this will happen as we become more at one with the tissues and harmonise with them.

- Instead of forcing the tissues out of that state (the bad parent pulling the child out of the cupboard), we work with the tissues, creating the perfect matching of the compression (like the wise parent sitting next to the child giving reassurance).

- Wait for the still point at the point of resolution! The wise and perceptive parent notes this point too, as it happens just before the child relaxes.

- The tissue changes and restorations then occur, with an improved quality of involuntary motion, along with a greater connectivity to the wholeness and health of the physiology. The child leaves the safe hiding place and goes to the kitchen with the parent.

CHRONIC OR ACUTE TISSUE QUALITY?

Is this the primary area of the problem or a secondary effect?

Questions of chronicity compared with the acute patient are important in practice. We frequently get asked by our patients: 'How long will it take to cure me/get me better?' I call this the dreaded question because the only true answer is to say: 'It depends, and depends on many, many factors.' Remember, as osteopaths we are not the primary practitioner, that is the patient themselves. We are at best the assistant. However, we must still do our best to answer the patient's natural curiosity. Their question may be underlying another but to them important, unspoken question: 'How much is this going to cost me?' That is assuming you are in private practice, where the patient has to pay your fees, and you are not covered under some insurance scheme. For example, nearly all patients in the UK do not have insurance cover to pay osteopathy fees. This is an important question for many patients. Truthful but careful answers are required. Clearly the more chronic their condition, the longer the prognosis will be, and the patient needs to be advised accordingly.

Gaining a diagnostic database in your awareness of the differences between a chronic issue and a more acute one comes from practitioner experience. However, time-based qualitative differences are usually quicker for a practitioner to develop compared with some other qualitative differences.

If working with a tissue, what is the fluid quality within that solid tissue?

Irrespective of the tissue type, we need to assess the fluid quality within that tissue. Generally speaking, healthy cells and tissues need good fluidity for high quality diffusion of nutriments and excretion of waste products. Dehydrated tissues are more at risk of becoming toxic. However, it is important to differentiate between a good fluid state and an oedematous tissue state arising from active inflammation. A good example would be an oedematous spinal disc with the patient in acute pain. This quality although fluid, is clearly not a healthy state. This differentiation palpation skill develops from repeated experience of such tissues.

What is the potency level and quality within the fluids and tissues?

When teaching, I often hear students say: 'The potency is much greater now' or 'The potency has increased after doing x, y, z, [a CV4, a lateral fluctuation or some other therapeutic input] to my model at the table.' It should always be borne in mind that potency never increases in the body! It is always infinite, it is our Life Breath, it is the Universal Energy within us – some may even say it is the 'Breath of God' within us.

In my opinion, what happens when we get physically or mentally stressed, or ill for any reason, is that the brilliant inner radiance of our potency gets covered by layers of sheets and blankets. Whether it is one sheet, several sheets, one blanket or many blankets with each illness, will depend on the severity of the illness or stress factor (of any type). Over time, with a variety of life events, the sheet and blanket layer thickness increases. This then covers, blocks, or masks the incredibly powerful inner light of the potency, and it no longer expresses fully in our tissues. As a consequence of this poorer expression of the potency, the tissues feel dull, have poorer involuntary motion, and feel exhausted, sick, depressed, and lacking in vitality and health.

All good treatments remove some of the layers from the system. Treatment allows the inner light, which was always very bright, to shine through the now thinner layers, and therefore the potency can now be more fully expressed to our palpation. The tissues then feel healthier to us as practitioners, and the patient feels healthier and has more vitality.

Centring is an effective way to remove some of our own sheets and blankets! We too have many of them, not just our patients. I recommend practising this for a while (20 or more minutes if you have the time) each day and always 20 to 30 seconds minimum before commencing any treatment with patients. Our own blankets annoyingly distort our perception and appreciation of the real diagnosis and the most effective way to engage therapeutically with our patients. Unfortunately, our ego is blind to perceiving our blankets and does not realise they need to be gradually removed during our lifetime, and may often say to you: 'There is no time to centre ourselves now, so let's just get on with the treatment or other things I need to do.' So, my advice would be to centre yourselves anyway, no matter what your thoughts tell you!

In conclusion to the chapter, I would consider the most important factor for you to consider when palpating is: 'Am I working from an "ego-based fulcrum"?' An ego-based fulcrum is where we assume we are right, and this can be expressed in a number of different ways:

- Assuming that you are the person who gets the patient better, when in fact you are merely the assistant. Our patients may say that we made them better, but perhaps they do not fully appreciate their own self-healing abilities.
- 'Knowing' in advance what you are going to feel, based on the case history. The reality may be something different.

- Not listening to the body, which is giving us advice on how best to give a treatment.
- Our ego wanting to get the person better so much that we over treat them. This risk is even greater if treating a close friend or family member.

Every patient can add to our knowledge of the physiology. In reality we all only have a limited understanding of the human physiology. If we are without ego, we then realise that the more we know, the more there is still to know. Humbly consider what each patient attending our clinic is teaching us. The best way to avoid working from an ego-based fulcrum is to practise centring on a regular basis.

REFERENCES

Brooks, R.E., 1997. Learning to listen. Excerpts from various lectures by Dr Becker. In: Brooks, R., ed. *Life in Motion, The Osteopathic Vision of Rollin E. Becker DO*. Portland, OR: Rudra Press, p. 149.

Cambridge University Press, 2021. Vitality. Cambridge Dictionary. Available from: https://dictionary.cambridge.org/dictionary/english/vitality.

Lewis, J., 2012. Mind. In: *AT Still: From the Dry Bone to the Living Man*. Blaenau Ffestiniog: Dry Bone Press, p. 268.

Still, A.T., 1902. *Philosophy and Mechanical Principles of Osteopathy*. Kansas City, MO: Hudson-Kimberly Pub Co. Reprinted, Kirksville, MO: Osteopathic Enterprises; 1986.

Still, A.T., 1908. *Autobiography of A.T. Still*. Kansas City, MO: Hudson-Kimberly Pub Co. Reprinted, Kirksville, MO: Osteopathic Enterprises; 1981.

Still, A.T., 1910. *Research and Practice*. Kansas City, MO: Hudson-Kimberly Pub Co. Reprinted, Kirksville, MO: Osteopathic Enterprises; 1986.

Part 2

EMBRYOLOGY AND DIFFERING ANATOMICAL AREAS OF THE PHYSIOLOGY

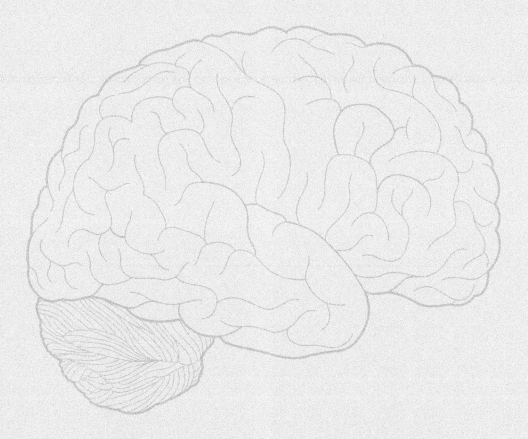

CHAPTER 4

Embryology and its Inner Relevance to Osteopaths

TISSUE TYPES

As we know, embryology is the study of development of the body. This is a fascinating study which will enrich your osteopathic abilities significantly. The three original tissue types are the ectoderm – the outermost layer, the mesoderm – the middle layer, and the endoderm – the innermost layer. It is worthwhile remembering which tissues derive from which layers.

The ectoderm
The ectoderm gives rise to tissues which function in relation to the external environment. These include the skin, nails and hair. However, our nervous system is significantly involved in our relating to the world around us and is also an ectodermal tissue. Our sense organs also relate to the outside world and are formed by ectodermal tissue. As such their epithelial lining, along with the lens of the eye, the nasal cavity, our sinuses, the mouth including the tooth enamel, and the anal canal, are also ectodermal tissues. The pituitary gland is another significant part of the physiology which has much influence on the physiology and is also derived from the ectoderm (Britannica.com 2019a).

Sadler describes these ectodermal tissues as those which 'maintain contact with the outside world' (Sadler 1995). I find Sadler's definition a useful way to remember the ectodermal tissues,

as the ectoderm is the outermost of the three layers and forms tissues with that function, that of relating to the external environment. This helps us to understand why aforementioned tissues are all of ectodermal origin, as they all have a direct relationship to the outside world. We need to see the world around us along with our other senses hence it includes the eye, nasal cavity and our mouth. Even our anal canal is 'relating to the world' in adding to it when we defecate. We probably do not choose or wish to think of our anus in such a fashion, but the embryology developed before our cultural behaviours affected our behaviour and thinking! In Chapter 17 we will look further at inter-tissue relationships, which will include ectodermal tissue relationships.

The endoderm
The endoderm by comparison with the ectoderm, forms the tissue covering layers of the body, the epithelium. Within the head the endoderm forms the lining epithelium of the auditory tube, and in the neck, the pharynx, larynx, tonsils, thyroid and parathyroid glands. In the base of the neck/thorax, the endoderm forms the thymus, trachea and lungs. The endoderm forms the lining of the digestive tube from the oesophagus to rectum, along with the bladder and the urethra, plus the vagina in females (Britannica.com 2019b).

We tend to associate the endoderm with just the gut tube and may forget that the endoderm also forms the organs within the throat and neck, in addition to the tracheal, lung tissue and other non-digestive tract pelvic tissues.

The mesoderm

Without having to create an exceptionally long list, the mesoderm creates all other tissues. These include all muscles, bones, joints, heart and blood vessels, as well as the fascial system.

THE OSTEOPATHIC RELEVANCE OF EMBRYOLOGY

As the late Dr James Jealous said to me in some of his lectures: 'The forces of embryogenesis become the forces of growth and development, healing and repair' (Jealous 1998). The study of embryology gives us great insight into the fulcra within tissues. Erich Blechschmidt showed in his studies and writings that the mechanical forces acting on the developing embryo strongly influence its growth and development:

> The knowledge of developmental movements leads to the conclusion that differentiation is an undivided biodynamic process that occurs during development and includes the chemical processes as well. Biomechanical features never occur beside biochemical features, but they always implicate the latter. A biochemical synopsis would be impossible unless one has a fundamental knowledge of the morphology as well as the biokinetics of the organic structures. (Blechschmidt and Gasser 1978)

Quite clearly Blechschmidt and Gasser would have approved of our osteopathic thinking and the significance of mechanics affecting structure and biochemistry.

I was recently having a conversation with a colleague about embryology and its osteopathic relevance when palpating. He summed it up rather beautifully in one sentence: 'Feeling the embryology is feeling the development of form and function' (Gosset 2021).

Embryology is a vast topic and I do not intend to go into great detail of the whole body in this chapter. I will, however, demonstrate how an embryological understanding can enhance our therapeutic skills. Hopefully in this manner you will be inspired to venture further into this rewarding field of study. For your reference, at the end of this chapter there is a table of the embryological times of bone formation of the skull base and vault.

USING EMBRYOLOGY IN A THERAPEUTIC CONTEXT

In the early 1980s, I was highly fortunate to have had Dr Robert Fulford (one of Dr Sutherland's key students) as one of my table tutors when I was a student on a cranial course, and also as a fellow teaching colleague in the mid-80s after I had joined the postgraduate teaching faculty of the British School of Osteopathy. Dr Fulford was very keen on the use of timelines in his clinical work, and I have been incredibly grateful to have had his instruction on this approach.

The development and growth of any tissue or structure starts, in the author's current opinion, with an expression of potency in the electromagnetic field (or some other subtle physical force), as a blueprint for that future physical aspect of the physiology. The potency within the health of that growing embryo starts to manifest as an energetic field in the area about to develop. For example, the potency and electromagnetic field would become active around the C7 somite very shortly before the physical manifestation of the upper limb bud in the fourth week of intrauterine life (IUL). Then the physical forces (as inferred by Blechschmidt and Gasser) come into play, and the limb bud grows into this pre-existing 'potentised' electromagnetic field.

After birth and into adulthood, this potentised energetic field still exists. I consider this to be what James Jealous was referring to in the above quotation. By applying our knowledge of embryology, alongside our anatomy of the patient, we can tap into this potentised field, and thereby help to amplify the self-healing and self-repairing processes of our patient's physiology.

Let us look at some examples of how we can use our knowledge of embryology to enhance our therapeutic ability.

The limbs

The upper limb bud emerges at the level of the C7 somite during the fourth week IUL, and finishes at the end of the middle finger; the lower limb bud begins at L5 a few days later and ends at the second toe. In simplistic terms, the limb buds consist of an apical ectodermal ridge, with a zone of proliferation immediately behind this, and the remainder being mesenchymal tissue in the shape of a paddle, which later differentiates into the constituent tissues. Molecules secreted by the apical ectodermal ridge stimulate continued division of cells within the zone of proliferation. Within the mesenchyme, there is a zone of polarising activity which determines which parts of the limb will become anterior and posterior.

The growing limb bud has a high metabolic rate and so is very thirsty for nutrition and requires metabolic waste products to be removed. This results in a strong osmotic gradient in the fluids of the mesenchyme towards and from the apical region. This flow of fluid along these gradients leads to the formation of the blood vessels within the limb bud. The blood vessels grow due to a demand-led process. As the tissues grow and differentiate, so motor and sensory fibres are

required, and the respective nerve fibres grow into the limb bud. This creation of the neuro-vascular bundle becomes the physiological axis of the new limb.

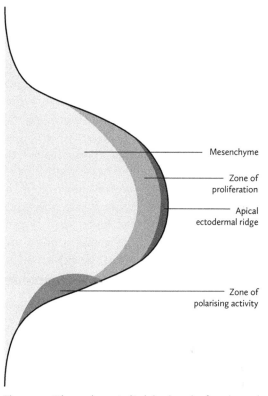

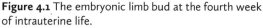

Mesenchyme

Zone of proliferation

Apical ectodermal ridge

Zone of polarising activity

Figure 4.1 The embryonic limb bud at the fourth week of intrauterine life.

Knowing the start and end points of the growth of the limb bud allows us to gain a sense (not the detail) of the whole process. We can gain a strong link to the potency of the limb by having our hand or finger contact on the origin and distal ends of the limb bud. When you do this, you may be able to get a sense of the potency flowing along this energetic 'pre-former' of the limb.

In Chapter 8: The liquid spine and limbs, there is an audio-based exercise helping you to feel the embryological development of the limb, but do not jump to that chapter quite yet – do work your way through the next few chapters first.

Osseous strains and restrictions in the cranium

When working with the cranial base or cranial vault bones, an understanding of the times of ossification is particularly useful. It should always be borne in mind that our bones develop relatively late in the embryological process. For example, consider this statement: 'Nothing ever goes through a bony foramen in the skull!' At an initial read of this sentence, it seems ridiculous. However, is it technically true? Because the relevant structure, the nerves or blood vessels, were present even before the bones existed! The bones developed around the pre-existing nerves and blood vessels.

So, now let us imagine we are working on a patient with a locked coronal suture between the frontal and a parietal bone, such as can occur with a trauma to the frontal bone, or the vertex. If the bones are locked, the expression of the potency within and between them will be reduced. We can use our awareness of the embryology to increase our palpation of the potency within the bones. From the ossification details at the end of the chapter, we can see that the frontal bones start to ossify from membrane at about the eighth week of IUL and the parietal bones at the seventh week of IUL.

Please note that cranial vault bones embryologically derive from membrane whereas cranial base bones derive from cartilage precursors, this being the deciding factor as to which are called base or vault bones. Do remember that the coronal suture is not fully formed until 18 to 24 months after birth, with the closure of the anterior fontanelle.

In Chapter 15 there will be much more on the topic of embryology along with practical exercises. However, it is important that you work your way through all the chapters in sequence, rather than jumping ahead to that chapter now.

An interesting patient

A lady in her late 40s complained of pains that had recently developed in her left glenohumeral joint with symptoms radiating to the left humerus. She had a history of tennis elbow on the left side ten years previously, and a long history of recurrent of pain and tenderness to the cervicodorsal region throughout her childhood and teenage years. There was no history of trauma. On gross assessment, there were no obvious mechanical postural tensions, though on cranial pattern assessment she did have a left side-bending/rotation and a sphenoid low pattern, both of which were well compensated for.

I was somewhat perplexed as I initially could not evaluate any logical reason for the onset of her symptoms. I then thought about the history of tenderness in her childhood years and decided to look at her timeline to assess if there were embryological or birth issues which could shed light on her current symptom picture. I then took the timeline approach to go back to the formation of the left upper limb. I recentred myself and then by bringing the fourth week of IUL to my awareness started to feel a gel like quality of this developing limb at C7. I started to feel a sense of this limb bud emerging and then felt a sense of shock and blocking of the growth process with the potency stopping just after it emerged at C7. My intellect kicked in, and I wondered if this could be the reason for the childhood cervicodorsal tension. Maybe, maybe not. Either way I felt I had to assist the potency of this developing limb bud.

I matched the incredibly delicate state of the mesoderm and kept my attention with this sense of shock to the potency, at the location of where it had just emerged from C7. I then very, very gently, mentally whispered to the potency inviting it to treat itself, if it wanted to, and waited, keeping as centred as possible. After a little while, there was a shimmering-like sensation within the potency and then a greater expression followed by a continued growth of the limb bud. A similar situation occurred when the potency and growth of the limb bud reached the position of what would become the glenohumeral joint and subsequently the left elbow. Each time I whispered an invitation to the potency to treat itself if it wanted to, it was followed by this shimmering and greater potency expression and continued growth of the limb bud. When the limb bud reached the tip of the middle finger, I stayed with the connection between C7 and the middle fingertip to ensure the potency flow was unhindered between the two ends of the limb bud.

I still did not know if this shock to the growing limb bud was the aetiology behind her symptoms. Childhood issues without any other obvious aetiology can be from birth trauma. Therefore, I then checked the birth process forces on the meninges via another timeline (more details on this approach in Chapter 15). I became aware of mechanical tensions associated with her birth, but having already done some deep work on her left upper limb bud, I decided to leave birth trauma treatment to her next visit. This was for two reasons: most importantly, because I felt her tissues were telling me that they had had enough for that day. Such messages must be acknowledged and followed. The second reason was because I wanted to know if, or how much, her symptoms would reduce by purely releasing her limb bud and without any other treatment being carried out on that visit.

She returned the following week exclaiming that her left shoulder and forearm 'felt radically different, much freer and somehow stronger'. At the treatment table I checked her left limb bud again to see how the potency quality was expressing, and it had maintained the quality after the previous treatment. I then did do some work on releasing her birth forces to the meninges and fasciae. She returned the following week symptom free.

I hope that this chapter has opened your awareness, if you did not have it already, of the significant benefit of gaining an understanding of embryology to our work. The above examples of the limbs and cranial vault are simple overviews of the embryology in these areas. As said above, this chapter cannot give a full embryological account as that would be a whole book in itself. However, I do strongly encourage you to delve much more deeply into this fascinating and rewarding topic.

Table 4.1 Embryological ossification dates for the cranial base and vault bones.

Ossification centres and dates			
Sphenoid	Formed prenatally, in cartilage *except for tips of greater wings*.		
	Body	This is formed in two parts (pre- and post-sphenoid) which remain ununited until the 7th or 8th month IUL.	
		Pre-sphenoid	Two ossification centres, one for the body and one for each lesser wing.
		Post-sphenoid	Two centres for the body, one for each greater wing peg.
	Greater wings		One for each centre.
	Pterygoid process		One centre for each.
	Pre- and post-sphenoid fuse at 8–9 months IUL.		

cont.

Ossification centres and dates		
At birth	When we are born, the sphenoid is in three parts: body and pterygoid unit, plus the two greater wings. In the first year after birth, the greater wings and body unite.	
Occiput	One centre for basilar part and one for each condylar part. Two centres for supra-occiput all formed in cartilage.	
	Two centres for interparietal occiput formed in membrane.	
At birth	When born, the occiput is in four parts: the basilar part, two condylar parts, and the squamous part, all united in cartilage. The condyles and basilar parts unite at 7–8 years. The squama and condylar parts unite at 3–5 years.	
Sphenobasilar symphysis	This fuses by the 25th year.	
Temporal bone		
	Squama	This ossifies in membrane from a centre at the root of the zygomatic process at the 7th to 8th week IUL.
	Petromastoid	This ossifies from several ossification centres which appear from the otic capsule at the 5th month IUL. These otic centres fuse by the end of the 6th month IUL.
	Tympanic part	This ossifies in membrane from a centre which appears at the 3rd month IUL. By the time of birth this becomes a ring, the *tympanic ring*, which is incomplete superiorly.
	Styloid process	This develops from the cranial end of the second visceral (hyoid) arch.
	Unification	The tympanic ring unites with the squamous part shortly before birth.
		The petromastoid fuses with the squamous part during the first year.
		The proximal root of the styloid fuses with the main part of the temporal bone during the first year.
		The remainder of the styloid does not fuse until after puberty, though sometimes it does not fuse.
The ethmoid	Ossifies from cartilage in three centres.	
	Perpendicular plate and crista gali	These begin to ossify in the first year after birth.
	Lateral masses (labyrinth)	One centre for each side appears between the 4th and 5th months IUL.
	Unification	The three centres fuse at the beginning of the second year.
The frontal bone(s)	These ossify in membrane from two centres which appear in the 8th week IUL in the region of the superciliary arches.	
	From each of these two frontal bones, the ossification spreads to the rest of each half of the bone, separated from its partner by the metopic suture.	
	Unification	The metopic suture begins to ossify in the second year after birth, and usually fuses by the 8th year, although the metopic suture can remain patent into adulthood.
The parietal bones	Each parietal bone develops from two centres one above the other at the parietal boss around the 7th week IUL in membrane.	
	Unification	These two centres unite early and ossification spreads towards the periphery of the bone, so the angles are the last to ossify, and these are locations of the fontanelles.

IUL, intrauterine life.

REFERENCES

Blechschmidt, E., & Gasser, R.F., 1978. Introduction. In: Burdi, A.R., ed. *Biokinetics and Biodynamics of Human Differentiation*. Springfield, IL: Charles C. Thomas, p. xiii.

Britannica.com, 2019a. Ectoderm. Encyclopaedia Britannica. Available from: https://www.britannica.com/science/ectoderm.

Britannica.com, 2019b. Endoderm. Encyclopaedia Britannica. Available from: https://www.britannica.com/science/endoderm.

Gosset, N., 2021. Conversation with Timothy Marris. 26 April.

Jealous, J., 1998. Conversation with Timothy Marris. June.

Sadler, T.W., 1995. Embryonic period (third to eighth weeks). In: Sadler, T.W., ed. *Langman's Medical Embryology*. 7th edition. Baltimore, MD: Williams and Wilkins, p. 87.

CHAPTER 5

The Inner Approach: To Be the Bone

The word bone is deeply associated with our profession: we are after all 'osteo' paths. To many (and also to me for many years), the meaning of osteopath is derived from bone plus the 'path' of pathology, thus 'bone pathology'. Pathology is the study of disease, but we as osteopaths do not treat bone diseases such as osteomyelitis of bone cancer. We, as practitioners are *par excellence* at reducing bone dis-ease, removing the 'dis' to leave the 'ease'! When working, we are feeling subtle, and at times gross, strains and tensions within the bone structure, and with treatment, are reducing the mechanical forces acting on and within the bone, resulting in greater ease.

Dr James Jealous once said in a lecture I attended: 'The "path" in osteopath can also come from the Greek "pathos" which can mean "feeling"' (Jealous 1997). The dictionary definition of the word pathos is: 'The quality or property of anything *which touches the feelings or excites emotions and passions*, especially that which awakens tender emotions, such as pity, sorrow, and the like; *contagious warmth of feeling, action, or expression*; pathetic quality' (Your dictionary, 2022). (N.B. The italics are mine as these definitions seem particularly relevant to us as osteopaths.)

When working as osteopaths we should be expressing that 'which touches the feelings or excites emotions and passions', and most of the time we do feel highly passionate about our work, our desire to help our patients. We also 'feel touched' not only in the afferent palpatory sense, but also 'emotionally moved' or 'touched' by the incredible wisdom of the human body when we work with our patients.

So, as osteopaths, we should not associate ourselves with the commonly used negative aspect of pathos, that which means disease. Andrew Taylor Still himself made this very apt statement in his book, *Philosophy of Osteopathy*: 'To find health should be the object of the doctor. Anyone can find disease' (Still 1903). So quite clearly, when Still coined the word Osteopathy, he did not do so thinking of ill health or disease, as he had health primarily in his awareness when treating his patients.

'Bone is the second most fluid tissue in the body after blood!' (Watt 1984). This is a quote from the late Dr John Watt, a retired professor of physiology at the medical school of Edinburgh University, who used to be one of my students on cranial courses, many years ago. This quote truly reflects the quality of bone in accordance with the 'inner approach'.

If we add Dr Watt's definition of bone to the above definition of pathos, then we have a tissue which ranges in its expression from the most hard and dense tissue to the second most fluid after blood, 'which touches the feelings or excites emotions and passions' of us as osteo-pathos practitioners. This for me is something of which we can, and should, all be truly proud!

BONE TISSUE

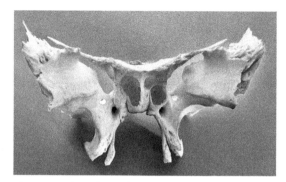

Figure 5.1 The sphenoid bone.

Bone stem cells are formed from osteoprogenitor cells and are important for bone repair and growth. These osteogenic cells are mesenchymal in origin and develop into bone spindle cells. As the bone develops, the cells become more numerous to allow bone remodelling (Nahian and Davis 2021). In simple terms, the osteoprogenitor cells are the stem cells of bone and form osteoblasts. These in turn create the osteocytes (mature bone cells) which build bone tissue, and the osteoclasts which breakdown osteocytes.

Osteoblasts carry an important role in bone metabolism, and are vital for bone formation and remodelling. Osteoblasts are layered inside and outside adult bone structures, encasing mineralised bone matrices. Together with osteoclasts, osteoblasts remodel bone in response to mechanical tension (Bourdieu and Hirschi 2019). Mechanical tension is what we as osteopaths are palpating within body structures, and we are continually adding it to our diagnostic data, when at the treatment table.

So, if osteoclasts and osteoblasts are remodelling bone in response to mechanical tensions, and we in our osteopathic work are reducing mechanical tensions on the physiology, can we change bone shape? More on this later in the chapter.

Let us look in turn at the different layers of bone.

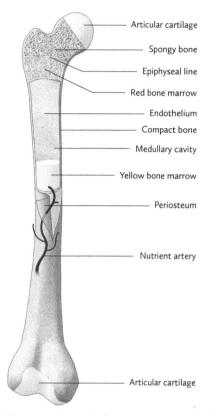

Figure 5.2 The right femur showing the differing layers and bony constituents.

Periosteum

When you consider bone as a tissue, how often do you consider the periosteum? It is the outermost layer of the bone and hence the first aspect to become damaged or distorted (even at a subtle level of force) from disruption coming from outside the bone. Only pathology such as a bone tumour can interfere with the periosteum from within. It is frequently useful when considering a tissue or an organ to consider the container in addition to the contained tissue or organ, as they have strong interrelationships.

In later chapters we will be looking at the capsule of the kidney, the pericardium and the pleura, each being a container of an organ. Even the three layers of the meninges, key tissues in our work with the involuntary mechanism, should be considered as the containers of the brain.

The periosteum is a thick, fibrous vascular membrane covering the bones, except at their extremities, the growing ends. It consists of an outer layer of collagenous tissue containing a few fat cells and an inner layer of fine elastic fibres. It is permeated with the nerves and blood vessels that innervate and nourish the underlying bone. Consequently, it is highly pain sensitive and easily inflamed. Tissues which are highly pain sensitive are either incredibly important tissues for the body physiology or are themselves protective tissues for the vital organs underneath.

As we will see in a later chapter, the outer layer of the pleura is very highly innervated with pain fibres as it is the protective layer for the lungs. As soon as these highly pain sensitive areas become even slightly damaged or threatened with damage, the brain receives the pain signals and puts an emergency action into service, so that we move away from the threat! Frequently our patients see pain as a bad thing, something to be eliminated at all costs. Vast fortunes go to the pharmaceutical industry from the sales of analgesics. I am not totally against analgesic medications, only they should be used to reduce pain to a tolerable level, rather than attempting to eliminate the pain. Pain gives us a warning of when we may be injuring ourselves by our actions and so should perhaps be considered 'a good thing'.

The periosteum becomes thinner and less vascular as we age, reflecting that the physiology of bone becomes less active as we get older. However, it remains a storehouse of osteoprogenitor cells ready to be activated subsequent to injury to the bone. It also remains vital to the health of the bone, and bone that loses its periosteum repairs more slowly and to a poorer quality. The periosteum also contains osteoprogenitor-based stem cells. These are essential for bone development embryologically and postnatal fracture repair (Wu *et al.* 2015).

The progenitor cells are located in the inner of the two layers of the periosteum. The outer layer is the fibrous layer containing mainly collagen, fibroblasts and elastin, along with the nerves and blood vessels. The inner (cambium) layer contains osteoblasts, fibroblasts and sympathetic nerves, which give the periosteum its regenerative ability. As we get older, there is a reduction in the number of osteoblasts, which results in a reduction of the thickness of this cambium layer (Lin *et al.* 2014).

Being easily inflamed due to its highly vascular state, the periosteum is very dynamically active. If, due to trauma or from a tumour, the periosteum is lifted away from the cortical bone, the osteoblasts underneath are consequently stimulated to lay down bone tissue as a protective mechanism in such cases of bone injury.

As you will discover as you progress through the chapters of this book, each tissue of the body has its own unique quality. This is due to the unique function of that tissue. We know that muscle, ligament, bone and fascia all have their unique palpatory qualities. Our perception of these qualities allows us to differentiate between tissue types. Muscle is firm but soft, bone is hard and dense, ligaments and tendons feel stringy, fascia feels like a sheet of sinew rather than string-like. Our brains instantly make these differential assessments because we have been experiencing these tissue qualities since starting out on our osteopathic journey. As we progress through this book you perhaps will be experiencing tissues you have not felt before. When feeling a new tissue, you have no database of what this new tissue feels like compared with tissues with which you are already familiar. This is where our anatomical awareness is essential.

Our anatomical knowledge is our road map or sat nav, an essential piece of kit when going on a journey to a new or unknown destination. However, our map is only as good as the software that runs the sat nav to give detail on the page of the screen. Road maps can show towns and differentiate between motorways, highways, main roads and local roads. This information is fine if travelling by car, but if going for a walk off-road into a national park, it will not help very much! For such a journey you need details such as contour lines, footpaths, streams and rivers, whether the trees are deciduous or coniferous, etc., so that you can navigate this more complex and demanding territory. Only then are you more likely to reach your desired destination.

Exercise on palpating the periosteum
N.B. Do remember the points from Chapter 2 on centring, matching and the osteopathic toolbox!

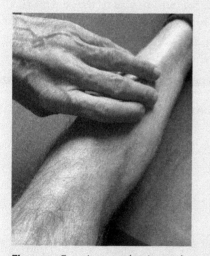

Figure 5.3 Exercise on palpation and treatment of the periosteum

https://youtu.be/-wZDtdlSL7Q

However, the map or sat nav cannot give you the experience of the place, only its topography and its distance from other locations. It does not tell

you what the flowers look like, whether the soil is wet, moist, or dry. Nor will it show you the quality of the reflections in a lake, the beauty of the sunset, etc. In the same way, our anatomical knowledge will not tell you the quality of a tissue – it must be experienced. With repetition of palpating 'new tissue', its unique tissue quality becomes fixed into your mental database for accessing in the future.

To take our awareness to the periosteum, if we have not felt it before, we must start somewhere quite familiar so that we know where we are on 'the map'. Often in tourist destinations there is a map showing the area and a sign saying 'you are here' with a big arrow pointing to it. If we have never felt the periosteum before, we need that tourist map and arrow.

Bone cortex

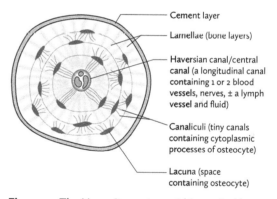

Figure 5.4 The Haversian system within cortical bone.

Cortical bone in long bones is sandwiched between the periosteum externally and the endosteum internally. It comprises the compact Haversian systems with the bone being laid down in a parallel manner, resulting in incredible strength for its size (to forces along the shaft).

In human anatomy, the femur is the longest and largest bone. Along with the temporal bone of the skull, it is one of the two strongest bones in the body. The average adult male femur is 48 cm (18.9 in) in length and 2.34 cm (0.92 in) in diameter and can support up to 30 times the weight of an adult. (Davis n.d.)

It is interesting to note from the above quotation that the temporal bone and the femur are the two strongest bones in the body for their size! By comparison, cancellous bone found at the growing ends is far less dense and, consequently, much lighter in weight. The spaces between the trabeculae contain fluid, blood and bone marrow. Being highly vascular they offer a higher level of cellular nutrition than the shaft.

When looking at an anterior X-ray of the pelvis, look at the direction lines of the trabeculae. They tell the tale of the forces acting on the bone at that specific time. If you look carefully, you will see that the lines of the trabeculae in the sacrum and innominate bones, along with the head and neck of the femur, all appear as if continuous through the joints and ligaments. The trabeculae demonstrate the dissipation of the forces within the bones as transmitted to them by the ligaments and the joints.

We must remember that bone tissue is a highly dynamic tissue, being continually broken down by osteoclasts and rebuilt by osteoblasts. The rebuilding which occurs will be taking place under the strains, shears and stresses which a person's body is experiencing *at that time*. These mechanical forces may be from recent or old accidents and injuries such as birth, road traffic accidents, falls and sporting injuries. They may also occur from postural insults or psychological stresses causing soft tissue compression leading to bone compression, either locally or globally within the body. It goes without saying that the more severe the force, the greater degree the bone trabeculae have to change and adjust to the input.

This phenomenon of bone being highly active, not passive, is often overlooked by practitioners. When we see a patient with an arthritic knee joint, for example, we tend to think that we cannot change the tibial plateau, so we need

to work to get symptomatic relief for the joint capsule, ligaments and associated soft tissues. However, if we remember that bone is continually modifying to the mechanical forces acting upon it (see above quote), it therefore means that if we change the mechanical forces acting on the bone, there is the possibility for the bone shape to change.

Normally the body slowly changes as mechanical tensions (postural or traumatic) tend to increase with age. However, as osteopaths we can and do reduce mechanical forces in the physiology. Many patients, for financial or other reasons, stop seeing us soon as, or shortly after, their symptoms disappear (in the UK most patients do not have private health insurance, and their osteopathic fees are not paid by the government). However, if patients are prepared to return for regular treatments when symptom free, in my experience, bone shape change can occur (see Case study: Margaret later in this chapter).

Endosteum

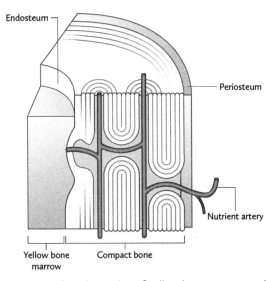

Figure 5.5 The relationship of yellow bone marrow and endosteum to compact bone.

As has been mentioned above, the endosteum is the inner covering of the cortical bone, sandwiched between the cortex and the bone marrow. The endosteum along with the periosteum and marrow contains the cells associated with the production, maintenance and modelling of the osteocytes. The endosteum comprises a single thin layer of mature osteoblasts. These surround the bone marrow which is at the centre of the shaft. Where there are areas of active bone resorption, osteoclasts are also found within the endosteum (Fuchs *et al.* 2009).

Like the periosteum, the endosteum is a vascular thin covering of the cortical bone through which the blood vessels pass, between the bone marrow and the hard cortical bone. Part of the role of the endosteum is the reabsorption of bone by osteoclastic activity to prevent the bone becoming too thick and solid. Consequently, the endosteum is an important aspect of bone remodelling.

Bone marrow

In rats, bone marrow accounts for 3 per cent of the adult body weight (Travlos 2006). Admittedly we cannot assume that the same ratio applies to humans, but nevertheless it does indicate the importance of bone marrow to the physiology. Red bone marrow (also referred to as myeloid tissue) is a soft and gel-like tissue which is located in the spongy or cancellous regions of the bones. Yellow bone marrow on the other hand is located within the shaft of the long bones. Marrow is either red or yellow depending on the level of haematopoietic cells in the red marrow, or fatty tissue which gives its colour to the yellow marrow.

Bone marrow has a phenomenal role in the haemopoietic system. According to Nichols, bone marrow produces 200 billion new red blood cells every day, along with white blood cells and platelets (Nichols 2017). Such a high metabolism requires a rich blood supply. These come from vessels within the marrow in the case of yellow marrow and from within the trabeculae of the growing ends for the red marrow.

The lymphocytes are formed in the yellow marrow and then they mature in the lymphoid tissues: the thymus, spleen and lymph nodes of the body. The function of yellow bone marrow in addition to lymphocyte formation is part of the fat storage system within the body. However, if there is a severe injury and loss of blood, or the body is in a state of high fever, the yellow marrow may be converted to red bone marrow to help maintain the level of red blood cells. The rest of the blood is synthesised in the red bone marrow. In addition to the synthesis of red blood cells, the red bone marrow along with the liver and spleen is involved with the destruction and clearance of the old red corpuscles which are no longer efficient in their physiology.

At birth, all bone marrow is red, reflecting the need for synthesis, and removal, of red blood cells. As we mature into adulthood, the ratio of red to yellow marrow changes as fat tissue replaces the red marrow. Consequently, in adults, red marrow is only present in the vertebrae, scapulae, innominate bones of the pelvis, sternum, ribs, skull and in the proximal ends of our long bones of the extremities. The other cancellous or spongy bones of the body are filled with yellow marrow.

As been mentioned above, bone marrow has a rich blood supply, created by a demand-led development of blood vessels. It has been found that arterial capillaries are present within the Haversian canals, which return to the bone marrow cavity and then on to the venous sinuses present there. This creates a circulatory blood flow within the bone marrow from its centre to its periphery, then returning to the centre of the marrow (Travlos 2006).

The bone marrow includes all the precursors of bone itself in addition to the haematopoietic function of the marrow. Fibroblasts, macrophages, adipocytes, osteoblasts, osteoclasts and endothelial cells are all present in the bone marrow. The macrophages, in addition to their immune system function, also contribute to the development of red blood cells as they contribute iron, which is essential for haemoglobin synthesis. The endothelial cells present are responsible for the formation of the small blood vessels within the bone.

Exercise on palpating the endosteum and bone marrow

https://youtu.be/aasuY9naJZ8

EMBRYOLOGY

In the previous chapter we looked at limb bud formation, but let us now consider bone formation in a little more detail.

If we consider embryology and how in the embryological phase of development, bone develops after nearly all other tissues, in a developing limb bud (commencing at the four-week stage) there is no bone as we know it, no hard structure. The limb bud is an extension of the basic mesenchymal, undifferentiated stem cells. We know that bone is developed having undergone a chondrogenesis stage, before undertaking the transformation into a hard bone tissue. In the last chapter we undertook a palpatory exercise to feel the quality of the pre-bone state, as if we were able to travel back in time and palpate the physiology. So, let us look at bone embryology.

Embryologically bone formation begins with the condensation of mesenchyme cells into chondrocytes, which then form a model for the respective bone. Into this cartilaginous bone model, blood vessels enter to supply the oxygen and nutriment at the regions near to the osteoblastic activity in the growing ends (the epiphyses). The chondrocytes within the shaft undertake hypertrophy thereby mineralising the cartilaginous matrix. The growth of the long bones then continues throughout childhood and our teenage years and is sustained by the increasing numbers of fibroblasts (Duke Medicine 2012).

If we were to imagine the pre-chondrocyte stage when the mesenchyme cells are aggregating around the future bone location within the limb bud, yet before development of true chondrocytes, there would be a gel-like state with all the precursors present for the development of the chondrocytes and the future bone. This point of development prior to the cartilage formation would, in my opinion, be quite analogous to the gel-like quality of bone marrow. The fact that bone marrow contains fibroblasts, macrophages, adipocytes, osteoblasts, osteoclasts and endothelial cells, to my mind, makes this analogy even more intriguing. When palpating the bone marrow, could we be feeling the quality of the four-week-old embryo limb buds?

From the above we can see the incredibly vital role of the marrow cells within our bones, how the marrow is an incredibly vital aspect of the haematopoietic system of the body, and how the bone core's function is about blood not skeletal structure. Likely the above information will not necessarily be new to you the reader, as it will have been covered in your undergraduate training and subsequent studies. However, when working with bone as a tissue in your patients – joints of long bones, vertebrae, the cranial base, pelvis, cranial vault, or scapulae – do you consider the haematopoietic role of the bone marrow within the bones?

BONE AND TRAUMA

Falls and injuries of all kinds happen to us from the time we are born. Birth itself is highly traumatic, then we start learning to crawl and walk, with subsequent falls in our learning process. As we go through childhood we experience greater injuries. Finally, as teenagers and then adults our activities and pursuits become more ambitious, often involving faster motion activities such as skiing, horse riding, cycling and also motor vehicle activities. Many physical sporting activities are exciting and exhilarating because they take us to the limits or even beyond our perceived ability. This gives an endorphin rush and makes us feel amazing. For example, skiing allows the (good) skier to move at speeds well beyond his or her running ability without added motor assistance; horse riding does the same, aided by the horse. As we stretch ourselves to get more and more exhilaration from the activities we pursue, the injury risk increases proportionately.

With bone being the densest tissue in the body, it will tend to hold onto the tissue memory of the injury longer than other tissues, which is what we frequently experience with our palpation. When we hold a limb and feel its quality, we become aware of the strain patterns in the bone both recent and old. These patterns may still be present in the fasciae and soft tissues, but to a different quality.

When working on traumatised bone, in addition to feeling the inappropriate mechanical forces still present within the dense cortical bone, remember that those same forces also went through the periosteum, endosteum and marrow. In our diagnosis, we seek to understand how the dynamic biomechanics of the cortical bone has been disturbed and how the physiology is having to cope (to a greater or lesser degree) with the disturbed state. When you next see a patient and feel a bone within a limb, in addition to feeling the hard bone quality, take your awareness to the periosteum, endosteum and marrow and see if their function is working well, or has also been disturbed.

INTRAOSSEOUS STRAINS

At this point I would like to discuss the importance of assessing intraosseous strains. I have found over the years that less experienced practitioners can easily overlook tensions within the bone structure, within the cortical bone, and have difficulty understanding why their treatments to symptomatic joints do not resolve. When seeing a patient with recurrent joint symptoms, we correctly assess the joint(s) involved and evaluate the stresses acting on the joints from the perspective of the muscles, ligaments and fasciae, and also note any other involuntary strains or shears from the body patterns.

What may be overlooked are tensions within the bones which comprise the joints. If such bones do have shears and tensions within their structure, then these will create forces into the joint structure, separate from those caused by the above factors. If these bones express heavy compression within themselves, either side of the joint, they lose their pliability, their plasticity. In such cases the joints then have to compensate for this lack of pliability by having to move more than perhaps they would prefer, possibly becoming hypermobile.

If you have a patient who suffers from hypermobile joints globally, then you have to consider what could be causing a global bony intraosseous tension. This may be from birth forces (more on this in Chapter 15), or it can be from chronic psychological tensions (see Chapter 16), or events within the womb.

CASE STUDY: MARGARET

I once had a lady who came to see me aged 62 complaining of pains in her left ankle and knee. She lived on her own, was divorced from her husband, had no financial worries, was overweight, and had no other symptoms nor medical history. She came across as a happy lady (only on the surface I later realised).

Her left tibial plateau was significantly larger than her right knee, to the point of instability and significant tension on the capsule and ligamentous attachments. She had a classical osteoarthritic knee joint, affecting the way she was having to walk to avoid pains; it also affected her left ankle joint mechanics. She also had degenerative changes to her lumbar spine, tension in her diaphragm and poor cervical mechanics. From a cranial perspective, she had much chronic intraosseous compression in her pelvis and sacrum, a strong left side-bending/rotation strain to the sphenobasilar symphysis, resulting in fascial and dural pulls from the cranial base on the left side of her pelvis, along with a deep compression of her central nervous system tissue.

In addition to treating to reduce the mechanical forces around and within her left lower extremity, I also worked to ease the significant compression in her brain tissue (which I felt had been there since the time of her divorce some ten years previously). I worked to ease the compression in her diaphragm and pelvic congestion, which soon became more apparent after the initial session.

After two or three treatments, she said: 'You're not just working on my leg, are you!' When I asked what she meant by that, she said: 'Because I can feel that I'm changing (for the better) as a person! Can we carry on with the treatments after my knee and ankle feel better?'

Her perceptiveness that I was working on her in totality, not just her musculoskeletal symptoms, opened the door for me to continue to treat and help her significantly beyond the point where her symptoms abated. She came about once a month thereafter. After about four to six months her weight started falling away. The treatments had reduced the compression in her brain tissue. She was genuinely much happier, not just the 'coverup' happiness she expressed in the beginning. It is a well-known medical fact that some people overeat to compensate for their inner psychological distress, resulting in their becoming overweight. Her pelvis became less compressed, partly from better sacral mechanics but also from the reductions in psychological distress. In my experience, a negative state from marital relationship/intimacy issues may cause pelvic tissue compression in our patients. I did not discuss these findings with her. With the treatments, the circulation in her pelvis and lower extremities also showed signs of good improvement.

As the months went by, the mechanics of her left lower extremity went through further and further changes, and tension became less and less through the femur, tibia and foot. As it did so, gradually the shape of her tibia and tibial plateau changed. She started looking younger as she expressed greater vitality. Her classical arthritic knee joint started improving!

When I last saw her (before she moved to a different part of the UK having found a new boyfriend) I had been seeing her for about two and a half years, her appointments being roughly monthly. Her left knee was as slender as a normal knee. Very sadly, this patient came to see me before the days of smartphone cameras, and I did not have my 35mm camera with me, and so I did not take 'before and after' photos. Very few patients have the insight to keep coming for treatment well after all their symptoms have disappeared, and so usually we do not get the opportunity to see such radical bone shape changes occurring from osteopathic treatment. However, all that happened with this patient was a reduction in the mechanical and psychological causes of her tensions, by treating my tissue findings. This changed the mechanics to the bone and soft tissues of the lower extremities and the bone steadily responded by remodelling to the new reduced mechanical tensions.

N.B. We are osteopaths not psychotherapists. If we keep to our professional training of diagnosing and treating tissue states, not asking verbal questions into the psychological causes of those tissue states of our patients, then we are keeping to our professional ethics and standards of osteopathic care. Even if we do come to realise what *may* (we do not know for certain) have caused such tissue tensions, it is not our role to enquire about them. (In Chapter 18 we will discuss this aspect of tissue consciousness further.) Should a patient ask (although unlikely) if their pelvic tensions could be from x, y or z (relationship issue),

I would recommend answering with a true but non-committal statement such as possibly or maybe, so as not to open up a can of psychological worms. Whatever the psychological cause, by keeping our professional osteopathic focus on tissue states, we can help such tissues.

> Do remember that if working in or near a delicate area of the physiology, e.g., pelvis, the chest (on women), mouth, eyes, face, sacrum and coccyx), be mindful of your hand position: give a simple explanation as to why you need to work on that part of the body and get verbal agreement from the patient that they are happy for you to do so.
>
> We must remember that gaining informed consent is professionally required for medicolegal reasons in our osteopathic clinics.

HORMONES AND BONE

Bone tissue is very much affected by the balance of certain hormones. Let us look briefly at each of these in turn.

Parathyroid hormone

There are four small parathyroid glands that are situated at the four anterior corners of the thyroid gland. According to University of Michigan Health, each parathyroid gland is normally about the size of a grain of rice (about 3–5 mm in diameter and 30–60 mg in weight) (University of Michigan Health 2022). The glands secrete parathyroid hormone (PTH), which regulates blood calcium levels. Under normal circumstances the parathyroid secretes additional PTH when the blood calcium levels drop and secretes less PTH when the blood calcium levels rise. From a clinical perspective, if a patient says they have a high calcium level in the blood, do bear in mind the high likelihood of

a tumour: 'If you have high calcium, you almost certainly have a parathyroid tumour' (Parathyroid. com 2022). Parathyroid hormone causes the breakdown of bone and the release of that calcium into the blood. This increases the ability of the body to absorb calcium from food and increases the kidney's ability to hold calcium which would otherwise be lost in urine. In addition, it also causes increased levels of vitamin D.

The body requires calcium for many reasons, including muscle contraction, oocyte activation, building strong bones and teeth, blood clotting, nerve impulse transmission, regulating the heart-beat and fluid balance within cells (Piste *et al.* 2012). Calcium is vital to the whole-body physiology and is therefore considered one of the most important physiological minerals. So, although the parathyroid glands are small, they are key to our health and wellbeing.

Oestrogens

Subsequent to the menopause, oestrogen levels drop in the body. Many post-menopausal women have lower calcium levels within their bones and are diagnosed as having osteoporosis. Naveh-Many and colleagues explain that:

> Oestrogens have a direct action on the parathyroid to increase parathyroid hormone gene expression and parathyroid hormone secretion. Osteoporotic patients have a decreased parathyroid hormone secretory response to changes in serum calcium, supporting the experimental data that oestrogens have a direct effect on the parathyroid. (Naveh-Many *et al.* 1995)

At of the time of writing, there is ongoing debate as to the pros and cons of oestrogen hormone replacement theory (HRT) for post-menopausal women. According to Cancer Research UK, research now shows that HRT does slightly increase breast, uterine and ovarian cancer risks, with the risks increasing the longer HRT is taken by the patient. However, many lifestyle factors affect cancer risk more, such as unhealthy weight, smoking and alcohol intake. Consequently, risks of HRT should be considered against the severity of the person's symptoms:

> Most types of HRT increase the risk of breast cancer. But the risk is higher for those using combined HRT, which uses both oestrogen and progesterone.
>
> Both oestrogen-only and combined HRT slightly increase the risk of ovarian cancer. But when HRT is stopped, the risk starts to go back to what it would have been if HRT wasn't taken. (Cancer Research UK 2021)

Therefore, if you have a patient considering HRT, do make sure they have a full discussion with their medical practitioner about the benefits and possible side effects.

Growth hormone

Along with the hormones mentioned above, bone is also considerably affected by growth hormone (GH) during childhood and our teenage years. Growth hormone is secreted by the anterior pituitary under regulation by the hypothalamus. GH often works in the body in conjunction with insulin-like growth factor 1 (IGF-1). Both GH and IGF-1 have significant effects on the regulation and control of bone growth and metabolism, and consequently they influence bone mass.

Throughout all our growing years the bone mass is steadily increasing, and the mass continues until our mid-20s. Following that time there is a slow decline in bone mass, though this loss of bone mass accelerates as we enter the later years of life. GH along with IGF-1 stimulates the increase of osteoblast cells with resulting bone development. These hormones also increase osteoclast action and hence bone reabsorption. Should there be an absence of GH, there is a reduction of bone remodelling and a loss of bone mineralisation. It is the effect of GH on the chondrocytes at the growing ends which results in bone growth (Olney 2003).

It should be remembered that growth hormone is developed and then released by the pituitary after the hypothalamus has secreted growth hormone releasing factor. Also remember that IGF-1 is mainly synthesised in the liver. Hence it can be seen that GH and IGF-1 are important hormonal factors in healthy bone growth, and deficiencies may reduce the ability for normal bone growth. Consequently, when working with children who are not as tall as would be expected for their age, it may be worth assessing the hypothalamus (see Chapter 12) and pituitary function (see Chapter 13), alongside assessing the liver (see Chapter 9).

I hope that I have opened your eyes a little further when looking at bone. Yes, bone is primarily considered by osteopaths for its musculoskeletal function and joint involvement, but I hope that you will now see bone with a new inner approach when in your clinic. It is incredibly important for its function in the haematopoietic system (working alongside the spleen and liver), and its relationships to hormones.

REFERENCES

Bourdieu, A., & Hirschi, K., 2019. *Encyclopaedia of Tissue Engineering and Regenerative Medicine, Vol 2*. Elsevier.

Cancer Research UK, 2021. Does hormone replacement therapy (HRT) increase cancer risk? Available from: https://www.cancerresearchuk.org/about-cancer/causes-of-cancer/hormones-and-cancer/does-hormone-replacement-therapy-increase-cancer-risk.

Davis, L., n.d. Body physics: motion to metabolism. Open Oregon Educational Resources. Available from: https://openoregon.pressbooks.pub/bodyphysics/chapter/stress-and-strain-on-the-body/

Duke Medicine, 2012. Limb development. Duke University Medical School Embryology Learning Resources. Available from: https://web.duke.edu/anatomy/embryology/limb/limb.html.

Fuchs, R.K., Warden, S.J., & Turner, C.H., 2009. Bone anatomy, physiology and adaptation to mechanical loading. In: Planell, J.A., Best, S.M., Lacroix, D., & Merolli, A., eds. *Bone Repair Biomaterials*. Woodhead Publishing, pp. 25–68.

Jealous, J., 1997. Conversation with Timothy Marris. 22 November.

Lin, Z., Fateh, A., Salem, D.M., & Intini, G., 2014. Periosteum: biology and applications in craniofacial bone regeneration. *J Dent Res*. 93(2): 109–116.

Nahian, A., & Davis, D., 2021. Histology, osteoprogenitor cells. In: StatPearls [Internet]. Treasure Island, FL: StatPearls Publishing. Available from: https://www.ncbi.nlm.nih.gov/books/NBK559160/

Naveh-Many, T., Epstein, E., & Silver, J., 1995. Oestrogens and calcium regulatory hormones: potential implications for bone. *Curr Opin Nephrol Hypertens*. 4(4): 319–323.

Nichols, H., 2017. All you need to know about bone marrow. Medical News Today. Available from: https://www.medicalnewstoday.com/articles/285666.

Parathyroid.com, 2022. Parathyroid glands, high calcium, and hyperparathyroidism. Norman Parathyroid Center. Available from: https://www.parathyroid.com/

Olney, R.C., 2003. Regulation of bone mass by growth hormone. *Med Pediatr Oncol*. 41(3): 228–234.

Piste, P., Sayaji, D., & Avinash, M., 2012. Calcium and its role in human body. Available from: https://www.researchgate.net/publication/274708965_Calcium_and_its_Role_in_Human_Body.

Still, A.T., 1903. *Philosophy of Osteopathy*. Kirksville, MO.

Travlos, G.S., 2006. Normal structure, function, and histology of the bone marrow. *Toxicologic Pathology*. 34(5):548–565.

University of Michigan Health, 2022. Parathyroid disorders. Available from: https://www.uofmhealth.org/conditions-treatments/endocrinology-diabetes-and-metabolism/parathyroid-disorders#:~:text=Each%20parathyroid%20gland%20is%20normally,system%2C%20their%20functions%20are%20unrelated.

Watt, J., 1984. Conversation with Timothy Marris during Sutherland Cranial Teaching Foundation Course. 19 September.

Wu, S., Lin, Z., Yamaguchi, A., & Kasugai, S., 2015. The effects of periosteum removal on the osteocytes in mouse calvaria. *Dent Oral Craniofac Res 1*. Doi: 10.15761/DOCR.1000134.

Your dictionary, 2022. Pathos definition. Available from: https://www.yourdictionary.com/pathos.

CHAPTER 6

Fascia and Cells with an Inner Approach

Fascia is an enormous and under-rated area of the physiology which I cannot hope to fully review here. I will review some microanatomical and histological aspects and then discuss osteopathic insights to this fascinating tissue. As with other chapters I additionally recommend you do your own studies on this topic.

WHAT IS FASCIA?

There has been much scientific debate as to what is fascia and what is not fascia. In the book *Fascia: The Tensional Network of the Human*, Robert Schleip and colleagues quote definitions of fascia given to the Fascia Research Congresses which are worth quoting in full, as the definition indicates the pervasiveness of fascia and how it affects almost all tissues of the body:

> The term fascia here describes the 'soft tissue component of the connective tissue system that permeates the human body'... The complete fascial net then includes not only dense planar tissue sheets (like septa, joint capsules, aponeuroses, organ capsules or retinacula), which may be also called 'proper fascia', but also encompasses local densifications of this network in the form of ligaments and tendons. Additionally, it includes softer collagenous connective tissue like superficial fascia or the innermost intramuscular layer of the endomysium. The cutis, a derivative of the ectoderm, as well as cartilage and bones are not included as parts of the fascial tensional network. However, the term fascia now includes the dura mater, the periosteum, perineurium, the fibrous capsular layer of the vertebral discs, organ capsules as well as bronchial connective tissue and the mesentery of the abdomen. (Schleip *et al.* 2012)

Clearly this definition of fascia is significantly comprehensive. The inclusion of the dura mater is intriguing, as we who work in this cranial field consider the Sutherland Fulcrum, the area around the straight sinus in the skull, as the fulcrum of the meninges and fascia, and were doing so quite some years before this inclusion of the dural meninges as a component of fascia.

Fascia is now also being acknowledged for its role in the development and maintenance of the extracellular matrix: 'The body consists of cells and the matrix outside, between the cells, the extracellular matrix (ECM). The cells in the fascia produce, control, and maintain all the complex ingredients of the ECM' (Nordin 2020). Nordin's definition of fascia as including 'cells that create and maintain the extracellular matrix' brings with it a whole new realm of responsibility and significance to fascia. The ECM itself contains vital components for the health and wellbeing of the physiology at the cellular level. We will look at these aspects in further detail in this chapter.

We know from our osteopathic training that we should look at the whole body, not just specific parts, but on occasions when we are running short of time or perhaps when a patient arrives late for their appointment, it is easy to focus on the area of symptoms. I expect we have all done that at some time in our practice. Even without the role relating to the ECM, fascia is the most pervasive tissue in the body after blood, so we need to pay attention to its fluid quality in addition to any strain patterns which may be prevalent. As you will have noted in your clinical work, many of our patients have relatively dehydrated fascial systems.

TENSEGRITY

As osteopaths we cannot discuss fascia without considering tensegrity. The word 'tensegrity' is derived from 'tension' and 'integrity' and was coined by the architect Buckminster Fuller in his paper: 'Tensegrity: looking at the interrelationship between tension and compression in architectural design' (1961). Tensegrity structures are those which have an integral structure such that it spreads the tensional forces over the whole. Let us consider a dome tent, for example. These tents are the type taken on extreme expeditions where the weather forces can be extraordinarily strong.

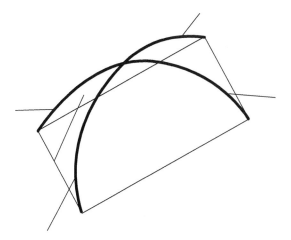

Figure 6.1 A dome tent is a great example of a tensegrity structure. Because of the dome-shaped poles and tension lines, all the wind forces against the tent are distributed against the whole of the fabric of the tent. This makes this type of tent ideal for mountain conditions/expeditions.

The nature of the tent poles, the flexibility of the tent fabric sheets, and the guy ropes' directions to the pegs cause the forces of the wind to be spread as evenly as possible across the whole tent structure. Consequently, by sharing the force there is less risk of damage to any one area and the occupant is more likely to get a restful night's sleep! Modern bridges often use tensegrity principles, for example suspension bridges, which make them far lighter than older solid stone and concrete bridges.

Another example would be a traditional full-masted sailing ship. Such old-style sailing ships, used before the days of steam ships, had several high masts, each with many ropes going from the masts to the hull of the ship. The masts each had several flexible, large sails. Each sail also had rigging ropes connecting to the cross members of the masts and to the hull. Consequently, instead of having a high pressure at their bases, the heavy masts transmitted their gravitational force (added to by the force of the wind) across the whole hull of the ship. Of course, this also importantly ensured that the force of the wind in the sails moved the ship instead of breaking the mast! These ships beautifully demonstrate the tensegrity principle.

The human physiology is also a tensegrity structure. We have a skeleton, our bone structure. This is the equivalent to the tent poles or the masts and cross beams of the ship. Our rigging, our guy ropes and our flexible sails are the muscles, fasciae and ligaments, all of which, *when the physiology is in a good state of balance*, spread the forces acting on the body in multiple directions. However, when the body mechanics are not in good balance, the tensegrity system starts to fail and excessive pressure gradually begins to develop in differing areas. These are the areas which we in this cranial field call 'compression', and if sustained, lead to varying levels of poor function and pathology. This would be like cutting one of the guy ropes of a tent or some of the rigging on a sailing ship. The tent or the ship would not fail completely, but its effectiveness and efficiency for its purpose would certainly be compromised.

As osteopaths we are highly efficient at palpating when the tensegrity structure is less than efficient and is resulting in mechanical tensions. As we all know, we pick up on tensions and strains of which the patient is totally unaware – they only know about the areas of symptoms. Likewise with tensegrity structures such as the ship, the symptoms, a cracking of a cross beam or a tear of a sail, could appear quite some distance away from the rigging tensioners that are out of balance, perhaps even next to the hull of the ship.

I suggest that you take a mini break from reading at this point, and do the following exercises before continuing the chapter.

Tensegrity exercises
Part A: The stack of bricks
Part A clearly demonstrates how the medical model (of many medical practitioners who do not look at the body as a whole) is quite wrong when assessing the spine – as if the vertebrae are like a stack of bricks. The exercise demonstrates *experientially* how patients can and do develop strains and tensions within their tissues. Just knowing the theory is totally different from *experiencing* how some patients have been living their life

for many years, consequently creating their current symptoms.

PART A EXERCISE ON THE STACK OF BRICK ANALOGY

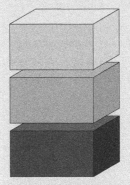

Figure 6.2 Does your body feel like a stack of bricks?

https://youtu.be/XjpV1kG6A4c

Part B: The tensegrity body
Part B, the tensegrity body exercise, is highly therapeutic and feels hugely different to the stack of bricks.

PART B EXERCISE: ON DISSIPATING TENSION AWAY FROM AREAS OF YOUR BODY

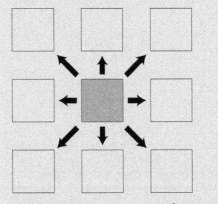

Figure 6.3 Spreading the tension from one cell to all its neighbours.

https://youtu.be/0906gDr6bL4

We gradually become like a tense stack of bricks (part A) when the body mechanics are not functioning properly, perhaps after an injury or accident, or the mechanical forces which have accumulated in the body over the years have become too much, failing the tensegrity system. Do not forget that psychological issues also cause powerful mechanical damage to the tensegrity system, thereby significantly adding to the aetiological factors.

When you felt the heavy stack of bricks pushing down on your spine, pelvis and lower extremities, it was probably quite easy to imagine how this would develop into arthritic degeneration, if left unattended for many years. It is also easy to conceive how living in such a state would make you tired, fatigued and, if chronic, could possibly make you a bit depleted and depressed, because all movement is such hard work. This would then lead to lack of or reduced exercise, with all the ensuing issues to the physiology which can then occur.

The tensegrity 'weightless body' exercise (part B), is close to how the body should be working all the time. The body is designed to spread its tension, to minimise it to such a degree that it is zero or negligible. When this occurs, the mind and body both feel lighter, freer, more effortless. Consequently, you will feel more energised throughout the day and your thinking will be clearer, as less tension is being transmitted to the head, resulting in more successful action. Remember, the quality of our thoughts results in the quality of our actions and hence the quality of life. In other words, this is how life should be lived and experienced!

Part B is an effortless exercise. It is greatly beneficial for our patients, as they can apply the principles to any activity they choose to undertake. It can be done standing, as suggested; however, it can be done in any position. Some patients may prefer to do it lying down, or sitting, or before and even during different types of exercise (though this will take a bit of time and practice). It is extremely valuable when working at a computer or in other situations which are posturally challenging. We all see patients where their occupation puts a lot of demand on their body mechanics. Teaching them this exercise will help to improve their body fluidity and their general wellbeing.

As we all know, osteopathic treatment is a powerful means of restoring the correct balance within and between tissues of the physiology, so that the inbuilt tensegrity mechanisms can be restored to full function and the energy and health of the person consequently increases, relative to the starting level of health. If someone is at what I call 'health level 1' which is like 'death warmed up', osteopathic treatment can perhaps ease their ability to cope with their condition, but may not change their condition. We are, after all osteopaths and not miracle workers, contrary to what some of our patients say!

FASCIAL STRUCTURE

As osteopaths we work with fascia all the time. It is almost impossible to place your hands on an area of the body without at the same time being on a fascial tissue. We have fascia between tissues, fascia covering tissues and fascia inside tissues. The quality of the fascia will depend on the quality of the extracellular matrix within. Bone periosteum is a modified connective tissue, a fascia that is quite different in quality to superficial fascia, for example. These differences will much depend on the relative ratios of collagen fibres and elastin fibres, along with the extracellular matrix of each. Tendons contain mainly collagen fibres whereas cartilage contains mainly polysaccharides, which then compress to form a firm gel surface for the joint. Where fascia ends and a different tissue begins opens another can of worms for the anatomist.

Extracellular matrix

If we consider the extracellular matrix (ECM) in closer detail, we find that it has close links to the cell walls of adjacent tissues and structures. This matrix comprises the space between cells, and binds the cells and tissues together. Within the matrix are secreted proteins and polysaccharides which are composed of tough fibrous proteins, mainly collagen, which is the most common protein in the body. Type 1 collagen is the most abundant protein in the physiology. This collagen assists in the maintenance of a significant number of tissues via its action on their cell surfaces. It also affects the molecules within the extracellular matrix along with cellular growth and differentiation (Di Lullo *et al.* 2021).

These collagen fibres can link together aspects of the matrix with the adjacent cells. Within the matrix, the fibres are embedded in a jelly-like polysaccharide ground substance. In addition to collagen, other significant constituents of the matrix are elastin fibres, giving varying degrees of elasticity, and the adhesion proteins,

fibronectins, glycosaminoglycans (GAGs) and laminin. These glue-like adhesion proteins can attach cells to the matrix in addition to holding the matrix components together.

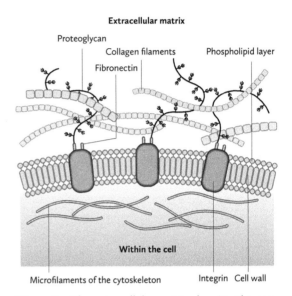

Figure 6.4 The extracellular matrix showing the connectivity from the matrix fibres to the microfilaments within the cell.

The role of the ECM is scientifically recognised to have profound influences on adjacent cells. The matrix influences the cell structures, signalling through to the cell, and even affects the gene/protein synthesis mechanisms. The ECM has been found to influence the essential morphological structure along with the physiological function via growth factors (GFs). It has also been shown to even influence signal transduction and gene transcription via its influence on cell surface receptors (Frantz *et al.* 2010).

The cytoskeleton connects to the integral proteins (integrins) and is found throughout the cell and even passes through the nuclear wall into the nucleus.

The GAGs (which are large molecules) attach themselves to carbohydrate polymers within the matrix, forming proteoglycan molecules (PGMs). These PGMs, being negatively charged, then attract to themselves positively charged sodium ions (Na^+). Via this mechanism the PGMs can then attract water molecules (attracted by osmosis to the sodium ion molecules), and thereby keep the matrix and any cells within it fully hydrated. According to Pankov and Yamada, who researched the cell binding properties of fibronectins:

> Fibronectin has a remarkably wide variety of functional activities besides binding to cell surfaces through integrins. It binds to a number of biologically important molecules that include heparin, collagen/gelatine, and fibrin... Fibronectin mediates a wide variety of cellular interactions with the extracellular matrix and plays important roles in cell adhesion, migration, growth and differentiation. (Pankov and Yamada 2002)

The fibronectin molecule binds to the cell membrane spanning receptor proteins, integrins which effectively hold onto the cell. They also can bind to collagen, fibrin and other GAGs. Consequently, they are involved in the repair process and can move cells within the matrix. Furthermore, it is now considered that this protein is even involved at the embryological stage of development: 'Fibronectin extracellular matrix is essential for embryogenesis... We therefore propose that it be considered a cell-cell communication event at the same level and significance as growth factor signalling during embryogenesis' (Gomes de Almeida *et al.* 2017).

These above papers indicate that the matrix around the cells of our body is not only an integral aspect of holding our body together at the cellular level, it also has a significant physiological influence. Further studies by Muscolino indicate another intriguing quality to us as osteopaths. He found that myofibroblasts within the ECM are now considered to have a contractile influence on the whole body. They are key in tightening up the tissues around a point of a wound, bringing the tissues together to allow healing at the point of damage. Muscolino explains:

> As great and greater tensile forces are placed upon the fascia, more and more myofibroblasts develop from the normal fibroblasts of the fascial tissue. For this reason, myofibroblasts are also known as 'stress fibres.' These myofibroblasts can then create an active pulling force that the fascial tissue is experiencing. For this reason, myofibroblasts are found in the greatest concentration in fascial tissues that have been injured and are undergoing wound healing. Fascial tissues with high concentrations of myofibroblasts have been found to have sufficiently strong force to impact musculoskeletal mechanics – that is, their active pulling forces are strong enough to contribute to movement of the body. (Muscalino quoted in Fitz-Simon n.d.)

Muscalino's statement that these myofibroblasts have the ability of being strong enough to contribute to the movement of the body indicates that the ECM could be an active part of the motion system of the body operating alongside the musculoskeletal system. Certainly, the compressive tensions we palpate around tissues in a negative state may be created by these myofibroblasts within the ECM.

The cytoskeleton

The cytoskeleton – microtubules and microfilaments within the cell – also has a fascinating role. It was not until the 21st century that science started to understand that the cytoskeleton is not just a cellular skeleton, but also has significant roles for cell function. For example, Kumeta and colleagues also found that the cytoskeleton enters the nucleus and can play a role in signalling within the cell:

In addition to nuclear import via classical nuclear transport pathways or passive diffusion, some large cytoskeletal proteins spontaneously migrate into the nucleus…accumulation or depletion of the nuclear populations thereby enhances or attenuates their nuclear functions. We propose that such molecular dynamics constitute a form of cytoskeleton-modulated regulation of nuclear functions which is mediated by the translocation of cytoskeletal components in and out of the nucleus. There is increasing evidence, however, that many types of cytoskeletal proteins are localised to the nucleus, suggestive of their direct involvement in the transmission of nuclear signalling and the regulation of nuclear functions. (Kumeta *et al.* 2012)

This indicates there is a continual interplay of information and regulation either side of the nucleus wall.

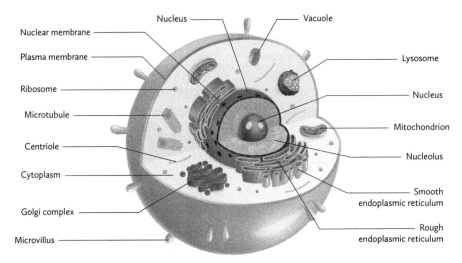

Figure 6.5 Internal cell structure.

So, we have established that there is a meshwork of fibres running throughout the ECM: collagen and elastin, with adhesion molecules acting on them and attaching to the integrins, the molecules which penetrate the cell membrane. As we know well as osteopaths, collagen transmits forces through the body and into the cells. Alberts and colleagues discuss how the matrix receptors, adhesion proteins, link to the cytoskeleton within the cell:

The linkage of the extracellular matrix to the cell requires transmembrane cell adhesion proteins that act as matrix receptors and tie the matrix to the cell's cytoskeleton. Although we have seen that some transmembrane proteoglycans function as co-receptors for matrix components, the principal receptors on animal cells for binding most extracellular matrix proteins – including collagens, fibronectin, and laminins – are the integrins. (Alberts *et al.* 2002)

It is increasingly becoming clear that integrins both bind cells to the ECM and also act as prime responders to the ECM. If cells are responders to the ECM, should we then consider the ECM as a primitive nervous system, a means of fundamental intercellular communication? In 1998, Donald Ingber discussed the tensegrity principle described by Buckminster Fuller within the physiology in his paper 'The architecture of life'. Ingber not only referred to the tensegrity of our musculoskeletal system but, as discussed below, included intracellular tensegrity:

Inside the cell, a gossamer network of contractile micro-filaments – a key element of the cytoskeleton – extends through-out the cell, exerting tension. In other words, it pulls the cell's membrane and all its internal constituents toward the nucleus at the core. Opposing this inward pull are two main types of compressive elements, one of which is outside the cell and the other inside. The component outside the cell is the extracellular matrix; the compressive 'girders' inside the cell can be either microtubules or large bundles of cross-linked micro-filaments within the cytoskeleton. The third component of the cytoskeleton, the intermediate filaments, are the great integrators, connecting microtubules and contractile micro-filaments to one another as well as to the surface membrane and the cell's nucleus. (Ingber 1998)

Here, Ingber clearly states that the extracellular matrix is in direct continuity with the cell interior, the cell cytoskeleton. We know from our experience with treating patients and from anatomy and physiology that our osteopathic work operates not only with gross tissue structures, but also with the fluids within such tissues including the matrix. Most practitioners who work with Sutherland's approach have experienced how compressed tissues feel dry within, and healthy tissues are permeated with fluid. Sutherland spoke of our treatments in agricultural terms, since he lived in a farming community, as 'irrigating the withering fields'. Here Sutherland is talking about increasing the fluidity within and surrounding the tissues including the extracellular matrix.

In the same paper, Ingber continues:

In addition, they act as guy wires, stiffening the central nucleus and securing it in place. Although the cytoskeleton is surrounded by membranes and penetrated by viscous fluid, it is this hard-wired network of molecular struts and cables that stabilizes cell shape. If the cell

and nucleus are physically connected by tensile filaments and not solely by a fluid cytoplasm, then pulling on receptors at the cell surface should produce immediate structural changes deep inside the cell. (Ingber 1998)

Andrew Maniotis, in association with Ingber, conducted further research on the effect of mechanical forces on the cell membrane and the effects on the cytoskeleton and the cell nucleus:

When we pulled fibronectin-coated pipettes that were initially bound to the cell surface many micrometres away from the nucleus, extensive changes in nuclear structure were observed, including evagination of the nuclear boundary and elongation of nucleoli along the principal axis of the tension field. These results indicated that cells and nuclei are literally built to respond directly to mechanical stresses applied to cell surface receptors, such as integrins. (Maniotis *et al.* 1997)

They go on to state that these mechanical links from the integrin molecules in the cell wall to the cytoskeleton and into the nucleus are likely to be signalling systems in addition to the chemical signalling systems:

The demonstration of direct mechanical linkages throughout living cells raises the possibility that regulatory information, in the form of mechanical stresses or vibrations, may be rapidly transferred from these cell surface receptors to distinct structures in the cell and nucleus, including ion channels, nuclear pores, nucleoli, chromosomes, and perhaps even individual genes, independent of ongoing chemical signalling mechanisms.

This type of 'mechanical signalling' (i.e., structural coupling) could serve to coordinate, complement, and constrain slower diffusion-based chemical signalling pathways and, thus, explain in part how mechanical distortion of the ECM (extracellular matrix) caused by gravity, hemodynamic forces, or cell tension can change cell shape, alter nuclear functions, and switch cells between different genetic programs. (Maniotis *et al.* 1997)

Here Maniotis and colleagues clearly consider that mechanical changes to the cell wall via the matrix can result in *altered nuclear function and change cells from one genetic program to another.* Goodwin and Nelson, in their more recent paper, also discuss how mechanical forces affect development of tissues: 'Developing tissues experience intrinsic mechanical signals from active forces and changes to tissue mechanical properties as well as extrinsic mechanical signals, including constraint and compression, pressure, and shear forces' (Goodwin and Nelson 2020).

In his paper 'Mechanics of the nucleus' Lammerding also discusses how the nucleus is disturbed by cell mechanics and can result in disease conditions:

> Research on diverse cell types further demonstrates how induced nuclear deformations during cellular compression or stretch can modulate cellular function. Pathological examples of disturbed nuclear mechanics include the many diseases caused by mutations in the nuclear envelope proteins lamin A/C and associated proteins, as well as cancer cells that are often characterized by abnormal nuclear morphology. (Lammerding 2011)

Let us pause a moment and consider just what the above papers mean to us as osteopaths. If one cell is connected to the matrix and that matrix is connected to cells within it and adjacent to it by collagen and elastin fibres via fibronectin (adhesion proteins), then this means that there is a direct mechanical transmission pathway for mechanical forces from one cell to another. In addition, the forces via the fibres in the matrix and the adhesion proteins connect to the integrins, and they in turn with the microtubules and microfilaments, connect to the cell skeleton fibres. These fibres are also shown to penetrate the nucleus and affect its function. We can now appreciate that mechanical forces from without will affect the cell nucleus and nuclear function, the synthesis of proteins, for all cell functions.

Goodwin's paper states that mechanical forces can affect cell development which is strongly linked to the function of the nucleus. Now, I am certainly not implying that we can treat conditions which arise from disturbances of the nucleus such as cancer with osteopathy. However, if we can reduce the mechanical tensions on the cell membrane and hence on the nuclear membrane and its contents, we may on a subtle level have a positive influence on the nucleus function and the overall health of the cell.

The internal structure of the nucleus comprises a nuclear membrane, also known as a nuclear envelope. The nucleoplasm (karyoplasm) contains the chromosomes and central nucleolus. The nucleoplasm and the cytochromes fill the space between the nuclear envelope and the nucleolus; it is the matrix present inside the nucleus which responds to mechanical forces affecting the cell. In addition to the above, when we add the action of myofibroblasts, which are now known to have 'muscular' qualities within the extracellular matrix which can exert forces on the physiology, we can now see that a whole new world of microphysiology is becoming available to us as practitioners.

Both Still and Blechschmidt in their different ways discussed how structure and function are interrelated in the physiology, and we as practitioners experience this clinically every time we see a patient. We now know that mechanical forces do influence the internal cell structure, even into the nucleus of the cell. Therefore, we can surmise that as a disturbance to the nucleus physiology can and does occur from mechanical forces to tissues, then an osteopathic resolution of that disturbance will improve the nucleus function. We should now be appreciating that we are taking the level at which we are working as osteopaths to the cellular and nuclear levels, not just that of gross tissue (see more on this topic in Chapter 18).

I acknowledge that the reader at this point may be thinking this is absurd, thinking that Tim (the author) has 'lost it, gone crazy', or 'lost the plot'! I ask you to hold back those thoughts and feelings until you have gradually worked your way through this book. In Chapter 18 we will be looking at the cell membrane and intracellular organelles. I do not suggest you skip chapters and go there now, as your skills and perception may need some refinement before you could appraise it properly. Please take your time and work through the osteopathic palpation exercises in each chapter. You will then find that your skill and perception ability will make significant strides forwards as you progress through the book. As this occurs, you will find yourself being able to feel aspects of the physiology which perhaps you cannot at present. That is, after all, the aim of this book!

Interstitium

Benias and his colleagues, in their paper about the interstitium, state that: 'Freezing biopsy tissue before fixation preserved the anatomy of this structure, demonstrating that it is part of the submucosa and a previously unappreciated fluid-filled interstitial space, draining to lymph nodes and supported by a complex network of thick collagen bundles' (Benias *et al.* 2018). This revelation that interstitial fluids within the extracellular matrix also exist in the adjacent interstitial space was reported on by the press as … researchers are calling this network of fluid-filled spaces an organ, the interstitium. However, this is an unofficial distinction; for a body part to officially become an organ, a consensus would need to develop around the idea as more researchers study it, Theise told Live Science. A 'new organ' is not implied in the research paper, though it does highlight the importance of fluid in the tissues adjacent to fascia.

Fascinatingly for us who acknowledge the cranial involuntary mechanism, the paper also discusses how this interstitium occurs in areas of the body where compressive and rhythmic motion takes place:

> All of the organs in which we have detected this structure are subject to cycles of compression and distension, whether relatively constant (lungs, aorta) or intermittent (digestive tract after a meal, urinary bladder during micturition, skin under mechanical compression, fascial planes during action of the musculoskeletal system). (Benias *et al.* 2018)

In the article the authors are referring to intermittent or rhythmic compression with reference to the bronchial tree in the lungs, muscles, digestive system, etc. As osteopaths who work with Sutherland's approach, we know that the whole body undergoes a rhythmic flexion and extension shape change, what Sutherland called the involuntary mechanism (IVM). Although not compression in the classical sense, we theorise and can palpate in our clinical work that this shape change of the IVM assists the physiology of fluid permeation in the fasciae and adjacent tissues, the interstitium. Osteopathically, we are working at this level all the time. When we assist the body to restore good fluctuation of flexion and extension of the body fluids and tissues, we actively feel under our fingers this increase in fluid dynamics within the physiology resulting in an enhanced level of health and wellbeing.

FASCIA AND ITS QUALITIES

Fascia consists of the superficial fascia, deep fascia and the visceral layer of fascia. The superficial fascia lies immediately under the skin. However, we may forget that the skin is the largest organ of the body so consequently the superficial fascia is a considerable size. Deep to the superficial fascia lies the deep fascia, this being the layer which holds everything together, particularly in the limbs and neck, but it is less well defined in the torso and face.

Modern science is now looking more closely at the fascia and not just seeing it as 'the bits that get in the way of the surgeon and anatomist'. Some, as shown in the quote from Helene Langevin below, consider that fascia contains a communication system within its functional repertoire:

It is proposed that these types of signals generate dynamic, evolving patterns that interact with one another. Such connective tissue signalling would be affected by changes in movement and posture and may be altered in pathological conditions (e.g., local decreased mobility due to injury or pain). Connective tissue thus may function as a previously unrecognized whole-body communication system. Since connective tissue is intimately associated with all other tissues (e.g., lung, intestine), connective tissue signalling may coherently influence, and be influenced by, the normal or pathological function of a wide variety of organ systems. (Langevin 2006)

Gatenby in his paper also comes to a similar conclusion:

The fluctuation of an ion concentration within the cytoplasm adjacent to the membrane channel can elicit an immediate, local response by altering the location and function of peripheral membrane proteins. Signals that affect a larger surface area of the cell membrane and/or persist over a prolonged time period will produce similarly cytoplasmic changes on larger spatial and time scales. We propose that as the amplitude, spatial extent, and duration of changes in cytoplasmic ion concentrations increase, the information can be communicated to the nucleus and other intracellular structures through ion flows along elements of the cytoskeleton to the centrosome (via microtubules) or proteins in the nuclear membrane (via microfilaments). These dynamics add spatial and temporal context to the more well-recognised information communication from the cell membrane to the nucleus following ligand binding to membrane receptors. (Gatenby 2019)

This concept of the fascia being a whole-body communication network fits in perfectly with our osteopathic principles and with our clinical and therapeutic experience. It is amazing that the scientific studies and theories referred to above verify the thinking of our founder, Andrew Taylor Still, over 100 years before. Still definitely was a true visionary!

Exercise on palpating the fascia in the forearm and the extracellular matrix

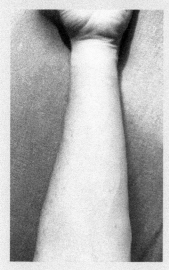

https://youtu.be/CeDO57TXB8k

REFERENCES

Alberts, B., Johnson, A., Lewis, J., *et al.*, 2002. Integrins. In: *Molecular Biology of the Cell.* 4th edition. New York: Garland Science.

Benias, P.C., Wells, R.G., Sackey-Aboagye, B., *et al.*, 2018. Structure and distribution of an unrecognized interstitium in human tissues. *Scientific Reports.* Available from: https://www.nature.com/articles/s41598-018-23062-6.

Buckminster Fuller, R., 1961. Tensegrity. Available from: http://www.rwgrayprojects.com/rbfnotes/fpapers/tensegrity/tenseg01.html.

Di Lullo, G., Seweeny, S., Korkko, J., Ala-Kokko, L., *et al.*, 2021. Mapping the ligand-binding sites and disease-associated mutations on the most abundant protein in the human, type 1 collagen. *Journal of Biochemistry.* Available from: https://www.jbc.org/article/S0021-9258(20)87534-6/fulltext?legid=jbc%3B277%2F6%2F4223&cited-by=yes#cited-by.

Fitz-Simon, W., n.d. Fascia, the body's connective tissue, can contract! ACAT. Available from: https://www.acatnyc.org/blog-posts/2014/04/03/fascia-the-bodys-connective-tissue-can-contract.

Frantz, C., Stewart, K., & Weaver, V., 2010. The extracellular matrix at a glance. *Journal of Cell Science.* Available from: https://journals.biologists.com/jcs/article/123/24/4195/31378/The-extracellular-matrix-at-a-glance.

Gatenby, R.A., 2019. The role of cell membrane information reception, processing, and communication in the structure and function of multicellular tissue. *International Journal of Molecular Sciences.* 20(15): 3609.

Gomes de Almeida, P., Pinheiro, G., Nunes, A., Gonçalves, A., *et al.*, 2017. Fibronectin assembly during early embryo development: a versatile communication system between cells and tissues. *Developmental Dynamics.* 245(4): 520–535.

Goodwin, K., & Nelson, C., 2020. Mechanics of development. *Developmental Cell.* 56(2): 240–250.

Ingber, D.E., 1998. The architecture of life. *Scientific American.* Available from: http://time.arts.ucla.edu/Talks/Barcelona/Arch_Life.htm.

Kumeta, M., Yoshimura, S., Hejna, J., & Takeyasu, K., 2012. Nucleocytoplasmic shuttling of cytoskeletal proteins: molecular mechanism and biological significance. *International Journal of Cell Biology.* Available from: https://www.hindawi.com/journals/ijcb/2012/494902/

Lammerding, J., 2011. Mechanics of the nucleus. *Comprehensive Physiology.* 1(2): 783–807.

Langevin, H.M., 2006. Connective tissue: a body-wide signaling network? *Medical Hypotheses.* 66(6): 1074–1077.

Maniotis, A.J., Chen, C.S., & Ingber, D.E., 1997. Demonstration of mechanical connections between integrins, cytoskeletal filaments, and nucleoplasm that stabilize nuclear structure. *Proc Natl Acad Sci USA.* 94: 849–854.

Nordin, C.R., 2020. Fascia guide: the components in fascia. Available from: https://fasciaguide.com/fascia-anatomy-physiology/the-components-in-fascia/

Pankov, R., & Yamada, K., 2002. Fibronectin at a glance. *Journal of Cell Science.* 115(20): 3861–3863.

Rettner, R. 2018. Meet Your Interstitium, a Newfound "Organ". [Online]. [1 May 2023]. Available from: https://www.scientificamerican.com/article/meet-your-interstitium-a-newfound-organ

Schleip, R., Findley, T.W., Chaitow, L., & Huijing, P., 2012. *Fascia: The Tensional Network of the Human Body.* Edinburgh, UK: Elsevier, p. xvii.

CHAPTER 7

The Inner Approach to the Cerebrospinal Fluid and the Meninges

Much has been written by Sutherland and others on this topic which I will not repeat. My hope here is that this chapter will add further insight and take your skills to a more profound inner level. We will commence with the fluid body, then look at cerebrospinal fluid from differing perspectives and finally progress to the meninges.

THE FLUID BODY

Before we discuss the cerebrospinal fluid, I would like to comment on what has been termed 'the fluid body'. In their paper 'The biodynamic model of osteopathy in the cranial field', McPartland and Skinner discuss how Sutherland started talking about the fluid body:

> Sutherland…compared the Breath of Life (BoL) to the cyclic, sweeping beam of light emitted from a lighthouse, 'lighting up the ocean but not touching it'.
>
> The BoL sweeps through the patient, enlightening the healing forces already present in the patient. This allows the 'Fluid Body' to emerge, where the whole body behaves as if it were a single unit of living substance. The Fluid Body represents the biodynamic model of osteopathy in the cranial field equivalent of a Bose-Einstein condensate, where individual molecules lose their identity and form a cloud that behaves as a single entity. (McPartland and Skinner 2005)

In Chapter 6 we looked at the qualities of the extracellular matrix (ECM) and the interstitium. You may have noticed with patients, as we take our attention to the finer aspects of the physiology and when we are centred within ourselves, that you have an experience of not feeling tissues any more. I used to call this a feeling of being 'beyond anatomy' as the physical anatomical tissues seem to disappear from the awareness of the practitioner but you are still palpating a deep level of the physiology. I would then verify to myself that I had not just fallen asleep! However no, I was feeling very clear within myself and highly aware in my consciousness, so this was not just my feeling drowsy.

Could this level of body awareness be described as the fluid body, being an experience of palpating at the level of the ECM and/or the interstitium? It would certainly fit in with being beyond anatomy, and the ECM is certainly the fluid continuum which pervades the whole physiology. We can gain a sense of the person's health and vitality, or potency, when sensing the physiology at this subtle level. The fact that the ECM interacts with the cell walls, the cytoskeleton and hence the nucleus would by definition give a sense of the wellbeing being expressed at the cellular level. By palpating at this level, a sense of the wellbeing of the whole person occurs.

Palpating the fluid body

Depending on your current experience level, you may already become aware of the fluid body when palpating your patients. Hopefully, from the previous few chapters you will be moving your perception to not only feel fascial and mechanical strains and shears within tissues, but now also letting your perception settle onto the more refined levels of the fluid body and the degree of vitality within it.

We will be discussing more about treating with potency in Chapter 19, however do become aware of the vitality and potency within the fluid body, the fluid throughout the body. With some patients they may have a high vitality and energy level expressed in a balanced manner. However, some patients may have a high energy level, yet this can be expressed in a distressed or anxious manner, not health at all. Others can have a low potency/vitality level, often a symptom of chronic fatigue and low wellbeing. Having some awareness of this level whilst helping your patients will also give you a sense of how well they will respond to your treatments (the body treating itself) and hence be more able to determine their prognosis.

THE CEREBROSPINAL FLUID (CSF)

The founder of our profession, Andrew Taylor Still, was a visionary in many respects. He certainly did not hold back on his views of the importance of the CSF. He wrote:

> A thought strikes him that the cerebrospinal fluid is one of the highest known elements that are contained in the body, and unless the brain furnishes this fluid in abundance, a disabled condition of the body will remain. He who is able to reason will see that this great river of life must be tapped, and the withering field irrigated at once, or the harvest of health be forever lost.
> The fluids of the brain are of a finer order than any fluids supplying the whole viscera. (Still 1902)

Many practitioners within our osteopathic profession have a negative view of Still, because of his style of writing. However, we must accept that his writing style was probably chosen for the reader of that time, which is quite different from the scientific perspective of today. We can ignore the style (if not happy with it) and consider the content – his meaning cannot be ignored.

CSF formation, function and absorption

Having taken Still's hint on its importance, let us now look at the physiology of CSF formation, function and absorption. For over a century the CSF, following research on animals by Dandy in 1919, was considered to be only synthesised within the choroid plexuses, lying within the ventricles of the brain. However, in recent years research has challenged this long-held medical theory. Here we will look at some of the more modern research on CSF and then consider the osteopathic relevance.

Orešković and Klarica investigated this long-held theory and revealed its shortcomings:

> Because of universally poor results, choroid plexectomy was abandoned by neurosurgeons as a treatment for hydrocephalus, and today it is an operation of historic interest only and has no place in the treatment of hydrocephalus. But the failure of choroid plexectomy to cure, or at least ameliorate progressive hydrocephalus was incompatible with the thesis that the choroid plexuses are the main source of active CSF formation. (Orešković and Klarica 2010)

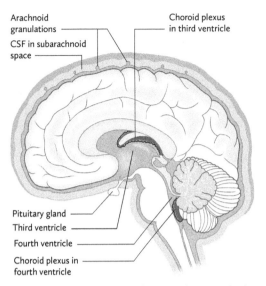

Arachnoid
granulations
CSF in subarachnoid
space
Choroid plexus
in third ventricle
Pituitary gland
Third ventricle
Fourth ventricle
Choroid plexus in
fourth ventricle

Figure 7.1 Sagittal section diagram showing the location of the midline choroid plexus positions within the brain. There are choroid plexuses also within the lateral ventricles (not shown).

In the same paper they further reference another experiment, stating:

> Moreover, the lateral ventricle became markedly dilated, which indicates that hydrocephalus can occur rapidly and progressively in the plexectomised ventricular system, and that the choroid plexus is not essential as a source of CSF secretion... Furthermore, when the rate of CSF formation within the lateral ventricles, the third ventricle, and the Aqueduct of Sylvius were compared in control and bilaterally plexectomised animals, the rates in the plexectomised group were found to be on average about 70% of the norm...or CSF formation in plexectomised patients remained similar to that in hydrocephalus-free individuals. (Orešković and Klarica 2010)

Other studies also verified that coagulation of the choroid plexuses to prevent CSF production did not help hydrocephalus patients and that they still needed a shunt inserted: 'The ventricular size was not significantly reduced by choroid plexus coagulation and only 35% of patients achieved long-term control without cerebrospinal fluid shunts' (Pople and Ettles 1995).

Such studies in hydrocephalus patients and animals indicate that the choroid plexuses are certainly not the sole source of CSF production, otherwise their complete removal would result in a 100 per cent reduction of CSF volume, not just a partial reduction. So, if the CSF is not just produced in the choroid plexuses, where are the other possible sources? Sakka and colleagues found:

> CSF is predominantly, but not exclusively, secreted by the choroid plexuses. Brain interstitial fluid, ependyma and capillaries may also play a poorly defined role in CSF secretion...60 to 75% of CSF is produced by the choroid plexuses of the lateral ventricles and the tela choroidea of the third and fourth ventricles. (Sakka et al. 2011)

The main functions of CSF are those of support, shock absorbency, homeostasis, nutrition and also providing an immunity role. The roles of support and shock absorbency result from the fluid of the CSF both lying within and surrounding the brain.

Support and shock absorbency

According to Adigun and Al-Dhahir (2021), the CSF supports the weight of the brain, estimated at 1500 gm, and suspends it in neutral buoyancy to a net weight of about 25 gm. This neutral buoyancy dramatically reduces the gravitational force of the brain onto the floor of the cranial base.

One of my UK teaching colleagues, Ernest Keeling, once beautifully demonstrated during a five-day Sutherland Cranial Teaching Foundation course, the protective role of the CSF with regards to reducing brain damage. He placed a very ripe plum in a jar of water, filling it to the brim and excluding any air by closing the lid. On shaking the jar, the plum rapidly moved around inside and was damaged against the glass walls. He then took another jar of water, in which he had previously dissolved as much salt as possible. He again placed a very ripe plum into the full jar and replaced the lid so that there was no air. When he shook this second jar strongly, it was impossible to make the ripe plum even touch the glass walls, let alone become damaged. This was because the dissolved salt in the water changed the specific gravity to being closer to that of the plum. It was an amazing and powerful demonstration to all who saw it of how the CSF in an enclosed space can protect the brain tissue. It became reverently known after that, to the faculty who saw the demonstration, as 'Ernest's Plum'!

Homeostasis

The CSF role is to maintain brain temperature, biochemical constituents and electrolytes whilst maintaining the correct CSF osmotic pressure. In addition, the homeostatic role includes ensuring the removal of waste products and their final diffusion into the venous and lymphatic systems. Naturally, all of these homeostatic roles benefit good brain physiology.

Nutriment

The CSF contains glucose, proteins, lipids and electrolytes which provide nutriment to the brain. We must remember that the brain is a highly active tissue and a major energy demanding organ, so it needs a plentiful supply of these constituents for its physiological functions.

Immunity

This role of the CSF is undertaken by the immunoglobulins and mononuclear cells within the fluid. Being directly within the brain ventricles and adjacent to the pia in the subarachnoid space, the CSF has a significant role in reducing the risk of brain infection.

Absorption sites of the CSF

Traditionally, absorption of CSF was considered to be through the arachnoid granulations into the superior sagittal sinus. However, modern research has revealed a much wider absorption field: 'Cerebrospinal fluid (CSF) drains through the cribriform plate (CP) in association with the olfactory nerves. From this location, CSF is absorbed into nasal mucosal lymphatics' (Mollanji *et al.* 2002).

Sakka and his team found with respect to CSF absorption:

> CSF circulation from sites of secretion to sites of absorption largely depends on the arterial pulse wave. Additional factors such as respiratory waves, the subject's posture, jugular venous pressure, and physical effort also modulate CSF flow dynamics and pressure. Cranial and spinal arachnoid villi have been considered for a long time to be the predominant sites of CSF absorption into the venous outflow system. Experimental data suggest that cranial and spinal nerve sheaths, the cribriform plate and the adventitia of cerebral arteries constitute substantial pathways of CSF drainage into the lymphatic outflow system. (Sakka *et al.* 2011)

However, there is controversy as to the degree of nasal mucosa involvement, this being highlighted by a paper by Melin *et al.*, who studied CSF absorption via the cribriform plate and nasal mucosa in humans:

> Despite a strong enrichment of CSF tracer in CSF spaces nearby the cribriform plate, there was no significant enrichment of CSF tracer in nasal mucosa, as measured in superior, medial, and inferior turbinates, or in the nasal septum. Therefore, this in vivo study questions the importance of CSF drainage to the human nasal mucosa and emphasizes the need of further human studies. (Melin *et al.* 2020)

Although in this paper the authors question the CSF absorption in the nasal mucosa, they do say that there was significant CSF within the cribriform plate. We do have to remember that many studies are done on animals, including four-legged mammals with large nasal cavities and large nasal mucosal areas compared with humans. This could therefore lead to variations of animal physiology within their nasal apparatus compared with ourselves.

Ma *et al.* looked at CSF absorption in mice and found that the lymph vessels participate in absorption:

> Here, we utilise lymphatic-reporter mice and high-resolution stereomicroscopy to characterise the anatomical routes and dynamics of outflow of CSF. After infusion into a lateral ventricle, tracers spread into the para-vascular spaces of the pia mater and cortex of the brain. Tracers also rapidly reach lymph nodes using perineural routes through foramina in the skull. Using non-invasive imaging techniques that can quantify the transport of tracers to the blood and lymph nodes, we find that lymphatic vessels are the major outflow pathway for both large and small molecular tracers in mice. (Ma *et al.* 2017)

Here we can see that the role of the lymphatic system is significant in CSF absorption. Like the venous system, the lymph vessels are under very low pressure and so are easily affected by mechanical forces against the vessels, affecting the quality of flow along the lymphatic tube. Research, as shown by Khasawneh and his team, also indicates that there are twofold routes of absorption, in addition to the cervical lymphatics:

The first is along the subarachnoid space of exiting cranial nerves. This provides a direct route in which CSF may be transferred from the cisterns to the extracranial lymphatics. The second pathway by which CSF may reach lymphatics is along the Virchow-Robin space of arteries and veins penetrating brain parenchyma. (Khasawneh *et al.* 2018)

In the same paper, the authors further indicate the role of the dural venous plexus:

> In addition to the circulation of CSF into cervical lymphatics, there have been studies describing CSF reabsorption into the dural venous plexus. At birth, arachnoid granulations are not fully developed, and CSF absorption relies on the venous plexus of the inner surface of dura that is more robust in infants. Although not as extensive in adults, the dural venous plexus is still believed to play a role in absorption. Adult and foetal cadaver dissections and animal models with intradural injections have all been shown to demonstrate filling of the parasagittal dural venous plexus. (Khasawneh *et al.* 2018)

It should be borne in mind that CSF production balances the absorption, their having to keep in harmony. Perhaps this is why there are a variety of CSF absorption sites, to ensure that as much as is possible, absorption stays within healthy parameters.

OSTEOPATHIC CONSIDERATIONS

From an osteopathic perspective, the production of the CSF being not only within the choroid plexuses, but also from the brain interstitial fluid, may be clinically significant with some patients (see Sakka *et al.* 2011). Sakka and his team put the volume of choroid plexus production of CSF at a total of 60–75 per cent; whilst this is a significant majority, it still leaves 25–40 per cent being created elsewhere.

The brain interstitial fluid is quoted as being

a site of CSF production. It is that fluid which surrounds the parenchyma cells: neurons, astrocytes and microglia, along with the microglial cells adjacent to the basal lamina up against the endothelial cells. If we take our palpatory awareness to the brain tissue (see exercise at the end of this chapter), in many patients we can feel tension directly within the CNS tissue, often associated with psychological tensions. In my opinion it would be naïve, though not proven, to consider such tensions as not having an effect on the physiology at this level, and hence on CSF production. Equally, compressive forces and compressed brain tissue states also create a negative mechanical force on the choroid plexuses and the ependymal layers of the brain (sites of CSF production).

With regard to CSF absorption, there are a number of ways in which osteopathic treatment can help and facilitate this process. The arachnoid granulations, which for many decades were considered the only site of CSF absorption, empty into the superior sagittal venous sinus. This sinus lies directly below the sagittal suture between the two parietal bones. Consequently, almost any injury to the vault, especially if to the vertex region, will have a detrimental effect on the sagittal suture, often creating a locking up of the suture, and thus affecting the physiology of the underlying superior sagittal venous sinus.

The cribriform plate of the ethmoid and the underlying nasal mucosa is now being considered as a site of CSF absorption. Even if the nasal mucosa involvement is now being questioned, the CSF being present around the cribriform plate is not doubted. Being part of the ethmoid, the cribriform plate is therefore a part of the cranial base. I personally consider the delicate ethmoid bone as being like a fine tuner to the actions of the sphenobasilar symphysis, as the coccyx is a fine tuner to the sacrum and the xiphoid bone a fine tuner of the sternum. As we all know, mechanical tensions within the cranial base are quite common, and most of these tensions are tolerated and adapted to by the cranial mechanism. However, mechanical forces beyond the tolerance/adaptation level can and do result in suppression of the involuntary motion of the cranial base.

Colin Dove (a close friend and colleague who sadly died in 2021) brought the teaching of cranial osteopathy to the UK whilst he was the principal of the British School of Osteopathy. Colin once said to me: 'Many practitioners in my opinion forget to look at the ethmoid when evaluating the cranial base and in doing so may not get the tissue resolution they are seeking' (Dove 2019). So, if on honest self-assessment you could be one of those practitioners who sometimes forgets to assess the ethmoid when looking at the cranial base (as I have at times), do remember that not only could disturbances to the ethmoid cause mechanical issues to the frontal and facial bones and olfactory nerves, they also (if restricted) could be affecting CSF absorption.

The cervical lymphatics are now accepted as sites for CSF absorption. As low-pressure vessels, the lymph vessels can be distressed by mechanical forces to the head and neck, particularly if caused by a traumatic event where the compressive shock can remain within the superficial and deep fasciae for a long time (if not treated). So, when treating mechanical shocks and strains to the cervical area, do also consider that you may be working on the lymphatic vessels, a site of CSF absorption.

The subarachnoid spaces of the cranial nerves are now also considered amongst the drainage sites of CSF. Although these are small spaces, osteopathic treatment of the cranial nerves (see Chapter 11) may assist this process. The Virchow-Robin spaces (VRS), the perivascular spaces which lie around the blood vessels as they cross through the subarachnoid spaces, are now considered a possible CSF absorption site.

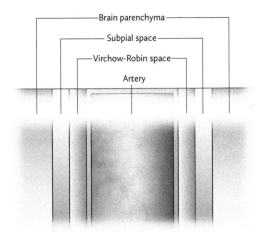

Figure 7.2 The location of the Virchow-Robin space in the brain, either side of a penetrating artery which originates from the subarachnoid space.

According to Ishikawa *et al.*, a study of perivascular spaces in the basal ganglia area revealed that these may be as large as 5 mm in diameter in healthy and aged individuals, and that the diameter increases with age in the basal ganglia and white matter. They also stated that the diameters in their control group ranged from 2 mm to more than 5 mm (Ishikawa *et al.* 2015). Clearly a 5 mm diameter VRS is less likely to get occluded than a 2 mm VRS, and these smaller ones could easily become affected by mechanical forces within the brain and so interfere with CSF drainage from those regions. Osteopathic treatment to the brain in such cases may improve the CSF flow.

CLINICAL ASPECTS OF WORKING WITH THE CSF

As you will have already completed some undergraduate or postgraduate training courses in working with the involuntary mechanism before purchasing this book, I will not be discussing techniques such as the CV4, lateral fluctuation or fluid drives in any detail. However, as you will already know, such approaches do have therapeutic benefit.

In nearly all therapeutic approaches when working with the involuntary mechanism, the tissues usually undergo some activity, some motion – what I refer to as 'the dance' – before settling themselves down towards and into a still point. During this still point, we as practitioners often feel an increasing expression of the potency (increasing *expression,* not an increased potency), as some of the 'blankets' are removed. The tissues or fluid then gradually return to flexion/extension or internal/external rotation with an improved quality.

With solid tissues, it is the fluids of the extracellular matrix within and the intracellular fluids which will be making these changes. The CV4

and lateral fluctuation techniques are approaches to bring this about in the whole physiology and can be especially useful if the body or a localised area feels dry, tight and non-responsive. The action of the CSF, even where the techniques are initially applied to the skull, should affect all fluids of the body. Therefore, these techniques should be done with the awareness on the whole 'fluid body', not just the cranium.

When seeing patients, the quality of the CSF within the cranium should always be evaluated as to whether it is flowing easily or feels more of a dry or sticky quality. As has become clear from the above, a poor-quality CSF will inevitably lead to a poorer physiology of the brain tissue. Fluid drive approaches are classically taught with an application to the occipitomastoid suture. However, I also find them very useful (as with a lateral fluctuation) when applied to the pelvis and hip joints, or to the shoulder girdle. A CV4 can be highly beneficial when applied via the sacrum or even a limb, though the latter approach takes a little while to get used to.

THE MENINGES

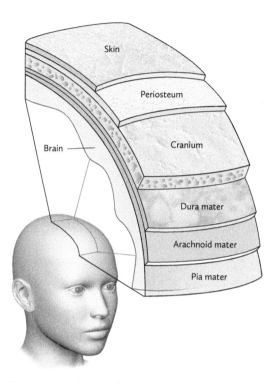

Figure 7.3 The layers of the meninges.

The meninges comprise three layers: the dura mater, arachnoid mater and pia mater. Between the arachnoid and the pia lies the subarachnoid space in which lies the cerebrospinal fluid (CSF). Embryologically the meninges were thought to arise from a mesenchymal sheath, the primary meninix, which then differentiated into the three layers. According to Dasgupta and Jeong, the neural crest cells within the cranium are key, taking on the role of the mesoderm:

> Histological observations in human foetuses also suggest that the cranial meninges originated from both the neural crest and the mesoderm. The most striking diversity of the neural crest derivatives is found in its cephalic domain where the neural crest replaces the role of mesoderm. The neural crest is a vertebrate-specific

migratory stem cell that generates diverse cell types and structures. (Dasgupta and Jeong 2019)

In their paper, Dasgupta and Jeong also discuss the differing origins of varying parts of the skull, indicating a strong dual origin of the dura mater with both ectodermal and mesodermal origins:

> For example, the meninges of the skull (which are considered to be fascial tissues) have an embryological derivation involving both the mesoderm and ectoderm; the dura mater that covers areas of the forebrain and caudal mesencephalon which derive from the neural crests (or ectoderm). The dura mater that covers the remaining hindbrain and midbrain derives from the mesodermal leaflet. The hypoglossal canal and the area of the sigmoid, transverse, and cavernous sinuses derive from the mesoderm; the falx cerebri and the falx cerebelli derive from the ectoderm, as does the dura mater covering the spinal cord. (Dasgupta and Jeong 2019)

So, in the above paper we see that the meninges have both ectodermal and mesodermal origins, when we tend to think of the meninges as just arising from the mesoderm. What is the significance for us as osteopaths? The skin is the largest ectodermal tissue. It is what we touch when palpating our patients (other than hair and clothing, unless doing internal work via the mouth or pelvis). So, the dura of some areas of the skull are 'cousins' of the skin as is the nervous system. (In Chapter 17 we will be looking in greater detail at interrelationships within the body from an osteopathic perspective.)

Research is also revealing that the meninges are important in the development of the skull, the sutures, the brain and even postnatally as stem cell niches, indicating that the relationship between the meninges and the adjacent tissues, the brain and skull, is much more interactive embryologically than previously considered:

> While genetic regulation of meningeal development is still poorly understood, mouse mutants and other models with meningeal defects have demonstrated the importance of the meninges to normal development of the calvaria and the brain. For the calvaria, the interactions with the meninges are necessary for the progression of calvarial osteogenesis during early development. In later stages, the meninges control the patterning of the skull and the fate of the sutures. For the brain, the meninges regulate diverse processes including cell survival, cell migration, generation of neurons from progenitors, and vascularisation. Also, the meninges serve as a stem cell niche for the brain in the postnatal life. (Dasgupta and Jeong 2019)

The above quotation contains some extraordinary statements for us as osteopaths. Saying that the meninges regulate cell survival of the brain, the generation of neurons from progenitors, and vascularisation of the brain adds significantly to the potential of osteopathy. This is especially true when working with babies and young children in whom the brain is still growing and maturing. Add to this the fact that the meninges are now found to have a stem cell function for the brain in postnatal life. This may be an issue of even greater significance in the area of the osteopathic treatment of the newborn (see Chapter 14).

Blechschmidt and Glasser in their introduction to *Biokinetics and Biodynamics of Human Differentiation* indicate that the biomechanics, the forces acting on the physiology at the time of change and development, affect the change process occurring during embryological development:

> The knowledge of developmental movements leads to the conclusion that differentiation is an undivided biodynamic process that occurs during development and includes the chemical process as well. Biomechanical features never occur beside biochemical features, but they always implicate the latter. A biochemical synopsis would be impossible unless one has a fundamental knowledge of the morphology as well as the biokinetics of the organic structures. (Blechschmidt and Glasser 1978)

As all osteopaths know, Andrew Taylor Still, our osteopathic founder, gave us a profound insight that osteopathy is based on the principle of structure influencing function. A wheel rolls smoothly along the road because of its shape. Blechschmidt was truly an osteopathic thinker, even though he may not have heard of osteopaths. He realised that shape is determined by the biomechanics present at that specific moment of formation. This is what we feel at every moment of palpation of our patients. We feel living change as we palpate the involuntary mechanism. If we take the thoughts of Still and Blechschmidt together, then the morphology of tissues should perhaps be considered an expression of their function.

The dura mater

Within the meninges, the dura has a strong fibrous quality. There are many collagen fibres within the dura tissue, giving it significant strength with pliability. This is required to give the brain a powerful protective layer within the skull. It is like the crumple zone of a vehicle which takes the impact of forces to a car, to offer maximum protection to the people within the passenger compartment – it being better to damage the engine or boot/trunk of a car than you or your passengers.

Compared with its 'embryological second-cousins', the arachnoid and pia (these being effectively embryological sisters), the dura has a reduced vascularity. Consequently, it becomes inflamed less easily, requiring a much greater distress before expressing vascular and irritable negativity. This can be felt osteopathically.

In the book of Sutherland's lectures, *Contributions of Thought*, he talks about the 'core link', the dural connection between the cranial base and sacral base (Sutherland 1967a).This core link, we know from our clinical experiences, can be a key factor in helping our patients. Dural tensions from trauma and strain patterns, especially if expressed in the cranial base, sacrum, or pelvis and coccyx, affect the whole spine via the dural attachments. Professor Frank Willard found that: 'The fibres of the dura embed deeply into the osseous tissue of the sacrum at the level of S2' (Willard 1989). This verifies Sutherland's theory and clinical findings.

The dura mater, both within the cranium and with respect to the dural sleeve around the spinal cord, is a significant conveyor of mechanical strains and stresses from one part of the central nervous system and spine to another. To ensure a full understanding, I recommend the reader to revise their knowledge of the patterns of function (see Chapter 3) and also read Sutherland's own writings, *Teachings in the Science of Osteopathy* (Sutherland and Wales 1990).

The arachnoid mater

The arachnoid lies immediately underneath the dura. As stated above, embryologically the arachnoid is more akin to a sister to the pia mater but a second cousin to the dura. The palpatory quality of the arachnoid is highly different from that of the dura. Like the periosteum (see Chapter 5), the arachnoid feels very dynamic and active, and consequently it is highly reactive. Therefore palpation at this level of the meninges commands deep respect from the practitioner. It is not the place to be if one's practitioner ego is 'out of the box' and looking to gain ascendancy! Total centredness, humility and respect are required when palpating the arachnoid mater.

In my clinical experience, the arachnoid can express states of physical disturbance in the head or spinal canal and disturbances to the psyche, especially those of feeling mentally pressurised

and irritated. When the arachnoid is irritated for any reason, it can be helped but *only* if you can keep totally centred whilst working. It is not a tissue to underestimate, nor to treat unless you truly know your ability to be without ego when at the treatment table (you also need to be without ego when making this assessment). If you are unsure, I would strongly suggest referring the patient to a more experienced osteopath.

Here are two highly abbreviated versions of clinical examples which may help to clarify such circumstances. I have changed patients' names to keep anonymity.

CASE STUDY: SARAH

Sarah was a bell ringer (campanologist) at her local church. She was in the process of bell ringing when she mistimed her rope pulling action with a heavy church bell. This resulted in a sudden extension movement of her lumbar spine as the rope pulled quickly upwards whilst she was holding it firmly (instead of allowing it to slide upwards and away from her hands). The result was a severe whiplash of her upper lumbar spine and a severe L1/2 disc herniation and prolapse. She was taken to hospital and after diagnostic evaluation, after a week or so, underwent surgery. The surgery was only partially beneficial, and much severe pain remained. She had a second surgery to reduce the scar tissue which occurred following the initial surgery, which was again only partially helpful.

When I saw Sarah for the first time, she had not sat down for 18 months and had to eat all meals standing up. She had not left her upstairs apartment in all that time. She was in too much severe pain to be able to carry out any spinal motion assessment and so all physical examination had to be passive. But, any normal spinal passive movement was also out of the question due to the severity of her symptoms! Any testing of the cranial base patterns either via the head or elsewhere in the body was also contraindicated as the tissues were screaming: 'No, don't do anything!'

All I could do was to allow my mental awareness, my third hand, to be with the tissues at each segmental level in turn, whilst staying centred and not 'doing' anything. From this experience I was then able to make a surprisingly accurate segmental analysis. It was when I brought my palpatory awareness to the level of L1/2 that I encountered the most extraordinary level of irritation and inflammation I have ever experienced in my whole professional career. I could feel irritation specifically to the arachnoid mater at that level. I can only describe that experience as 'palpating a volcano', an explosive and highly active one. I then realised that with Sarah there was nothing I could 'do' without risking making her feel very much worse. I then had a lightbulb moment!

There was nothing I could 'do' so the treatment had to be without me doing anything! *Everything* had to come from her physiology, not mine. I realised that my role was just to be totally centred (way beyond anything I had done before whilst treating patients), observing whilst having a sense of compassion for what the tissues were having to cope with, this volcanic activity!

For six weeks (weekly sessions) I just sat there doing nothing except being totally centred, being 'with the tissues', and listening. No symptomatic change occurred each time although after about 25 minutes I had this intuitive sense of needing to 'come off' and finish the session. Sarah had come to the end of the line in terms of medical help, she had nowhere else to turn for further help and having been recommended by her pain clinic consultant to see a cranial osteopath, she had an amazingly high level of trust in my skill and ability. So, despite no change symptomatically, she was happy for me to continue seeing her. At the sixth or seventh session I felt a small

amount of change and that the intensity of the volcano marginally reduced. After eight weeks from the commencement of my visits, she said she could sit for two minutes at a time in a dining chair to eat, for the first time in nearly two years!

After about three months of these treatments (my doing nothing except being centred and expressing a sense of compassion to the tissues), I started to feel that the volcano had reduced to a forest fire, and Sarah was able to leave her apartment to step outside for a little while and get some fresh air!

In all I treated Sarah over a two-and-a-half-year period (until I moved to another area of the UK), during which time her life became more normal, though she still had to be very careful with limiting her activities and movements and also to avoid getting tired.

What is the difference between purely doing nothing, and being centred with a sense of compassion for Sarah's tissue state? This is an especially important question which raises several further questions. First, is it possible to be purely doing nothing, without influencing the result? 'In experimental psychology and clinical research, there is overwhelming evidence that experimenters' attitudes can influence the outcome of experiments' (Sheldrake 1998).

In my experience of teaching the cranial osteopathic approach, and that of many teaching colleagues, when a student has too much of their awareness on the tissues, wanting to get them better or make a powerful change, no positive benefit arises, and it can aggravate tissue states. It is even possible for the practitioner to impose a tissue state on a patient's tissues, and then diagnose that as the patient's problem. If there is too much practitioner intention or even imposition of a tissue state, then the patient's tissues will shut down as a protective response to that 'unconscious' influence of the practitioner.

It is extremely important that the practitioner

must have their attention with the tissue state, without interference from excess attention or excess desire to get the patient better; only then does the desired therapeutic change occur. By being centred, the practitioner ensures that they are in the state of least ego, the most neutral state, a state of not wishing to impose anything upon the tissues. This act of being centred is very different to simply doing nothing. I like to describe it as 'actively doing nothing'. The action comes simply from the action of being centred!

This is why I consider osteopathic treatment to be so profound – we put what Sutherland called our 'feeling, thinking, seeing fingers' to work (Sutherland 1967b). In his later lectures and presentations, Sutherland uses the term 'THINKING, FEELING, KNOWING FINGERS'. Anne Wales, as the editor of Sutherland's writing, specifically chose to have these words printed in capital letters, indicating the strong emphasis Sutherland put on them as he spoke. Notice he does not use the word 'doing'. We need to have fingers that are aware, that can feel (proprioception) and know: this encompasses much more than merely thinking about the anatomy and physiology.

Being compassionate towards the tissues

Treating Sarah made me realise how important it is to become aware of how the tissues in any situation are coping with having to live in a certain state (I discuss this fully in Chapter 18). Becoming aware of this state, which I call 'cellular or tissue consciousness', gave me a big breakthrough in my therapeutic skills and has taken them to a whole new level.

CASE STUDY: RICHARD

Richard is a 42-year-old senior manager in a large corporation. His complaint was of headaches and head tensions, especially around the occiput and forehead regions, which he had had for around nine months. His home life is well balanced, and he is reasonably healthy. However, he said that he is in a very stressful job and does not get on well with his immediate line manager. His immediate boss took up his position within the company a couple of months prior to the onset of Richard's headaches and head tensions.

On examination, apart from some minor postural imbalances and mild spondylotic changes to his cervical region, his spine was relatively normal with no excessive mechanical strains nor tensions. He had mild cranial base patterns which were not affecting his cranial mechanics in any significant manner. However, when I evaluated his meninges, it revealed some significant findings.

The quality of the dura mater was very tight and felt like a tortoise shell, as if it wanted to keep the world out and protect him. The arachnoid mater was very, very irritable throughout. The quality of this irritation to the arachnoid was of a very different quality to that of Sarah in the previous case study. Here there was no significant force vector from any direction, however it had the quality of chronic anger and psychological distress. It felt on palpation as if the arachnoid was 'pissed off' (please excuse my bluntness with this phrase, but these were actual words that came to my mind, as if from nowhere, as I palpated his arachnoid – more on this when you reach Chapter 18). From experience I could tell that this arachnoid state had been present for around eight to nine months (see Chapter 15 on timeline diagnosis and treatment). It was as if the dura mater was attempting to keep his boss away, while the arachnoid had just had enough distress from his boss.

His brain tissue was doing the opposite of the dura mater. Whereas the dura was keeping strong and felt as if wanting to 'push outwards', keeping the world out, his brain was energetically compressing and shrinking inwards away from the world, as if wanting to hide. Again, like the arachnoid there were no external force vectors, only that of 'implosion'.

There was a sense of the dura and central nervous system (CNS) tissue slightly fighting against each other as each wanted to express in directions 180 degrees from each other. The arachnoid was irritated by these two tissues responding as they did to the events happening from his work situation.

My treatment included specific acknowledgement of his arachnoid mater and the cause of its distress, along with acknowledging the 'keep out' role of the dura and the retreating (hiding) CNS. N.B. This did not require talking to the patient about his work environment during his consultations, I was simply working just at a palpatory tissue level.

After 5–6 sessions his headaches and tensions disappeared, and he then had the clarity of mind to address the underlying work-related cause. These treatments again involved compassionately acknowledging the frightened state of the brain tissue, the 'pissed off' state of the arachnoid, and the dura having to be a shield to keep the world (his boss and office) out. I then invited the tissues to treat themselves, by actively doing nothing, except being highly still and centred within myself.

Although I have never seen another patient quite like Sarah since that time, I have seen a number of patients very similar to Richard, the exact cause of psychological stress being unique to each patient. I am sure you will have seen similar patients in your own practices and, hopefully, this chapter will give you new insights on how to treat them.

The pia mater

The pia mater is vastly different from its second cousin, the dura mater, and different from its sister, the arachnoid mater. Like its sister the arachnoid, it is a very delicate tissue compared with the dura mater. Although it is less severe in its irritable reactions than the arachnoid, the pia nevertheless can and does express irritation.

Pia irritation is more like a high-pitched buzzing feeling on palpation. However, compared with the arachnoid it feels much gentler and silkier in its texture. The Latin translation of its name is 'tender mother', and this silky quality on palpation certainly makes it feel very tender. This title is quite amazing as I am sure the person who named it never palpated it as a tissue!

Because of this tender quality and the fact that the pia mater is in direct contact with the neural tissue, the pia (as with irritability of the arachnoid) also commands total respect from the practitioner. When palpating the pia, you need to be totally centred and still within yourself to ensure you do not disturb it in a negative manner. The pia follows all the contours of the brain, and it is impossible to surgically separate the pia from the grey matter. The pia could be considered the 'skin' or 'periosteum' of the brain, but a different tissue from the brain. I have noted that the pia mater does become irritated in fear states or excessive mental pressure. This expresses itself as a subtle but present buzzing quality within the pia mater. Like the dura and arachnoid, the pia mater can become disturbed or irritated specifically or in conjunction with changes to the other meningeal layers.

During 2020, 'the Covid lockdown year', I was not working for several months. When I restarted seeing patients once again, I detected a quality that I have not ever felt before – it was present *in all adults but not in any children under the age of about 14*. At first, I could not understand what this could be, then after a week or so I realised what this was. On the British news at that time (as I am sure was the same everywhere), every broadcast was 99 per cent about the fears of Covid and how it was affecting countries all over the world. This was not just over a few broadcasts, but continually throughout the day, every day of the week, and it had been that way for six months by that time. In other words, all adults were being exposed to the fear of developing a serious illness from Covid.

Children on the other hand were not interested in watching the boring news with the grown-ups; they would much rather be playing a game with their friends or siblings. So, the adults had been bombarded with negativity about Covid for six months and this was still continuing. The pia irritation was from that fear bombardment. The under-14-year-old children did not have that fear as they were not interested in watching the news, and for many even if they did, they would not fully comprehend the fear of Covid. They just knew that they could not go to school. This fear in the adult population, and the subsequent pia irritation, gradually reduced when the UK vaccination programme involved significant numbers of the population.

I know that some people have concerns about the Covid vaccination programme. I am not commenting on the success or possible negative aspects of it. I am only commenting that the programme did seem to reduce the fear in many adults within the population, and that the media started to reduce the time allocated to fearful Covid broadcasts.

As a practitioner you can differentiate between the meningeal layers by the quality under your fingers to help you diagnose which layer or layers you need to help.

We will make further palpatory explorations of the regions of the brain at the treatment table in Chapter 12.

Like all osteopathic learning, our palpatory databank in respect to the three layers of the meninges and CNS requires repeated experience. With time, you will gradually be able to ascertain which layer or layers of the meninges are the primary tissues needing your osteopathic help. Being highly specific in where you take your osteopathic skills (part of the purpose of this book) will significantly increase your success rate with patients. Merely having 'the meninges' in your awareness will not bring about the same level of therapeutic change as having your awareness

directed to the layer or layers of the meninges which are requiring help. It is as if the patient's body knows when you fully understand exactly which specific tissue needs treatment and its exact anatomical location, and it then consequently responds more profoundly.

Meninges palpation exercise

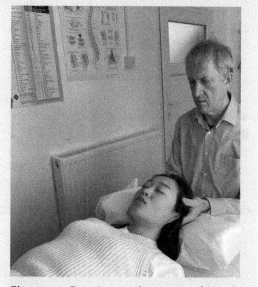

Figure 7.4 Exercise on the journey from the occiput through the 3 layers of the meninges to the brain.

https://youtu.be/oem6loC6jag

In the above exercise, we only focussed on the anatomy with respect to which layer you were palpating. I purposely did not talk about the anatomical location, other than at which bone you were going to start. I did not want you to have too much to think about other than tissue quality during the exercise. Once you become more at home with palpating and diagnosing tissue type differentiation, then you can combine that with your anatomical location diagnosis. This will enable you to decide where in the skull, or spine, and with which of the meningeal layers, if any, you will need to work on.

A word of caution regarding the above case study of Sarah. I discussed how I felt it would be wrong to apply any cranial osteopathic technique to her arachnoid mater, for fear of aggravating her condition. When doing the exploration exercise, you will have noted how the arachnoid can easily be disturbed. For this reason, if you feel that your patient's arachnoid is asking for help, just stay very centred, acknowledge (with compassion) its irritability and then 'do nothing'. Whisper mentally and very politely to the tissue, the arachnoid in this case, asking if it wishes to treat itself. It will probably reply 'yes', and you probably will shortly feel the activity of a self-treatment occurring. Just accept that the body will make whatever changes it wants to, but only if it wants to.

This will not be your choice but that of the patient's physiology. I have known cases where the tissues say: 'Thanks for the invitation, but actually I don't want to treat myself at the moment.' In such circumstances, always respect that response and do not question it. The patient's physiology will always know more about its needs and requirements than any practitioner. The practitioner makes an educated guess, whereas the patient's physiology knows, and doesn't need to guess!

In his writings, Sutherland does not mention the arachnoid mater nor pia mater. I cannot say for certain, but I am sure he could palpate and differentiate between these tissues. Maybe, this is because he felt these tissues were too delicate for the level of palpation skill of these early pioneers of our work. To put this in context, Sutherland would spend two whole weeks just teaching his students how to do a Compression of the Fourth Ventricle (CV4) technique. This is very different to the modern day, where it is sometimes the subject of just one lecture and a practical session within a teaching course.

Do remember, that all cells of the body are expressing inherent motility, not just the brain and spinal cord. Some practitioners I have taught misunderstood the physiology by thinking the brain motility causes the motion of the membranes and subsequently the motion of the bones of the skull and sacrum between the ilia. If that were the case, there would be a minor, but definite, time lag between these elements. Such a time lag would cause a degree of chaos in the physiology. Each cell of the whole physiology is always undergoing flexion and extension at the same time, unless there is a compressive/pathological state somewhere, preventing or reducing flexion and extension at that location. Therefore, each cell of the dura in the connection to the sacrum from the cranial base (the 'core link') is flexing (shortening and widening) and extending (lengthening and narrowing) at the same time.

We will be looking at the sacrum in Chapter 8 to discuss this further.

THE SUTHERLAND FULCRUM

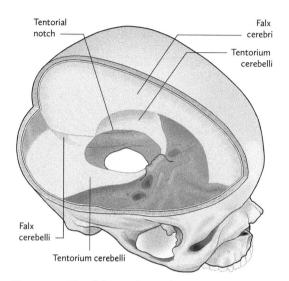

Figure 7.5 The falx cerebri and tentorium cerebelli showing the Sutherland Fulcrum at their junction.

At this point we should acknowledge the so-called Sutherland Fulcrum (SF). This is an area (not an exact point) in the region of the straight sinus, the venous sinus which runs along the junction between the falx cerebri (frequently just called the falx) and the tentorium cerebelli (likewise frequently just called the tent). The Sutherland Fulcrum is the fulcrum of the dural meninges, the point at which the forces acting on the meninges are being resolved, to the best of the physiology's ability at that moment.

This is not a fixed anatomical location, because as we move our body position, our fascial system adjusts its mechanics, and the SF accommodates to these mechanical changes. As has been mentioned in Chapter 6, the dura mater is now considered part of the fascial system. We, as practitioners of Sutherland's work, find that the Sutherland Fulcrum has a profound relationship to the functioning of the fasciae of the whole body. If it feels blocked or locked to some degree, which can occur for a variety of physical or emotional reasons, the fascial system loses varying amounts of its adaptability to the body's demands.

Shears through the falx cerebri or tentorium cerebelli

During development, the falx and tent are formed by the layers of the dural coverings of the brain meeting each other as the brain folds into its adult shape. The dura covering the medial aspect of the left and right cerebral hemispheres meet each other in the midline as the hemispheres expand in size. The meeting of the two layers thereby creates the falx cerebri. Likewise, when the dura covering the cerebellum meets the dura covering the occipital lobes of the cerebellum, the two layers form the tentorium cerebelli.

As the falx and tent are comprised of two layers, it is possible in certain situations for a shear to occur between the two layers. It can be quite easy for practitioners to overlook such mechanical strains as they may or may not fit with the patterns of function (strain) associated with pattern testing. The falx can have shears within it of an anterior and posterior type or even a torsion between the two layers. These may be reflections of such strains in the cranial base. However, the tentorium can have a shear where the upper layer is shearing to one side (e.g., to the left), and the lower layer is shearing to the opposite side (e.g., to the right). Such a finding is not in harmony with any standard strain pattern. Equally there can be an anterior shift of one layer (e.g., the superior layer) and a posterior shift of the other layer (e.g., the inferior layer). Again, such a finding does not harmonise with a standard strain pattern. Because findings such as these do not harmonise with the standard types of patterns accommodated by the sphenobasilar symphysis, these states tend to 'lock up' the dural system.

Tensions within the falx and tent as described above are, in my experience, quite common. However, you can get other tensions and strains within them – the tent especially can have a combination of tensional forces between the layers. If these strains and shears between the two layers of the falx and tent are not carefully resolved, then you may find that the patient's symptoms do not fully respond to your treatments, because the tensions between the layers will be causing tension and compression within the falx, the tent or both.

The venous sinuses

We need to be mindful that the venous sinuses within the skull have an intimate relationship to the cranial bones and the dura mater. Where the dura reflects to form the tentorium or the falx, it creates a small gap which fills and becomes a venous sinus during our embryological development. The superior sagittal sinus, the transverse sinus and the sigmoid sinus are all formed in such a manner. The straight sinus is formed by the meeting of the tentorium with the falx in the occipital area. So whenever we feel a state of tension within the dura mater, we must consider how that tension will be having an effect on the venous sinuses.

Of course, we need to also acknowledge that these venous sinuses are the venous drainage pathways for the brain tissue. Should there be any turbulence in venous flow, which would happen if the venous sinuses became pressurised by tensions within the dura mater, it would hinder good venous drainage away from the brain and possibly lead to degrees of cerebral venous congestion and consequent headaches. So do think about the venous physiology within the cranium when palpating the meninges of your patients.

I hope that this chapter has stimulated further thought when working with the CSF and meninges of your patients. Such a vast topic as the meninges could have filled several books, so this chapter hopefully will stimulate further self-study.

Treatment of intra-falx or intra-tent strains and shears exercise

Do remember to be very centred and match the tissue tone with your elbow fulcrum, forearm tone and third hand!

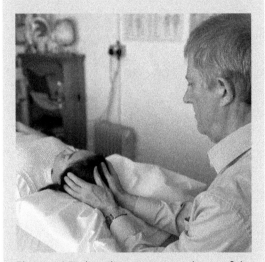

Figure 7.6 Feeling the two separate layers of the falx cerebri.

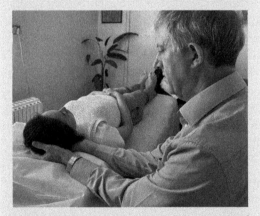

Figure 7.7 Palpating the upper and lower layers of the tentorium cerebelli.

https://youtu.be/6lH9AraHWKM

REFERENCES

Adigun, O.O., & Al-Dhahir, M., 2021. Anatomy, head and neck, cerebrospinal fluid. In: StatPearls [Internet]. Treasure Island, FL: StatPearls Publishing. Available from: https://www.ncbi.nlm.nih.gov/books/NBK459286/#_NBK459286_pubdet_.

Bleschmidt, E., & Glasser, R., 1978. *Biokinetics and Biodynamics of Human Differentiation: Principles and Applications.* Springfield, IL: Charles C. Thomas, pp. xiii–xiv.

Dasgupta, K., & Jeong, J., 2019. Developmental biology of the meninges. *Genesis.* 57(5): e23288.

Dove, C., 2019. Conversation with Timothy Marris. 28 July.

Ishikawa, M., Yamada, S., & Yamamoto, K., 2015. Three-dimensional observation of Virchow-Robin spaces in the basal ganglia and white matter and their relevance to idiopathic normal pressure hydrocephalus. *Fluids Barriers CNS.* Available from: https://fluidsbarrierscns.biomedcentral.com/articles/10.1186/s12987-015-0010-1#citeas.

Khasawneh, A., Garling, R., & Harris, C., 2018. Cerebrospinal fluid circulation: what do we know and how do we know it? *Brain Circ.* 4(1): 14–18.

Ma, Q., Ineichen, B.V., Detmar, M., *et al.*, 2017. Outflow of cerebrospinal fluid is predominantly through lymphatic vessels and is reduced in aged mice. *Nat Commun.* Available from: https://www.nature.com/articles/s41467-017-01484-6.

McPartland, J., & Skinner, E., 2005. The biodynamic model of osteopathy in the cranial field. *EXPLORE: The Journal of Science and Healing.* Available from: https://www.researchgate.net/publication/7001330_The_biodynamic_model_of_osteopathy_in_the_cranial_field.

Melin, E., Eide, P.K., & Ringstad, G., 2020. In vivo assessment of cerebrospinal fluid efflux to nasal mucosa in humans. *Sci Rep.* Available from: https://www.nature.com/articles/s41598-020-72031-5.

Mollanji, R., Ozanovic-sosic, R., Zakharov, A., Makarian, L., *et al.*, 2002. Blocking cerebrospinal fluid absorption through the cribriform plate increases resting intracranial pressure. *Am J Physiol Regul Integr Comp Physiol.* 282(6): 1593–1599.

Orešković, D., & Klarica, M., 2010. The formation of cerebrospinal fluid: nearly a hundred years of interpretations and misinterpretations. *Brain Research Reviews.* Available from: https://core.ac.uk/download/pdf/206068857.pdf.

Pople, I.K., & Ettles, D., 1995. The role of endoscopic choroid plexus coagulation in the management of hydrocephalus. *Neurosurgery.* 36(4): 698–701.

Sakka, L., Coll, G., & Chazal, J., 2011. Anatomy and physiology of cerebrospinal fluid. *European Annals of Otorhinolaryngology, Head and Neck Diseases.* 128(6): 309–316. doi.org/10.1016/j.anorl.2011.03.002.

Sheldrake, R., 1998. Experimenter effects in scientific research: how widely are they neglected? *Journal of Scientific Exploration.* Available from: https://www.sheldrake.org/research/experimenter-effects/experimenter-effects-in-scientific-research-how-widely-are-they-neglected.

Still, A.T., 1902. *Philosophy and Mechanical Principles of Osteopathy.* Kansas City, MO: Hudson-Kimberly Pub Co. Reprinted, Kirksville, MO: Osteopathic Enterprises; 1986.

Sutherland, W.G., 1967a. The core-link between the cranial bowl, and the pelvic bowl. In: Wales, A.L., ed. *Contributions of Thought: Collected Writings of William Garner Sutherland 1914–1954.* Kansas City, MO: Sutherland Cranial Teaching Foundation, pp. 90–92.

Sutherland, W.G., 1967b. Let's be up and touching. The osteopathic physician. In: Wales, A.L., ed. *Contributions of Thought: Collected Writings of William Garner Sutherland 1914–1954.* Kansas City, MO: Sutherland Cranial Teaching Foundation, p. 1.

Sutherland, W.G., & Wales, A.L., eds., 1990. *Teachings in the Science of Osteopathy.* Portland, OR: Rudra Press, pp. 153–164.

Willard, F., 1989. Conversation with Timothy Marris. 2 February.

CHAPTER 8

The Liquid Spine and Limbs

In this chapter we will enter the next stage of the book, looking at the body outside of the head from a regional perspective. We will look at the spine and the limbs, and in further chapters, explore the abdomen, pelvis and the thorax. I chose to name this chapter the liquid spine and limbs because we should envision the spine, limbs and their joints as being highly liquid and not bony, ligamentous and muscular. As has been discussed in Chapter 5 on bone states, bone in health is a very fluid structure. Similarly, healthy joints and muscles are both solid and fluid in their quality. It is when these tissues become acutely or chronically pressurised, usually from external traumatic forces or postural forces, that the fluid quality decreases and bones and joints feel hard and dry, and muscles become tight and fibrotic, leading to symptom development and eventually degenerative change.

EMBRYOLOGY

Perhaps for obvious ethical reasons, there are very few modern scientific papers indicating the appearance of somites in humans, as most scientific studies are done on chick embryos. In the paper by Orts-Llorca relating to human embryonic development of somites, it states that somitic segmentation takes place between stages 9 and 13, which is from 19–21 days to 28–32 days of gestation (Orts-Llorca 1981). This indicates that the whole process of somite development takes approximately 9–13 days from the end of the third week of intrauterine life (IUL), to the early or mid-part of the fifth week IUL.

These somites are effectively stem cells which can develop into a variety of essential structures such as the muscles, vertebrae, dermis of the dorsal skin, and vascular cells which then develop into the aortic formation and future spinal arteries. According to DeRuiter:

'The somites eventually diverge into sclerotome (cartilage), syndotome (tendons), myotome (skeletal muscle), dermatome (dermis), and endothelial cells, each corresponding to different regions within the somite itself.' The same paper continues: 'Because the somites are an essential part of the developing body plan of vertebrates, any disruption in the cycle of formation or segmentation can result in anomalies such as congenital vertebral defects' (DeRuiter 2010).

The somites develop into the segmental levels of the vertebral column with the future intervertebral discs and the emergence of the nerve roots occurring at the centre of the somite level; the vertebrae each consisting of part of the somites above and below. We should remember that in embryological terms, bones develop later than most other structures and tissues. Many practitioners (medical and osteopaths included) tend to think segmentally in terms of numbering of the vertebrae because this is standard anatomical referencing. Perhaps we should be thinking of the somite level, as when we name a nerve such as the L4 nerve, not the vertebra level when describing the vertebral column or levels within the thorax or abdomen.

In Chapter 15: Back to the time: an inner approach, we will be discussing how as osteopaths we can develop the skills to treat past conditions – or even prenatal tissue states – as though we are treating them at the time of the event. Once you gain this significant osteopathic skill, the time of formation and the development of somites become key points in time to remember. N.B. Please do not now rush ahead to Chapter 15 (even if tempted to do so), as it is wiser to continue working your way through each chapter and the osteopathic exercises within it, as many of the exercises sequentially require higher skill levels.

LIMB DEVELOPMENT

The relationship between the ectoderm and mesodermal layers results in an outgrowth which will become the limb bud. At the third week a swelling develops on the ventrolateral surface, which will become the lower limb bud. During the fourth week, two to three days after the true upper limb bud formation, the lower limb bud is properly formed (Mooney 2021).

Soon after the appearance of the limb bud, it modifies into what is described as a paddle shape. This has a leading edge of ectoderm, the ectodermal cap, with the core of the paddle as mesoderm. A differentiation within the leading aspect of the limb occurs creating the zone of polarising activity. This area then determines which part of the limb will become the anterior and posterior aspects. By the seventh week IUL there are indentations on the growing end of the limb buds indicating the differentiation into digital rays, which will become separate fingers or toes.

It is worth noting that the limb buds are not revealed on ultrasound until the eighth week, by which time the limb buds have become significantly developed and differentiated. The limb buds are growing and differentiating within at an extraordinary rate. This is possible due to the very high level of energy and vitality within their ectodermal cap and the mesenchyme. As osteopaths we can use this vitality and potency to increase the therapeutic potential within both child and adult limb tissues.

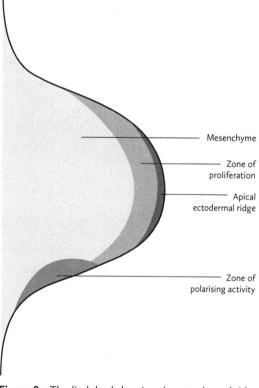

Mesenchyme

Zone of proliferation

Apical ectodermal ridge

Zone of polarising activity

Figure 8.1 The limb bud showing the ectodermal ridge and the zone of polarising activity.

The upper limb bud emerges from the level of the C7 somite around the fourth week IUL, and the lower limb bud a week later from the L5 somite. The final finishing point of the upper limb is the tip of the middle finger, and the lower limb finishes at the tip of the second toe. By harnessing the potency present during the limb development and growth stages, we can assist the body to restore and improve the physiological state of joints, chronic muscle issues and chronic ligament or tendon problems within the child or adult limb.

Although we will discuss going back in time in Chapter 15, it would be appropriate to borrow an approach from that chapter at this point.

Exercise using the enhanced potency of the limb bud in treatment

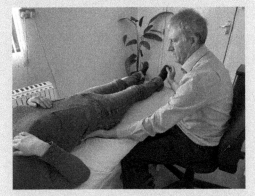

Figure 8.2 Working with the embryological potency of the limb bud. In the lower extremity the limb bud starts at L5 and finishes at the second toe. In an upper limb, the limb bud starts at C7 and finishes at the tip of the middle finger.

Here in this exercise, we will explore treatment of a limb using embryological potency. Do centre yourself as deeply as you can, without strain nor effort as *you cannot try to relax!*

https://youtu.be/NkxzQEbHUfU

Within the limb bud there is also a physiological fulcrum, which creates the flow of nutrients to supply the significant needs of the occurring growth. This process is a fundamental aspect of embryology, that of the formation of blood vessels. The cells within the mesoderm, and especially just behind the apical cap or ectoderm, are undergoing a phenomenal growth process, rapidly dividing and modifying as the limb growth occurs.

When a cell suffers low oxygen levels, it secretes a chemical called vascular endothelial growth factor (VEGF). This stimulates the endothelial cells to grow in the direction of the oxygen hungry cells and carry both oxygen and nutrients to them. This results in a rich capillary bed being formed in the growing end of the limb bud. With the restoration of oxygen to the cells, the VEGF levels are reduced. As the limb growth progresses, some of these capillaries start to coalesce and remodel, becoming larger arteries.

In this way, blood vessels are created by a demand-led process and not a push process, the hungry cells creating that demand. Veins are created due to the need to remove metabolic waste products and send them back to the very rapidly growing liver via the hepatic arteries. The nerves of the limb on the other hand, grow more like the growth of a tree, emerging from the neural tube and into the limb buds. However, the developing major blood vessels and the nerves growing into the limb bud are in a close arrangement, as there are no muscles nor bones at this stage.

If you think of the brachial nerve plexus, the subclavian artery runs through the plexus, creating a powerful and potent neurovascular structure for the upper extremity. As it grows and extends down the limb, this neurovascular bundle becomes the physiological axis for the limb growth. Later, as the muscular and joint development occurs, so the nutritional and oxygen demands within the developing limb cause the creation of side arteries within it, to supply those needs.

In the practical exercise you have just done, you felt the potency of the developing limb and brought this forwards into the present day to create a significantly increased therapeutic power for therapeutic change.

Exercise using the physiological axis of the limb

As an exercise, you may now wish to go to the treatment table and again feel the vibrant health, the potency of the growing limb bud. However, after you feel the potency, acknowledge that there is a physiological axis along the growing limb, that of the main blood vessel growth into the limb. Having an awareness of this physiological axis or therapeutic fulcrum seems to amplify the action of the potency when you invite the limb to treat itself, should it choose to do so.

When we stand, are our hip, knee and ankle joints touching? This may seem like a ridiculous question. Gravity acting on the weight of our body would obviously seem to cause joint surfaces to touch each other. However, 21st century scientific thinking may question this fact. Gerald Pollack, in his book *The 4th Phase of Water* (2013b), writes at length to describe how water molecules behave differently from 'normal' in certain circumstances. In simple terms, when water molecules contact 'Teflon'-type chemicals, the water molecules align differently and cause particles within the water to be pushed away by negative electric fields from the 'Teflon'-type surface. He calls the area where substrates within the water get pushed away the Exclusion Zone (EZ). He also published a paper on this topic in the *Journal of Physical Chemistry* the same year. Here he refers to work done verifying this phenomenon:

The aqueous region next to various hydrophilic surfaces was recently explored by two groups with extensive experience in optics. Both groups found that the refractive index of the interfacial zone next to Nafion and hydrogels was higher than that of the bulk water beyond, by up to 10%. This highly refractile zone extended some 50 μm from the material surface. Thus, the EZ has a higher refractive index than bulk water. (Pollack 2013a)

I was fortunate to be present when Gerald Pollack came to the UK in 2017 to give a presentation on his work, and to give a one-day workshop. During the workshop, we worked in pairs. First, one person lay down on the treatment table and we had to evaluate the knee joints and their quality, to feel if one lower extremity and particularly the knee joint had more tension than the other.

Then we were asked to feel the lower extremities, and in particular the knee joints of the same person when they stood upright. Rather than tell you what I felt, let's do this as an exercise for yourself working with a partner.

Initially, have your model lie down on the treatment table supine and then centre yourself.

https://youtu.be/c3-2U1rReew

What did you notice? Did you get any sense that on one or both of the lower extremities, it felt as if there was some repulsion sensation, pushing the tibial plateau away from the femoral condyles? I have found this with many people. Colleagues attending the workshop felt it on their partners with whom they were working, and nearly all the students on my courses, when doing this exercise, felt a sense of the cartilage surfaces of one or both knee joints pushing away from each other.

Perhaps you felt one knee showing greater indications of less joint touching than the other. If so, was the joint where the cartilage was touching the same limb expressing more mechanical tensions when you palpated the limb supine at the treatment table? I suspect most likely it was.

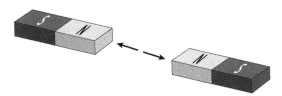

Figure 8.3 In healthy joints, even weight-bearing joints, the joint surfaces do not touch due to an electromagnetic repulsion force.

If this Exclusion Zone as named by Pollack results in an electromagnetic force pushing the cartilages (in health, good mechanical balance through that limb) away from each other, it would back up the palpatory experience. In my experience (and those of others I have discussed this with), I find that the limb with more mechanical disturbances is able to override the electromagnetic repulsion between the cartilages, presumably due to the disruptive mechanical forces present.

The implication then becomes that in health where there are minimal negative tensions and forces acting in and around joints, the joint surfaces should not be touching. In other words, we should be standing and walking on a cushion of fluid and electromagnetic repulsion, not on our cartilaginous joint surfaces. This would also mean that when strains and tensions acting on our joints become too great, the cartilage surfaces start touching each other, with the subsequent wear and tear over time leading to osteoarthritis. Conversely, joint surfaces that never touch each other will never wear out!

This comprehension makes our clinical findings much more understandable. What is even more exciting is that as osteopaths, we are excellent at reducing mechanical strains and shears within the body. So, by steadily reducing the mechanical strains acting on an arthritic joint we have the potential to reach a point where the joint surfaces again stop touching each other.

THE CLAVICLE

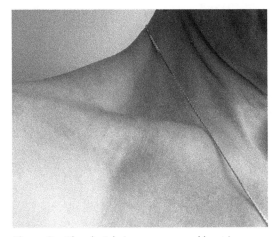

Figure 8.4 The clavicle is a very unusual bone!

The clavicle is a unique bone in the body:

- The clavicle is the first bone of the body to start its bony development and is one of the last bones in the body to fully ossify.
- It is formed by both membranous development and cartilaginous development.
- It is the only bony connection of the upper limb to the axial skeleton.
- It is classified as a long bone, but it has no medulla like other long bones.

Embryology of the clavicle

According to Hyland *et al.*, the clavicle undergoes development in a fascinating manner. The medial and lateral ends of the clavicle develop in differing manners embryologically. The sternal end forms via a cartilaginous precursor before ossification, whereas by contrast the lateral end of the bone forms via a membranous precursor (Hyland *et al.* 2022).

The area of bone onset – the lateral end of the clavicle – being formed by membrane, is also considered a dermal bone. Here the membrane is laid down near the ectodermal surface. This is comparable to the shell of a tortoise, which also is considered a dermal bone. Such bones develop by a process called accretion, the bone being laid down within the dermis by osteoblasts. Bones of the cranial vault are also considered dermal bones.

The 's' or sinusoidal shape of the clavicle is also formed in the embryological phase: 'The sinusoidal shape of the isolated clavicle of an 8.5-week foetus (CR length 35 mm) could be seen well under the dissecting microscope' (Ogata and Uhthoff 1990). It was originally thought that the bone develops its shape when much vigorous motion of the baby in the womb occurs much later, but this research shows that the curved shape is much more fundamental and its development is not yet fully understood.

One of the last bones to complete formation

The clavicle does not finish its formation until around our 23rd to 25th year: 'The medial clavicular physis does not fuse until 23 to 25 years of age' (Hughes *et al.* 2020). Considering that it is the first bone to start its ossification and is the last to finish its growth process, there must be a reason for this phenomenal length of development. Let's consider some of the reasons.

The clavicle is the only bone linking the upper limb to the axial skeleton, to the manubrium. We have to remember that the scapula only has a muscular sling attachment to the dorsal spine.

Consequently, we could consider the clavicle as a bony fulcrum for the upper limb. We should also remember that any mechanical force transmitted towards the torso from the hand, if the elbow is straight, is transmitted directly to the clavicle.

Think about your own past experiences: when you are about to fall forwards at any time, the first thing you do, almost by reflex action, is to put your hand out to break the impact of your fall. Such an impact to the hand drives the forces up to the clavicle and may in some cases result in a fracture of the bone. We know that the most adventurous times of our life are when we are toddlers, learning or having just learned to walk, involving many falls in that learning process. Or, perhaps when as teenagers or in our early adulthood we take up more exciting, but more dangerous activities and pursuits. Consequently, the clavicle is known to be the most commonly fractured bone in the body!

Perhaps a late ossifying bone allows for much adaptation for these mechanical bone injuries and compressions. If we also consider life in the womb, the growing baby moves its limbs and pushes against the uterine wall. Although such intrauterine forces are nothing like those in postnatal life, we must remember that the limb is far more delicate at that time.

Hyland also mentions that usually in the clavicle, unlike standard long bones, there is no medullary cavity and consequently no central artery to the bone. It does have a periosteal arterial supply but is considered to have its cortical supply from the nearby suprascapular, thoraco-acromial and internal thoracic arteries (Hyland *et al.* 2022). Perhaps this lack of a medullary cavity is due to its small diameter, and possibly from its mixed embryological origin. However, having three differing arteries supplying the bone, it heals well following a fracture. It should also be mentioned that it is the only long bone which is not immobilised within a cast following a fracture as the consequences to lung function would be too great (as with rib fractures).

From an osteopathic perspective this is a very important bone. It is a fulcrum for the upper extremity and is exposed to significant mechanical forces from falls. We should also be aware of its anatomical role in giving protection to the subclavian artery and vein, and to the brachial nerve plexus. As will be discussed in Chapter 10, the manubrium has very important vascular relationships. The sternoclavicular joint (SCJ) equally is very close to vital blood vessels. Mechanical tensions within the SCJ will therefore affect the manubrium and its mechanical relationship to the vessels underneath. The subclavian veins are significant veins of the body, draining into the superior vena cava. The whole lymphatic system drains into the subclavian vein at or close to its junction to the jugular veins in the neck. Bearing in mind that both the veins and lymphatic vessels are low pressure vessels, it means that their fluid flow can be disturbed by relatively minor forces to the respective vessel walls.

Often as osteopaths we tend to forget that the fluids travelling within our blood vessels and lymphatics can get disturbed by mechanical forces. Anyone who has a garden hose will know that if you accidently stand on the hose or it has a kink somewhere, the volume of flow out of the end of the hose is immediately affected and reduced in volume. Even a mechanical pressure on the side of an artery could potentially have a negative influence on the blood flow within the vessel. Whether this would have an influence on the tissues supplied by that vessel is open to question, much depending on the degree of mechanical tensions involved. However, as osteopaths we know that subtle tensions within tissues may result in pathological changes if sustained for many years. When feeling strain patterns in the body we can appreciate how they can become factors in our diagnoses, so we should not ignore mechanical influences on blood and lymph vessels.

Exercise on the clavicle

https://youtu.be/2v7LJiTylyU

THE SPINE

An osteopathic discussion on the spine could easily fill a large book, so I do not propose to go into great detail in this chapter. However, by discussing osteopathic principles, they can then be applied to many aspects of spinal treatment.

The core link

Sutherland used the term 'core link' to describe the dural link between the foramen magnum and cranial base, and the sacrum. As we have discussed in Chapter 7, the dura mater is highly collagenous and so as a tissue it is very effective at transmitting mechanical forces. Therefore, any forces imparted to the dural tube from either the cranial base or the sacrum will be transmitted to the other end. Clinically, we frequently see patients who have tensions on one side of the cranial base and get back pains in the pelvis. The forces would tend to be unilateral with, for example, a side-bending rotation pattern or to the opposite side if the patient has a torsional pattern. However, with the so-called non-physiological patterns (vertical and lateral shears), the forces are a bit more complicated.

Although the sacrum as a whole bone in general follows the occiput, I have found that within the sacrum, the intraosseous tensions appear as if the sphenobasilar symphysis is represented in the middle of the sacrum for expressing the vertical and lateral shear patterns. In a vertical shear, where the basisphenoid feels more superior than the basiocciput, it feels as if the upper segments of the sacrum want to be more superior and the lower segments more inferior, causing a tension within the sacrum. Equally with a lateral shear where the basisphenoid feels more to the left (if palpating a left lateral shear pattern), the upper segments of the sacrum feel as if they want to be more to the left and the lower segments more to the right. In other words, the vertical and lateral shears are reflected as shears within the sacrum as opposed to the side-bending/rotation and torsional strains, where the bone as a whole reflects the cranial base pattern.

I shall not attempt to describe here the palpatory quality of a multiple strain pattern in the sacrum, as these are not so easy to define, more of a feeling of the sacrum being locked up! Many patients do have more than one cranial base pattern being expressed at the same time.

The functional sacrum

Whilst on the topic of the sacrum, we should discuss 'the functional sacrum'. This is a term which (as far as I know) was coined by a UK cranial osteopathy teaching colleague, Nicholas Handoll. He used the term functional sacrum to describe the position where the sacrum was felt to be functioning from, rather than its anatomical location between the two iliac bones. When there is a trauma to the body, the shock wave is transmitted through the tissues, shifting the fulcrum under which they operate. In the cranial base, we have the so-called Sutherland Fulcrum, which is not an exact location, but is described as somewhere near the junction of the falx cerebri with the tentorium cerebelli. It is not an exact place as differing forces on the body tissues shift this fascia and dural fulcrum away from the straight sinus (the falx and tent junction). The Sutherland Fulcrum, by shifting its position in any of the three dimensions, makes for a better compensation by the body to whatever force entered the body, or whatever postural change has occurred.

Functional sacrum exercise

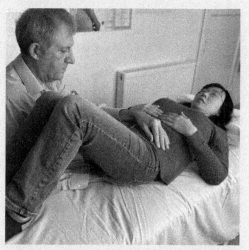

Figure 8.5 Exploring to find the functional sacrum.

https://youtu.be/HEHArvHZyB8

The sacrum also shifts its physiological function as the fulcrum for the two lower extremities, to the best place to accommodate the mechanical forces which have influenced the base of the spine and pelvis. In many cases where the person has not had any major injuries, the sacrum may well be functioning in or near its true anatomical position. However, this is not always the case. Bad falls, motor vehicle accidents, skiing injuries, horse riding injuries (this list could be endless), all will result in the lower limb fulcrum, the sacrum, needing to shift its 'working/functional' position, to accommodate the event(s).

In such cases you may find that when you put your hand under the sacrum, although you have your hand between the two ilia at the back of the pelvis, you find that the sacrum feels as if it is sitting or functioning from a different location. If this is the case, it is important that you evaluate as closely as possible the exact position of this 'functional sacrum' position. Wherever this happens to be, the anatomical tissue located at this position now has a functional sacrum energetically sitting on top of it, and consequently it won't be happy!

CASE STUDY: RACHEL

Whilst teaching a practical session on the functional sacrum, one of my osteopathic students was having some difficulty feeling where this functional sacrum was. She said it didn't feel like it was happy in its true position but could not detect it being anywhere different. When I put my hands on the student model lying down, in a manner that the student still had her hands under the sacrum (the model being supine), I could feel and agree with the student that the sacrum did not feel happy.

I then asked the student to become more centred within herself so that she could perhaps feel more accurately, as I could tell that the sacrum had shifted its functional position but not by very much. After the student had centred herself again, I asked her if she felt whether the sacrum could have shifted a little to the left or right. She paused and felt, then said: 'A bit to the right.' To make the student think more precisely, I asked her to say in centimetres how far to the right, to which she replied: 'about 2 cm'.

I then repeated the questioning in terms of superior/inferior and anterior/posterior. Again, after her initial response, by asking her to describe the movements in centimetres, her final conclusions were that the functional sacrum had shifted about 2 cm to the right, 1 cm anteriorly and just under 1 cm superiorly. I then asked her that if that was the case, what did the body of S2 now have functionally

sitting on top of it? She paused whilst thinking through her anatomy, then replied: 'perhaps the S1 intervertebral foramen on the right'.

I then guided the student to match accurately the tension in the sacrum tissues until they became softer, and then invited the sacrum to treat itself. Whereupon the sacrum went through a treatment process and gently shifted back to its true anatomical position. The model then said, in a surprised tone: 'Oh my God, my right-sided sciatic pains have just disappeared. I've had those for about five years and many osteopaths have treated me in the past, but to no benefit.'

My comment to both students was that yes, the functional sacrum was sitting on the S1 foramen and so the S1 nerve effectively had a sacrum sitting on top of it and didn't like it! The previous practitioners may have worked on the lumbosacral region and even may have felt the sacrum, but missed this slight shift of the functional sacrum, the true cause of her sciatic symptoms.

Sometimes I have seen patients in practice where the functional sacrum sits on top of the rectum or sigmoid colon. This results in chronic constipation. Again, the lower parts of the colon in these examples hated having the functional sacrum sitting on top of them, as they then found it more difficult to move stools further down the tube.

One of my patients experienced an extreme trauma, where she had fallen through the attic floor feet first, down through the bedroom ceiling and onto the floor below, a total fall of about 12 feet (3.65 metres). Such a fall onto the feet with straight legs puts a very severe shock through the sacrum. In her case the functional sacrum felt as if it was up around her heart. Luckily, she was only in her late 20s and had no existing heart issues (but then if she were older, maybe she might have been more cautious and careful when in her attic!). As I was able to treat her within two weeks of the accident, no serious consequences occurred to the heart. In a much older patient (and ignoring the risk to more degenerative limbs), to have a sacrum sitting on top of the heart would in my opinion lead to heart pathology if left untreated.

The Sutherland Fulcrum outside the body

How many times have you heard someone say, when not feeling well, 'I feel awful, I feel beside myself.' I have asked in several countries where I teach, and this phrase is also used in other languages when someone is distraught with anxiety or severe distress. The words 'I feel beside myself' are in my opinion a very true statement, because I have seen a number of patients in my professional career where the Sutherland Fulcrum lies outside the body.

The patients I have seen where the Sutherland Fulcrum is outside of the body are those who have experienced a very strong physical trauma, such as a high impact road traffic accident. The position of the Sutherland Fulcrum in the more severe cases was several metres outside of the body, the fulcrum shifting there by the power and direction of the impact to the body. In many cases of the Sutherland Fulcrum external to the body, the physiology is truly struggling to operate around this fulcrum and certainly needs careful help to 'bring the person back inside themselves'.

To treat such a finding, a practitioner needs to be highly centred. Then you need to have part of your awareness on the location of the fulcrum outside the body. This means that you need to get an impression of how far it is outside the body and the direction towards which it shifted. Without any level of trying, the more accurate you can be the better, but a rough guess without effort is better than trying to become highly accurate.

Having perceived the distance and direction of the current Sutherland Fulcrum outside the body, you will need to match the tension in the cranial base by adjusting your elbow fulcrum and forearm tone, to that point of softening.

Then have another aspect of your awareness, using what we call divided awareness, on the area around the junction of the falx cerebri and tentorium cerebelli, so that your awareness is on both the Sutherland Fulcrum outside the body and on the area where it would be much happier, its home position. Then very gently (because it is very uncomfortable where it is now located), invite the relationship between the outside of the body location and the home region of the Sutherland Fulcrum to treat itself if it wishes to.

In almost all cases, a shifting relationship occurs between these two areas, and the Sutherland Fulcrum starts moving in a direction towards the body. It may re-enter the body or even return to its home area. However, accept that it may only travel part of the way, and you may need to offer the patient another treatment to bring the fulcrum closer to home. I would suggest a gap of around one week before seeing the patient again to allow the body to adjust before the next treatment.

Treating spinal segments

I will now add a few words on treating spinal segments with an inner cranial approach. We all have patients where there is a disturbed mechanical finding – this may be affecting the apophyseal joints or the intervertebral discs, or the segmental postural muscles.

Sutherland described the use of direct action and exaggeration methods when offering any treatment. I would add to this 'inviting the body to treat itself'. Exaggeration is where we take the tissues further in the direction they have already travelled and is a common therapeutic approach. Direct action is to gently guide the tissues back in the direction from whence they came. With both exaggeration and direct action, the tissue guidance stays within the comfortable limits of the tissues.

Both of these approaches create a gentle level of confusion around the tissues, causing the body to reorganise itself back to a better physiology.

A useful approach to working on one or two localised segments of the spine is to slide your hands under the spine until the tips of your fingers are on the far side of the spinous processes, then slightly flex your fingertips so that they can exert a minor force to the spinous processes in a direction back towards you. Do this just to the point where around 70 per cent, but not all, of the slack is taken up. Adjust your elbow fulcrum and forearm tone until you feel some softening of the segments. Then, being centred, mentally invite these specific segments to treat themselves, if they wish. They usually do want to, unless the body wants you to treat somewhere else first, or the body has already had enough treatment during that session.

Severe spinal pain

You may have had patients with severely herniated disc problems or perhaps scarring from spinal surgery onto other tissues or other very painful conditions. With such patients, I would ask you to be even more highly centred. The reason is twofold.

First, the ego must be well and truly outside of the consulting room, because it is very easy to let the ego creep in and increase your desire to get the patient better, overshadowing the patient's tissues when they tell you that they have had enough treatment. Carrying on beyond when the patient's tissues have told you to stop results in over treatment. This can easily cause an increase in symptoms in the already delicate tissues (hence the pain levels), with the result that the patient may cancel all future appointments with you. This is clearly not good for the patient, nor for your professional reputation.

Second, our perception must be at the highest level possible, so that not only do we know when to finish the treatment, but we also ask the body to do the treatment for us. The more severe someone's condition, the easier it is to do something which may further irritate it. By simply asking the body to do the treatment for us, we remove any sense of pressure on ourselves to get them better.

It is also better not just to under treat that area, but also to under treat in terms of not treating too many places on the body during any one appointment. When in severe pain, the patient suffers a depletion of energy. Battling against severe pain is exhausting for them as a person in addition to the pain itself. Consequently, the patient's whole body, not just the site of pain, has poor vitality and therefore is easily irritated. If the person in severe pain happens to be a family member, I would highly recommend you refer them to an experienced colleague, as we become even more anxious and keen to get family members better than people we know less well.

REFERENCES

DeRuiter, C., 2010. Somites: formation and role in developing the body plan. *The Embryo Project Encyclopedia.* Available from: https://embryo.asu.edu/pages/somites-formation-and-role-developing-body-plan.

Hughes, J.L., Newton, P.O., Bastrom, T., Fabricant, P.D., & Pennock, A.T., 2020. The clavicle continues to grow during adolescence and early adulthood. *HSS Journal.* 16 (Suppl 2): 372–377.

Hyland, S., Charlick, M., & Varacallo, M., 2022. Anatomy, shoulder and upper limb, clavicle. In: StatPearls [Internet]. Treasure Island, FL: StatPearls Publishing. Available from: https://www.ncbi.nlm.nih.gov/books/NBK525990/

Mooney, E., 2021. Lower limb embryology gross morphologic overview of lower limb development. *Medscape.* Available from: https://emedicine.medscape.com/article/1291712-overview.

Ogata, S., & Uhthoff, H.K., 1990. The early development and ossification of the human clavicle: an embryologic study. *Acta Orthopaedica Scandinavica.* 61(4): 330–334.

Orts-Llorca, F., 1981. La somitogenèse chez l'embryon humain: apparition des myotomes [Somitogenesis of the human embryo: appearance of myotomes]. *Bulletin de l'Association des Anatomistes.* 65(191): 467–482.

Pollack, G.H., 2013a. Comment on 'A Theory of Macromolecular Chemotaxis' and 'Phenomena Associated with Gel–Water Interfaces Analyses and Alternatives to the Long-Range Ordered Water Hypothesis'. *Journal of Physical Chemistry B.* 117(25): 7843–7846.

Pollack, G.H., 2013b. *The 4th Phase of Water.* Seattle USA: Ebner and Sons Publishers.

CHAPTER 9

An Inner Evaluation of the Abdomen and Pelvis

INTRODUCTION

In this chapter we will look at the organs of the abdomen and pelvis and how osteopathic treatment may help their functions. Much of the abdomen is associated with digestion and assimilation processes, but the kidneys, spleen and adrenals are also vital components of the abdomen. I include the liver as part of the digestive system, even though not part of the digestive tract, as it receives the absorbed digestive nutrients from the gut tube, providing the building blocks for its chemical requirements. However,

as we shall see, the liver also has metabolic relationships with the spleen.

The diaphragm muscle can be considered an abdominal tissue and also a thoracic tissue. However, I will be discussing it here rather than in Chapter 10. In the previous chapter, aspects of sacral function such as the functional sacrum, and the core link to the cranial base, were discussed. Consequently, I will not be discussing the sacrum here at length, except in the relationship of the sacrum to the pelvic floor and pelvic organs.

THE DIAPHRAGM

Brief anatomy and innervation

The dome of the diaphragm rises much higher into the thorax than one would imagine, well above the xiphoid during exhalation. However, I researched many websites whilst writing this chapter, and, curiously, I could not find any references to the vertical height of the dome of the diaphragm in the exhalation phase.

We must at this point remember when looking at cadavers in the dissection room, or anatomical images online or in books, that the cadaver is dead! This may seem a silly statement to make, but our involuntary mechanism recedes into extreme extension at death, therefore the positions of the tissues in the cadaver are in the

extreme extension phase and so appear taller and thinner than when alive. Hence the dome of the diaphragm in dissections and diagrams is anatomically higher in diagrams than in real life.

The dome of the diaphragm has its origins at the xiphoid process, the costal margin and ribs 7–12, whereas the crura have their origins at the bodies of L1–L3 and also at the anterior longitudinal ligament. The muscle fibres arise at their origins, then blend with the fibrous central tendon at the apex of the dome.

The innervation of the muscle in terms of its respiratory role is by the phrenic nerve, which originates in the cervical spine at nerve roots C3, C4 and C5. However, this is not the only innervation. Young and his team found that the diaphragm crura is also innervated by the vagus nerve, which inhibits the crura to allow the food bolus to enter the stomach when stimulated. In the conclusion of their paper it states:

> We conclude that vagal sensory and motor neurons functionally innervate the crural diaphragm (CD) and phrenoesophageal ligament. CD vagal afferents show mechanosensitivity to distortion of the gastroesophageal junction, while vagal motor neurons innervate both CD and distal oesophagus and may represent a common substrate for motor control of the reflux barrier. (Young *et al.* 2009)

It seems highly logical that the oesophageal opening into the stomach should be under vagal control at this important junction of the digestive tube. Having a key digestive role, it does seem strange that for many years and in some places, even now, the phrenic nerve is the only nerve considered to innervate the diaphragm muscle, along with the intercostal nerves adjacent to the diaphragm. For example, the website 'Teach me Anatomy' states:

> The halves of the diaphragm receive motor innervation from the phrenic nerve. The left half of the diaphragm is innervated by the left phrenic nerve, and vice versa. Each phrenic nerve is formed in the neck within the cervical plexus and contains fibres from spinal roots C3–C5. (Jones 2020)

I have added this quote to emphasise that the vagal innervation of the diaphragm is still not being commonly taught.

The main role of the diaphragm, as is well known, is changing the volume of the thoracic cavity to cause air to enter and force air out of the lungs, both of which are assisted by the intercostal muscles and secondary muscles of respiration.

However, there are less well acknowledged roles such as the stimulation by gentle compression to the abdominal organs lying immediately inferior to the muscle. We must not forget that the stomach, liver, transverse colon and spleen, plus the aorta, inferior vena cava (IVC) and cysterna chyli, all have direct abdominal relationships to the dome, and the kidneys, adrenals and pancreas, along with the aorta and IVC, have relationships to the crura of the diaphragm.

It is difficult to say exactly how much this gentle and relaxing action of the diaphragm has on the function these organs. My thoughts are that such an action will have a relaxing effect on the organs when their digestive work has finished and they are dormant, awaiting their next digestive workload to arrive. The regular massaging action may also help to negate excessive sympathetic tensions should the autonomic nervous system be out of balance, a common finding in our patients.

Embryology of the diaphragm

The diaphragm develops embryologically from differing regions. The muscle tissue and its central tendon are derived from the septum transversum, which arises cephalic to the pericardial cavity. The diaphragm also forms from the pleuroperitoneal folds along with the somites (Merrell and Kardon 2013).

With the shape changes of the embryo due to the foregut invagination, the septum transversum then finds itself lying between the heart and the liver at week four of intrauterine life. The septum transversum becomes the central tendon of the diaphragm, and further embryological development comes from the pleuroperitoneal folds and the somites.

The diaphragm separates the thorax from the abdomen and is functionally a midpoint between the cranial base and the sacral base. Perhaps this, combined with emotional factors affecting the muscle, makes it exceedingly rare (in my experience) to find a diaphragm in good condition. (I will discuss the emotional aspect of the diaphragm muscle in Chapter 16: The inner relationship of mind, body and emotions, so I will not elaborate on that here, other than to say that the diaphragm is a highly emotionally related structure.)

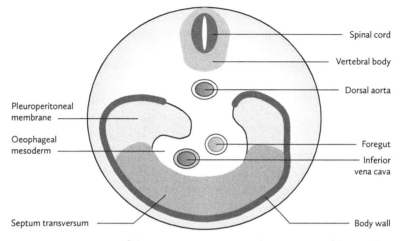

Figure 9.1 Superior view of the septum transversum, the precursor of the diaphragm.

Functionally the diaphragm tends to be strongly affected by cranial base patterns or sacral strains. For example, if there is a rotational pattern evident in the cranial base, then this tension seems to shift over the midline to the sacrum on the opposite side of the body. This then creates a torsion within the diaphragm. If the sacrum has compromising patterns being expressed compared with the cranial base, then it is the diaphragm which has to compensate between the two conflicting patterns. More physical tension within the physiology results in a reduced resistance to mental tension, causing emotional tensions within the body including the diaphragm.

Exercise on the diaphragm

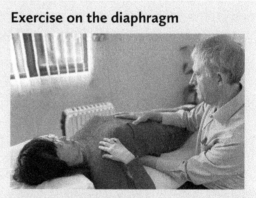

Figure 9.2 Palpating the diaphragm, which if necessary, is a good starting point to feeling the abdominal organs.

Centre yourself first, and match the tissue tensions with your elbow fulcrum, forearm muscle tone and your third hand.

https://youtu.be/h-tS_rsFTdo

THE GUT TUBE

The gut tube is approximately 9 metres (just 6 inches under 30 feet) in length from mouth to anus. It becomes quite surprising how most of that length fits into the abdomen and pelvis, while still giving space for the other organs. In this section we will look at the differing aspects of the gut tube and then have a practical exercise exploring the digestive tract.

The oesophagus

The oesophagus passes through the muscular right crus of the diaphragm, an elliptical sling. This opening, as has been mentioned above, has a separate innervation by the vagus nerve, which also controls the majority of the digestive tube to roughly two-thirds across the transverse colon (the exact point is somewhat variable). Having passed through the diaphragm, the oesophagus empties the food bolus into the stomach. (The main discussion of the oesophagus is in Chapter 10: The inner approach to the thorax.)

Stomach

The average size of the stomach is approximately 30 cm (12 inches) by 15 cm (6 inches) at the widest part. It is considered that the average (non-distended) stomach has a full volume of approximately 1 litre (1.75 UK pints/just over 2 US pints). The stomach is highly expandable and most papers written about the stomach do not mention maximum capacity. However, Wenzel *et al.* were doing research on the respiratory system and were looking to see the influence on the lungs of a stomach filled to total capacity: 'Respiratory system compliance was measured at pre-arrest, after return of spontaneous circulation, and after 2 and 4 litres of stomach inflation in the post-resuscitation phase; peak airway pressure was subsequently calculated.' (Wenzel *et al.* 1998).

Clearly Wenzel and his team were inflating the stomach to fill its maximum volume, as they were interested in the influence on the lungs, but it does give some indication that we wisely do not eat to our stomach's full capacity. When we feel full in our stomach, quite clearly from the above, this is not from the actual stretch of the stomach wall to true potential fullness. The sensation of feeling full is a vagal response to stretch receptors in the stomach wall. If, as happens with some people, the stomach wall becomes enlarged over a period of time, then the stretch receptors do not send the 'full' signals to the conscious mind until an even larger than normal volume has been reached, leading to over consumption and consequent weight gain.

The stomach is lined with a thick mucous lining, under which are the strong muscular fibres which move the food within the organ. The mucous lining is ridged to increase its surface area. The acidity of the stomach is very high, approximately pH 1–2. Clearly such acidity is highly protective against bacteria and viruses, with only the most resistant of them causing us health issues, should they be consumed on or in our food.

Compared with the time spent in the small intestine, food does not stay very long in the stomach. According to one paper, food stays in the stomach for approximately 40 minutes before passing through the pyloric sphincter (Shaikh 2021). During its time in the stomach, food is broken down and mixed with digestive enzymes. Carbohydrates are more easily and more quickly broken down than proteins, which is why a high 'carb' intake gives a faster energy rush compared with a 'heavier' high protein meal. When ready, food now in a liquid chyme state, enters the duodenum.

The duodenum

Most of the duodenum, along with the rest of the small intestine and large colon, is surrounded by the peritoneum, known as the mesentery. The mesentery is fixed firmly against the posterior abdominal wall, and the nerves and the blood vessels reach the digestive tract via the mesentery. The small intestine (jejunum and ileum) has its mesenteric attachment to the posterior wall in a diagonal arrangement from the superior end to the left side of the upper abdomen, to the inferior end lying to the right side of the lower abdomen.

The duodenum is approximately 25 cm (nearly 10 inches) long and is the widest part of the small intestine (duodenum, jejunum and ileum). The first part of the duodenum (that adjacent to the stomach) is within the peritoneal aspect of the abdomen, and then it moves behind the peritoneum to be firmly attached to the posterior abdominal wall. The initial section, like the stomach, has a strong mucosal lining, to insulate the wall from any stomach acids which may have passed through the pyloric sphincter, the muscular valve between the stomach and duodenum. Halfway down the descending aspect of the duodenum lies the sphincter of Oddi, a muscular ring which surrounds the papilla of Vater, also known as the major duodenal papilla. Some texts also refer to the minor duodenal papilla, a variation having a small opening into the duodenum just above the larger opening.

The ampulla of Vater opening into the left wall of the descending duodenum is for both the common bile duct and pancreatic duct. Bile is created by the liver and stored in concentrated form in the gall bladder, and is secreted into the bile duct to help the breakdown of fatty acids and aid digestion. The duct also secretes bicarbonate which is produced in the cells of the pancreatic ducts within the pancreas. This bicarbonate, being alkaline, helps to neutralise the stomach acid fluid and protect the duodenum, which at this point no longer has a protective mucous layer.

The pancreatic duct drains into the common bile duct to exit via the ampulla of Vater, but if present, it will drain into the minor duodenal papilla and not mix with the bile duct. The pancreas is a highly metabolic organ, with the exocrine cells producing digestive juices at a rate of approximately 1.5–2 litres per day (InformedHealth.org 2018). This is a phenomenal degree of activity for such a small organ and explains why it needs such a large blood supply (see section below on the pancreas).

These pancreatic digestive enzymes are synthesised within the exocrine acinar cells. The main enzyme types are amylase, lipase and trypsin. Amylases help to break down starch and convert large carbohydrate molecules into more easily metabolised simple sugars. Lipases help with the breakdown of fats. In this respect they are assisted by the bile which is secreted into the duodenum with the pancreatic enzymes. Trypsin assists with the breakdown of proteins. Protein breakdown commences in the stomach and continues in the small intestine. Trypsin is a proteolytic enzyme, formed as an inert enzyme trypsinogen, which becomes active in the duodenum.

The final part of the duodenum becomes narrower in its lumen as it becomes the jejunum.

The jejunum

This middle stage of the small intestine is approximately 2.5 metres long (just over 8 feet). It varies from its sister the ileum by having a very different internal structure. There are many folds within the internal surface of the jejunum wall, often described as a feathery because of its appearance on X-ray. These internal folds dramatically increase the surface area of the wall and also have a mechanical buffering effect which slows down the passage of the food chyme through the tube. Both the increased surface area and the mechanical slowing effect of the food chyme within the jejunum result in increased digestion efficiency. This results from an enhanced interaction between the digestive enzymes secreted and the food chyme passing along the jejunum.

The villi are found within the circular folds of the jejunum wall and are approximately 1 mm in length. These little hairs have the effect of increasing the absorption surface area of the gut wall. However, there are approximately 200 million of the miniscule microvilli per square millimetre of the small intestine wall. Although too small to even imagine, these have the effect of enhancing the surface area of the plasma membrane, which significantly enhances the food absorption process (Seladi-Schulman 2021).

200 million microvilli per square millimetre is a staggering number, especially if you multiply that by the length of the jejunum and also its circumference. To save your brain power, I have done the maths and that comes to 4,250,000,000,000,000 (4,250 trillion) microvilli along the jejunum wall! This incredible number demonstrates how important good digestion is for the physiology. During this journey along the jejunum, the wall along with the villi and microvilli are absorbing sugars, fatty acids and amino acids.

The ileum

This is the latter stage of the small intestine. It is about 3 metres long (just under 10 feet). Unlike its predecessor the jejunum, the ileum wall interior is smooth and not feathery. Functionally the ileum absorbs the remainder of the proteins, fats and sugars, and also importantly vitamin B12, as well as any bile acids which will then be recycled (Collins *et al.* 2022).

The large colon

The physiological function of the large colon is mainly the absorption of absorb water to prevent dehydration. It also absorbs electrolytes and vitamins, and synthesises some vitamins. It does these functions whilst at the same time moving faeces along the tube and into the rectum (Azzouz and Sharma 2022).

The ileocecal valve between the ilium and ascending colon is a powerful muscular valve which prevents backflow from the colon to the small intestine. 1.5 litres (just over 2.5 UK pints /3 US pints) pass through the ileocecal valve per day, much of this fluid being reabsorbed by the colon.

The appendix lies just inferior to the ileocecal valve on the wall of the ascending colon. It is associated with the immune system, though it could also serve as a storage site for healthy gut bio-flora. Although it is a poorly understood tissue for its role in the physiology, it is well known for the pain and inflammation it can cause, frequently leading to the need for surgical appendectomy.

The length of time food can reside in the large colon is perhaps much longer than you think, ranging from 4 to 72 hours, with an average of 36 hours (Science Learning Hub 2014). It is worth mentioning that when asking a patient if they have regular bowel movements, be specific – a patient of mine once said: 'Yes, I am very regular, I always go for a bowel motion, once every week.'

The large colon measures 1.5 metres in length, including the rectum, and about 5 cm (just under 2 inches) in diameter. The large colon includes the appendix and has sites where mechanical issues can cause disruption of good colon health. The hepatic and splenic flexures, where the colon takes right angle changes of direction, can often be places where gas that is produced may get stuck if mechanical issues occur in those regions. Likewise, the sigmoid colon, lying to the left side of the upper pelvis, has the shape of a side-lying 'S' and can be a site of mechanical disturbance. Disturbances to the pelvic mechanics, and as is quite common, having a functional sacrum energetically sitting on top the sigmoid colon, can result in bowel issues such as constipation.

The role of micro-organisms within the gut, especially the large colon, is now being acknowledged as significant in the health of the individual. In their paper in the *British Medical Journal*, Valdes and his team explored the role of the gut microbiota: 'Lower bacterial diversity has been reproducibly observed in people with inflammatory bowel disease, psoriatic arthritis, type 1 diabetes, atopic eczema, coeliac disease, obesity, type 2 diabetes, and arterial stiffness, than in healthy controls' (Valdes *et al.* 2018). This finding emphasises the need to have a good spectrum of 'friendly' gut bacteria from eating a healthy variety of foods. We all have patients who may have some of these conditions listed by Valdes, and if so, we should encourage them to ensure that they have a good and varied diet.

> Gut bacteria are an important component of the microbiota ecosystem in the human gut, which is colonised by 10^{14} microbes, ten times more than the human cells. Gut bacteria play an important role in human health, such as supplying essential nutrients, synthesizing vitamin K, aiding in the digestion of cellulose, and promoting angiogenesis and enteric nerve function. However, they can also be potentially harmful due to the change of their composition when the gut ecosystem undergoes abnormal changes in the light of the use of antibiotics, illness, stress, aging, bad dietary habits, and lifestyle. (Zhang *et al.* 2015)

It is worth pausing over the comment about 'stress' creating abnormal change in the gut eco-system. We will be discussing the gut more in its relationship to stress and anxiety in Chapter 16.

The gut nervous system – the enteric nervous system (ENS) – is a system of nerves, neurons and neurotransmitters which extends along the entire digestive tract from the oesophagus all the way to the anus. Its significance is highlighted in a paper by Rao and Gershon:

> The human ENS contains more than 100 million neurons, which dwarf the number of efferent fibres that reach the gut in the vagus nerves. The complexity of managing the behaviour of the bowel is sufficiently great that, in contrast to the remainder of the peripheral nervous system (PNS), evolution has endowed the ENS with the ability to manifest integrative neuronal activity (that is, uniting complex inputs into a coherent and purposeful behavioural output) and the ability to control gastrointestinal behaviour independently of input from brain or spinal cord... The gut–brain alliance has raised consciousness as a contributor to health, but a gut–brain axis that contributes to disease merits equal attention. (Rao and Gershon 2016)

Being able to operate without the brain within the gut wall, the enteric nervous system is now considered a second brain. Add to this the role of psychological interactions with the central nervous system and we see that the health of our gut tube is far more important than just being part of the nutritional system as previously considered.

The descending colon and the sigmoid colon have to be considered when thinking of the rectum. The movement of the colon contents can move with regular peristaltic motion like the small intestine, but also there can be bulk movements, known as high-amplitude propagated contractions. These high-amplitude propagated contractions start in the caecum and ascending colon, and the defecating process can begin as early as one hour prior to bowel motions occurring. During this time, the contractions become stronger up to the time of defecation (Bassotti 2021).

When food enters the stomach it causes stimulation, which as has just been described, can occur up to one hour before defecation occurs. These contractions are described as being like a toothpaste tube being squeezed at the opposite end from the nozzle. Unlike other mammals, humans have conscious control over bowel movements, enabling us to 'wait until the right time'. People with busy lives can put off this 'right time', leading to constipating habits.

The rectum

The rectum is the final aspect of the gut tube before the anus. It has two flexures in the anterior posterior plane, initially the sacral flexure which is concave anteriorly, then the anorectal flexure which is concave posteriorly. In addition, there are lateral flexures, three in total, which are folds of the internal wall of the rectum. These flexures allow for the rectum to be longer within a confined space.

The last part of the rectum is the ampulla. This is continuous with the anus and its function is to store faecal matter until the time is right. However, in constipated patients, the area of storage can back up much higher into the colon.

Anus

This is the final area around the anal ring. This is a powerful sphincter with two sets of muscles: the inner set is solely under autonomic control, and the outer, stronger ring is under conscious control. The purpose of the two muscular rings is twofold. The inner, unconscious ring keeps the resting tone of the sphincter at a safe level, so that nothing escapes until it is supposed to. The outer, conscious ring opens when the brain determines that it wants to evacuate the bowel. It is up to the individual to listen and choose to act on the signals saying: 'We need to empty the bowels.'

There is a ring of veins within the interior of the anal wall. These veins act as a soft cushion on the wall of the anus to soften the tension of the muscles. If a person has venous congestion for any reason, then these veins can become swollen and droop into the anal area, becoming haemorrhoids. In my experience, not many patients tell us that they have haemorrhoids, due to embarrassment, though I suspect quite a number do. Certainly, many patients do have pelvic congestion, some of which leads to venous congestion. I will discuss this more later in the chapter.

Exercise: Journey along the digestive tube

Please centre yourself before scanning the QR code/accessing the web link and match the tissue via your elbow fulcrum, forearm tone and your third hand.

https://youtu.be/iovXzF9-6pg

THE PANCREAS

The pancreas is a unique organ in that it secretes both exocrine and endocrine chemicals. The exocrine enzymes are secreted into the gut tube, whereas the endocrine hormones are secreted into the venous blood for distribution to the whole body.

The pancreas is 15 cm (6 inches) long and lies in a transverse position at the level of L1. It is retroperitoneal on the posterior abdominal wall and has a close relationship to the duodenum which surrounds the head of the pancreas. The head is also close to the right kidney and adrenal gland. As mentioned above, the pancreatic duct drains into the descending duodenum. The neck of the pancreas lies in front of the aorta, superior mesenteric artery and vein, and also lies directly in front of the portal vein. The body lies behind the stomach and in front of the left kidney, and the tail is against the spleen. The pancreas is innervated by the vagus nerve.

The pancreas has a rich blood supply, coming from the splenic artery, which runs in a tortuous fashion along the superior edge of the pancreas, and also has an anastomotic supply from both the anterior and posterior pancreaticoduodenal arteries. Any organ or aspect of the anatomy which has an anastomotic blood supply is clearly a highly important structure with a high metabolism (remember from Chapter 8 that blood is sucked by demand from the tissue to create the blood vessels, which then supply it).

The venous drainage of the pancreas, like that of the spleen, is the splenic vein and also the pancreaticoduodenal veins. These veins drain into the portal system, taking the venous blood to the liver (more on this later in the chapter).

Pancreatic hormones

I will only briefly discuss the endocrine secretions by the pancreas here, as the exocrine secretions draining into the pancreatic duct have been discussed above with the digestive system. The overview offered here may stimulate your appetite for further reading.

There are four main hormones synthesised within the pancreas: glucagon, insulin, pancreatic polypeptide and somatostatin.

Glucagon

A peptide hormone known as glucagon, is secreted by the pancreas in the alpha cells of the Islets of Langerhans. When the blood glucose levels drop to abnormal levels a state of hypoglycaemia develops. This is a powerful stimulant for the pancreas to secrete glucagon. The glucagon then stimulates glucose production by the liver to rebalance the blood sugar levels.

Glucagon in addition to glucose metabolism is involved in both amino acid and hepatic liquid metabolism. Glucagon also can have an effect of increasing resting energy levels of the body.

From the above description we can see that the peptide hormone glucagon should work as a metabolic partner to insulin in their combined role to maintain the correct blood sugar levels. So, it can be seen that pancreatic hormones have an effect on the liver and as such the pancreas secretions go into the duodenum and onto the portal system and thereby on to the liver.

Insulin

Following the breakdown of carbohydrates in the digestive tract, the processed sugars then enter the blood stream. In response to these raised glucose levels the pancreas secretes insulin, allowing that glucose to cross the cell walls, giving the cells access to the energy rich glucose.

Should blood sugar levels become excessive, then glucose is stored in the liver as glycogen, aided by insulin. When insulin levels drop, then glucose is released back into the blood. So, insulin is a powerful regulator of blood glucose levels. Chronic imbalance results in diabetes.

Pancreatic polypeptide

Pancreatic polypeptide is a complex digestive secretion containing 36 amino acids. The physiology secretes it when the body undergoes eating or fasting and also when exercising. Its action can inhibit the secretion of bile by the gall bladder and also inhibit pancreatic exocrine secretions. However, the action of pancreatic polypeptide in the digestive process is still not fully understood (Britannica.com 2019).

Interestingly, although pancreatic polypeptide is secreted by the pancreas, it is now being considered a factor in brain function and our behaviour, in addition to the function of the digestive system. Both anorexia and obesity are now also being linked to its physiological actions as it affects our appetite and body weight. Some consider it to be linked to types of cancer and diabetes (Yazdi 2021).

This is a hormone which affects a variety of functions. One of the most important is sending signals via the vagus nerve back to the brain, sending signals giving a sense of hunger or fullness. It can cause a feeling of fullness by reducing appetite in the brain, and in the digestive system it slows down the peristaltic movements, reducing the rate of flow of chyme through the digestive tube. Pancreatic polypeptide also has a relaxing effect on the gall bladder, stopping its ejection of bile and thus slowing down the digestion of fats. In addition, it reduces the secretion of digestive enzymes and pancreatic bicarbonate.

Pancreatic polypeptide is a very important substance regulating our desire to eat or not, and adjusting the efficiency of our digestion or not, depending on the physiological need at the time.

Somatostatin (growth hormone inhibiting hormone)

The functions of somatostatin are widespread, affecting the whole physiology, being secreted in a number of other locations in addition to the pancreas such as the hypothalamus and central nervous system. The physiological action of somatostatin reduces the secretions of the pancreas, both exocrine and endocrine, and also reduces pituitary secretions. In the central nervous system, somatostatin affects neurotransmission and our memory processes. Another effect of somatostatin is to reduce the development of new blood vessels, and it is considered to have an inhibiting effect on the growth of cancer cells (O'Toole and Sharma 2022).

Exercise on the pancreas

Please centre yourself before scanning the QR code/accessing the web link. Even though the pancreas is delicate and glandular, you will still need to match the pancreas, although very gently.

https://youtu.be/LD9Umq_Vl2l

THE SPLEEN

Anatomy

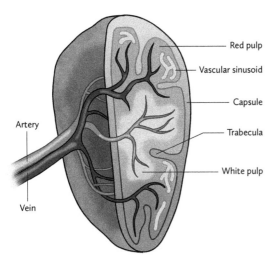

Figure 9.3 The internal structure of the spleen.

The spleen is a relatively small organ, lying within the peritoneum. However, it has vital functions for the blood physiology. Anatomically it lies between the 9th and 11th ribs, on the left side of the abdomen just underneath the diaphragm. It is adjacent to the stomach, pancreas and left kidney/adrenal gland. Considering its very important role for the blood, it is interesting that it lies just under the heart, only being separated by the thin diaphragm muscle and tendon.

The ventral surface of the spleen is indented by the stomach (the gastric surface) and a smaller area by the kidney, and possibly the adrenal gland, this latter indentation being the renal surface. At the very base of the ventral surface is a small, flattened area which lies up against the pancreas.

The spleen starts developing in the 15th week of intrauterine life (IUL), whereas the pancreas and the adrenals start developing much earlier, at the fifth week IUL. This would explain why although the pancreas and adrenals are much more delicate organs than the spleen, they still create a moulding of the adjacent (just forming) spleen. It is because the adrenals and pancreas form before the spleen exists that they are able to make an indentation into the spleen whilst it is in its early, highly delicate state. The kidneys and stomach both form during the fourth week IUL so again, the developing spleen has to fit in around these structures.

The spleen is an important aspect of the immune system, along with the thymus gland, which are the only two organs of the body to receive efferent lymph vessels. All the other lymph vessels only supply lymph back towards the heart via the subclavian veins.

Physiology

The basic function of the spleen is being a massive blood filter, to remove aged blood cells, and also a powerful organ of the immune system. The internal structure of the spleen comprises the white and red pulp. These colour differences indicate very different functions. The white pulp is made up of lymph tissue surrounding an arteriole. It mainly contains white blood cells. The inner area of the white pulp contains B cell lymphocytes, whereas the outer white pulp and the surrounding marginal zone contain the T cell lymphocytes. By contrast, the red pulp is composed of splenic cords and a significant volume of venous sinuses, which give it the red colour. The cords which are splenic cells supported by reticular connective tissue have two functions. According to Kapila and his team, the function of these cords are as follows:

The splenic cords provide the organ structure through reticulin and fibrils. The cords also contain a reservoir of monocytes to aid in wound healing. Splenic cords lead to splenic sinuses where macrophages respond to antigens and filter abnormal or aging erythrocytes out of blood flow. (Kapila *et al.* 2022)

The structure of the spleen makes it effectively a giant lymph node, being the largest part of the mononuclear phagocyte system (previously called the reticuloendothelial system). Monocytes, which are the largest of the leukocytes, have only a very short life span with the majority surviving only around 24 hours (Monie 2017). In contrast to monocytes, macrophages have a far longer life span which ranges from several months to even years (Van Furth and Cohm 1968).

Therefore, in addition to its important role for the immune system, the spleen enables macrophages to digest ageing erythrocytes, leukocytes and megakaryocytes when their functional life comes to a conclusion. The phagocytes within the spleen also play an important function in defending against micro-organisms such as mycobacteria, fungi, bacteria, protozoa and viruses, thus keeping the blood healthy, and where possible, stopping the spread of such organisms around the body. The venous blood from the spleen is sent via the portal vein (see more below) to the liver, so that the liver can recycle the iron from the digested and aged red blood cells.

In terms of its blood storage capacity, the spleen is a substantial organ. It keeps the blood in storage, being ready to release it when there is an occurrence of severe blood loss. In order to do this, between a quarter and a third of the body's erythrocytes are stored within the spleen, along with about a quarter of the body's platelet cells (Kapila *et al.* 2022). This is a very high volume of red blood cell and platelet storage for such a small organ. However, in circumstances when a severe injury with much blood loss occurs, the physiology does need an efficient blood cell reserve 'tank'.

Despite the significant role of the spleen to the blood health, the physiology can manage to function if the organ is removed. This may be a result of severe injury or from surgical splenectomy if serious pathology to the spleen is present. In such cases, the spleen's physiological roles are then undertaken by the liver.

Exercise on the spleen

Centre yourself first and remember to match the spleen tissue quality with your elbow fulcrum, forearm tone and third hand.

https://youtu.be/M6hTu3hkScA

THE HEPATIC PORTAL VEIN

The hepatic portal vein (more generally called the portal vein) is significant in terms of its anatomical size, and incredibly significant in terms of its physiology. The portal vein and its tributaries receive all the blood from the superior mesenteric, splenic, inferior mesenteric, left and right gastric, and the pancreatic veins. In other words, it receives the blood returning from the whole abdominal digestive tube (but not the pelvic aspect), plus the spleen and pancreas. It is about 7 cm (2.75 inches) long and it divides at its hepatic end into two veins, one for each lobe of the liver. As has been seen in the section on the spleen, the splenic venous blood is also taken to the liver in addition to the digested food from the gut, because the breakdown of blood is a role of both the liver and spleen.

THE LIVER

After the skin, the liver is the largest organ in the body. It lies in a highly protected position, underneath the rib cage, indicating its vital importance to the body. With its role as a phenomenal biochemical factory, it is no wonder that it receives all the blood coming from the digestive tract. It is considered to have over 500 physiological actions (Newman 2022).

There are two lobes of the liver (left and right) but these are comprised of very many small lobules, the working components. The liver contains an amazing number of individual lobules: 100,000. Each of these hexagonal shaped, individual lobules includes a central vein along with a hepatic portal vein located at each corner. A so-called portal triad is thereby formed by each of the portal veins running run alongside a hepatic artery and a bile duct (Van Grunsven 2017).

The success of liver transplant surgery is increasing in terms of longevity of the recipient. The UK National Health Service (NHS) claims that most people live for 10 years, with many living for 20 years or more following liver replacement (NHS 2021). Should you have a patient due to undergo a transplant, do advise them that it is a successful procedure. Hopefully such patients changed their lifestyle following the diagnosis, if toxication was the aetiology.

The liver is unique in the physiology because it is the only organ capable of self-regeneration after damage. This can happen following partial removal of the organ but also following damage from toxicity such as alcohol or ingestion of toxic substances. Oertel and Shafritz outline the mechanism by which this can happen:

> Hepatocytes constitute the first cell population to enter the cell cycle, followed by the biliary epithelial cells and then nonparenchymal cells. Serial transplantation studies have demonstrated an almost inexhaustible self-renewal capacity of hepatocytes, with calculations suggesting that a single hepatocyte is competent to give rise to many entire livers. (Oertel and Shafritz 2008)

The suggestion that just one hepatocyte can produce many entire livers is quite astounding. Not only does this show the amazing regenerative ability of the liver, but also that self-regeneration of the liver is a vital task, indicative of its physiological importance. The number of people worldwide who die of alcohol consumption is staggeringly high. Clearly it would be very much higher if it were not for this amazing ability of the liver to repair itself from the effects of toxic substances.

In 2016, alcohol use was ranked as the seventh leading risk factor for premature death and disability worldwide, and was the leading cause of death for people aged 15–49 years old (GBD 2016 Alcohol Collaborators 2018). According to the same study, globally, one in three people drink alcohol (equivalent to 2.4 billion people), and 2.2 per cent of women and 6.8 per cent of men die from alcohol-related health problems each year. These figures equate to 9 per cent of the world population dying from alcohol-related health problems per year.

In the UK, 8,974 deaths related to alcohol-specific causes were registered in the UK in 2020, equivalent to 14 deaths per 100,000 people (Office for National Statistics 2021). In the USA, it is estimated that 95,000 people (around 68,000 men and 27,000 women) die from alcohol-related causes annually, making alcohol the third-leading preventable cause of death (Centers for Disease Control and Prevention 2019). This equates to approximately 30 deaths per 100,000 population.

Clearly these figures for both the UK and the USA are significant and concerning. Many accidental deaths are caused by excess alcohol consumption. I am not intending to be authoritarian, nor am I against enjoying a drink, but clearly if we choose to drink alcohol, we should do so with respect and wisdom.

The functions of the liver

These are numerous (over 500 as quoted above), and highly significant for the health and wellbeing of the whole physiology. These comprise the synthesis, breakdown and storage of physiological chemicals, outlined as follows.

Synthesis

As mentioned in the section on the duodenum, bile assists in the digestion of fatty foods, acting as a surfactant and allowing the digestive enzymes to penetrate the fat molecules more easily. Some of the bile is then stored in the gall bladder in a concentrated form and the remainder is carried by the hepatic duct to the common bile duct and hence to the duodenum. In addition to bile, the liver has a role in the formation of some of the **blood plasma** proteins, the main protein being albumen.

The liver is also a synthesiser of cholesterol. The body produces cholesterol to assist the carriage of fats in the blood around the body. Harvard Medical School describes its role as follows:

> Since cholesterol is a fat, it can't travel alone in the bloodstream. It would end up as useless globs (imagine bacon fat floating in a pot of water). To get around this problem, the body packages cholesterol and other lipids into minuscule protein-covered particles that mix easily with blood. These tiny particles, called lipoproteins (lipid plus protein), move

cholesterol and other fats throughout the body. (Harvard Health Publishing 2017)

Briefly there are two types of cholesterol: good and bad. At excessive levels, bad cholesterol (low density lipoprotein (LDL)) increases the risk of heart disease by depositing on the blood vessels, resulting in atherosclerosis. Conversely, good cholesterol (high density lipoprotein (HDL)) reduces the risk of heart disease by absorbing the cholesterol and transporting it back to the liver, where the liver then breaks it down and removes it.

Foods which increase levels of HDL in the body are olive oil, whole grains, beans and legumes, high fibre fruit, fatty fish (salmon, mackerel, tuna, sardines and rainbow trout), flax, nuts, chia seeds, avocado and soy (Holland 2021). So do suggest to your high-risk patients that they increase these foods in their diet.

Storage

As has been already mentioned in the section on the pancreas, the liver converts glucose into glycogen as a safe form for storage until required. When the body undergoes a demand for energy, the liver reforms the glycogen back into glucose. The liver also synthesises proteins which it releases into the blood for usage as a building block by various other organs and tissues.

The liver is the 'graveyard' for haemoglobin molecules. As we saw when discussing the spleen, haemoglobin molecules have a relatively short lifespan and so need to be broken down when their efficiency for oxygen carriage within the blood reduces. The liver, when breaking down the haemoglobin molecules, stores the iron in readiness for use in the synthesis of replacement haemoglobin.

Breakdown

The liver has an important role in protein breakdown. One of the by-products of that process is ammonia, which is highly toxic to the body. The liver converts the ammonia into urea, a safe chemical to the body, before excreting it in the urine.

The liver has a significant role in clearing the blood of excess drugs and poisonous substances. Such chemicals may be food which has become toxic and should no longer be eaten, alcohol, substances classified as illegal drugs, or even medically prescribed medications which give the patient side effects in addition to their intended benefit(s).

The liver is highly involved in the regulation of our blood and its ability to clot when there is a breakage of a blood vessel. Clotting is caused by coagulation factors which the liver produces. Vitamin K is one of the important constituents of some of these coagulation factors. Vitamin K is absorbed as a fat-soluble substance, so the role of bile to help break down fats helps the release of vitamin K for the synthesis of coagulation factors.

The liver has a vital role in the immune system. As has been described, all the venous blood from the digestive tract is carried by the portal vein to the liver. Food is not always washed nor cooked to the degree where all bacteria and microbes have been destroyed; the liver is the first part of the physiology to deal with such a situation and reduce the risk of infection.

Anybody who has had a young child in their care may have witnessed the child putting something in their mouth, which you would certainly not do, and then eat it. It is amazing how frequently this happens, but the child has no or only mild symptoms. This demonstrates how the acidity of the stomach and then the immunity role of the liver can help the physiology.

The liver not only breaks down haemoglobin molecules from the blood, but also clears away the bilirubin from the red blood cells. Should this process not occur properly, a jaundiced appearance may result in the eyes and skin of the body.

Exercise on palpating and treating the liver

Please ensure you centre yourself and match the liver tone with your elbow fulcrum, forearm tone and third hand before scanning the QR code/accessing the web link.

https://youtu.be/qGG49EIIXAc

THE KIDNEYS

These bean shaped organs lie retroperitoneally, in a close relationship, being just lateral to the vertebral bodies of L1–L3, though the right is slightly more inferior due to the embryological influence of the large liver. The left kidney is in close relationship to the aorta, and the right kidney to the inferior vena cava on the posterior abdominal wall. The organs lie directly in front of the respective psoas major muscles with the left close to the pancreas and the right close to the liver. The adrenal (suprarenal) glands sit on top of each kidney.

Each kidney is covered in a fibrous renal capsule. This is a thin covering, yet it is extremely strong, containing many collagen and elastin fibres. These are highly protective for these vital organs and reduce the risk of damage. As osteopaths we can at times detect tensions within these renal capsules and if present, reduce such mechanical forces. There is an exercise demonstrating this at the end of this section.

Internally, the kidney is composed of pyramids with their apices directed towards the renal pelvis, where the urine aggregates before passing into the ureters. The renal arteries each transport a phenomenal volume of blood to the kidneys. Consequently, the renal veins need to deliver this filtered blood back to the inferior vena cava, which lies adjacent to the right kidney and a short journey in front of the aorta for the left kidney. The pyramids contain the working units of the kidney, the arterioles, venules, Bowman's capsule and the nephrons.

The arterioles are wrapped and squeezed around themselves like a small ball within the cup of the Bowman's capsule. This is the filtering unit, and the filtrate passes into the adjacent loop of Henle (LOH) and then to the proximal and distal convoluted tubules. Surrounding the LOH and convoluted tubules are anastomoses of efferent blood vessels having left the Bowman's capsules. The anastomoses, called the vasa recta, deliver oxygen and nutrients to these functioning aspects of the kidney, and remove water and solutes to prevent excess water loss. They also reabsorb the blood essential nutrients, that may have passed into the nephron tubes.

In brief, the roles of the kidneys are to:

- Excrete waste products which were in solution within the blood.
- Maintain the correct acid/alkaline balance of the blood – this being required as many of the body metabolic processes create acidity.

- Maintain the body water levels and also those of minerals such as sodium, calcium, phosphorus and potassium. Consequently, maintaining these mineral levels helps the nervous system and muscles. In addition, calcium helps maintain good bone physiology.
- Produce and eliminate hormones.

In their book *Hormones and the Kidney*, Park and Hirschberg outline the hormonal relationship of the kidney as follows:

> As producers of hormones the kidneys are an endocrine organ. Hormones that are produced in the kidneys include 1,25-dihydroxyvitamin D3, renin and angiotensin, and erythropoietin. The kidney also contributes to the circulating pool of growth factors such as insulin-like growth factor-1 (IGF-1). Moreover, the kidneys participate in the regulation of hormonal action by eliminating hormones from the circulation, primarily polypeptide hormones. Renal elimination contributes significantly to the degradation of many peptide hormones and, to a lesser extent, catecholamines and some steroid hormones. (Park and Hirschberg 2011)

The vital importance of kidney function is expressed by the volume of blood passing through the renal and accessory renal arteries. According to Knipe and El-Feky, the accessory renal arteries, though not always present, are very common, and are found in around 25 per cent of people, being bilateral in around 10 per cent of the population.

Triple and quadruple renal arteries are present in around 2.5 per cent and less than 1 per cent of the population, respectively (Knipe *et al.* 2022).

The blood volume passing through the kidneys is quite phenomenal. As described in *Vander's Renal Physiology*, renal blood flow is around 1 litre per minute, which represents 20 per cent of the resting cardiac output through tissue that constitutes less than 0.5 per cent of the body mass. Considering that the volume of each kidney is less than 150 millilitres, this means that each kidney is perfused with over three times its total volume every minute (Eaton and Pooler 2013). This staggering volume of renal arterial supply equates to all the blood in the body passing though the kidneys 40 times per day (Hoffman 2021). Clearly great effort is made to keep the blood well filtered by the kidneys.

Having given an overview of kidney anatomy, let us get to the treatment table for an exercise on the renal capsule and kidney.

Exercise on the kidney and kidney capsule
Do be well centred and match the kidney and also the kidney capsule when working in this exercise.

https://youtu.be/UYkybxih7ao

ADRENAL GLANDS

These small glands sitting on the superior aspect of the kidneys have a dual function. The outer cortex is the hormone-secreting aspect of the organ, and the inner medulla is a ganglion for the sympathetic nervous system. The cortex produces four main hormone types: mineralocorticoids, glucocorticoids, corticosterone and adrenal androgens.

Mineralocorticoids

The most important mineralocorticoid is aldosterone. This hormone is associated with controlling the body salt and water levels; consequently, it has a strong regulatory influence on the blood pressure. If the aldosterone levels become reduced, the kidneys lose an excessive volume of fluid, and there is a serious consequence to the body of dehydration.

Glucocorticoids (cortisol)

Cortisol is involved with many physiological functions (and named hydrocortisone when used as a medicine). The body has glucocorticoid receptors throughout the physiology and consequently the hormone affects most if not all tissues. These include the nervous system, the immune response, the circulation and cardiovascular system, the respiratory system, the reproductive system, the musculoskeletal system, and the skin with superficial fascia. Although the digestive system is not included in this list, it too will be affected by the nerve supply and the circulatory aspects.

The glucocorticoids have a number of actions in the immune system. For example, they produce apoptosis of proinflammatory T cells, suppress B cell antibody production and reduce neutrophil migration during inflammation (Thau *et al.* 2022).

The stress response is an action of the physiology which we see very commonly in our patients. We will look at this in greater detail in Chapter 16, but as an overview, let us consider the relationship between stress and cortisol. The physiology is continually being bombarded by external stimuli, some of which the psychophysiology rightly or wrongly interprets as a threat. This perceived danger stimulates the sympathetic nervous system, resulting in a multitude of hormonal and physiological reactions known as the fight or flight response.

Within the brain, it is the region of the amygdala which coordinates the psychological response to the real or perceived fears and threats. Where appropriate, the amygdala, which is the part of the brain associated with fear, then signals the hypothalamus to stimulate the sympathetic nervous system, reducing the blood flow to the less urgent tissues and increasing the flow to the aspects of the body which will be needed to get the body away from the fearful threat. The sympathetic system stimulates the adrenal glands to produce epinephrine which consequently increases the heart and breath rates.

If the real or perceived threat persists, then the adrenals are stimulated to produce cortisol, which keeps the physiology in a state of hyper alertness. A state of hyper alertness may be very necessary, for example to avoid a car accident when you see a vehicle coming towards you. However, where the threat is perceived rather than real, these sympathetic and high alert responses are not lifesaving but create a negative physiological imbalance. As osteopaths we certainly see patients where the musculoskeletal system is hypertonic due to the consequences of raised cortisol as the hormone is powerfully involved with the stress response.

Corticosterone

This hormone is not so much involved in the stress response in humans as in other mammals, but its main role is that of a precursor for the mineralocorticoid aldosterone, the regulator of body fluid levels.

Adrenal androgens (dehydroepiandrosterone (DHEA) and testosterone)

These are fairly weak male hormones which have an influence on male sex organ development during puberty, and also girls during puberty as they are involved in maintaining the sexual differences between men and women. The pituitary gland regulates the adrenal gland secretion via ACTH (adrenocorticotropic hormone) from the anterior pituitary.

The medulla of the adrenal gland contains chromaffin cells that secrete catecholamines, including epinephrine (adrenalin) and norepinephrine (noradrenalin), along with dopamine. These are all produced subsequent to sympathetic preganglionic stimulus. These hormones produce the stress responses of increasing the heart rate and blood pressure, constricting the blood vessels and gut tube, and raising the metabolism ready for the fight or flight activity.

THE PELVIS

The sacrum has already been covered in the spine section of Chapter 8, and the rectum and anus earlier in this chapter, so I shall not repeat those aspects of the pelvic anatomy here. In this section, I will be focussing on the pelvic diaphragm (floor), uterus and bladder.

The pelvic diaphragm/pelvic floor

This important sheet of muscles links the pubis to the coccyx, along with linking the two lateral aspects of the pelvis. It supports the bladder and the base of the uterus (in females) and the prostate in males. It also includes the anal ring, which has been discussed earlier in the chapter. In brief the pelvic muscles involved are: the pubococcygeus, puborectalis and iliococcygeus.

Anteriorly the pelvic diaphragm is attached to the posterior aspect of the pubis. Laterally it is attached to the tendinous arch of levator ani, and to the ischial spine. Posteriorly the diaphragm is attached to the inferior aspect of the sacrum and coccyx. In the midline the pelvic diaphragm forms a levator raphe.

Function

In addition to its supportive roles to the bladder and uterus, and the sphincter role around the anus, the pelvic diaphragm should play a role in relating to the body's other transverse diaphragms: the diaphragma sellae (above the pituitary gland), the tentorium cerebelli, the suprapleural membrane and the respiratory diaphragm. These transverse diaphragms help to move fluids. The pelvic diaphragm should play an important role in the return of venous blood and lymph through the pelvis and to the abdomen and back to the heart. Unfortunately, the pelvic floor muscles are frequently not in a healthy tone.

When the pelvic floor muscles are too tight or have an insufficient tone, they do not allow the natural diaphragmatic motion to occur. This can be a factor in the development of venous congestion. The venous congestion can be expressed within the pelvis or it can also be expressed as venous stasis in the lower extremities and varicosities. Where no varicosities or swelling of the ankles is expressed, there can still be hidden pelvic venous congestion around the bladder, uterus/prostate, and rectum. These structures have many veins surrounding them and when congested they become tortuous, and are visually expressed in various veins of the lower limb. Such pelvic venous congestion will have a detrimental physiological effect on the respective organ involved. If a patient's pelvis ever feels 'boggy', consider the presence of pelvic venous congestion and internal varicosities being present.

Uterus and ovaries

These lie posteriorly to the bladder in front of the rectum, the ovaries being lateral to the uterus, and the uterus curving slightly anterior to also be over the top of the bladder. If the uterus is prolapsed it can produce excessive pressure on the bladder and reduce the bladder capacity. From an osteopathic perspective the uterus and ovaries are supported by ligaments.

Uterine ligaments

- Broad ligament: this is a sheet of the peritoneum which drapes over the uterus, fallopian tube and ovaries. It is continuous with the fasciae of the lateral aspects of the pelvis.

- Round ligament: this starts at the junction of the fallopian tube with the upper body of the uterus and passes to the labia majora around the vaginal opening and inguinal canal.
- Cardinal ligaments: these pass from the cervix to the lateral wall of the pelvis.
- Pubocervical ligaments: these bilateral ligaments link the cervix to the posterior aspect of the pubic bones.
- Uterosacral ligaments (recto-uterine ligaments or sacro-cervical ligaments): these run between the cervix and the sacrum.

Ovarian ligaments

The broad ligament supports the ovary and fallopian tube. In addition, the ovary is also supported by:

- The ovarian ligaments: these connect the inferior aspect of the ovary to the side wall of the uterus.
- Ovary suspensory ligaments: these link the ovary to the lateral wall of the uterus. It is questionable as to whether they are separate ligaments or simply an aspect of the broad ligament.

Clinical consequences

Many women get pain in the pelvis prior to the onset of their menstrual cycle. Many have already been to the appropriate medical practitioner, only to be told that there is nothing wrong, and that it's just one of those things that some women have to accept (or something similar).

In the few days before menstruation, the uterus is at its largest volume and hence most heavy. This will therefore be the time when the tension on the uterine ligaments is at its greatest. The fascial thickenings or ligaments,

as with ligaments in other parts of the body, will be tender when over stretched. In these circumstances, if such women have mechanical strains and tensions in the pelvic bowl, then the pelvic ligaments around the uterus and ovaries will already be tense. Therefore, when the ligaments are under a second level of tension pre-period, it then results in symptoms. Many women have said, after mechanical tensions in the pelvis had been treated whilst helping a spinal condition, that their pre-period pains have gone away.

The bladder

The bladder is a muscular container to hold urine. It comprises a specialised muscle, the detrusor, and a urothelial lining. The muscle is smooth muscle with the fibres laid down in a spiral fashion, allowing contraction of the whole bladder wall at the same time. Its volume is estimated to be around 500–600 millilitres (0.88–1.0 UK pints/1.05–1.27 US pints). Under extreme circumstances the bladder can stretch beyond this, but a wise person empties their bladder regularly!

Bladder supporting ligaments

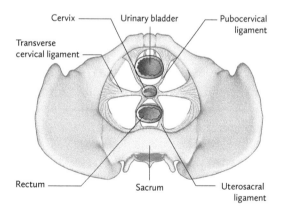

Figure 9.4 The female pelvis showing the bladder ligaments.

- The lateral ligaments pass from the inferior aspect of the bladder to the lateral pelvic wall fasciae.
- Puboprostatic ligaments comprise two

each side, and they run from the bladder to the prostate, stabilising the neck of the bladder.

- Lateral puboprostatic ligaments run from the tendinous fascial arch of the pelvis to the superior aspect of the prostatic sheath.
- Medial puboprostatic ligaments lie between the posterior aspect of the pubic bone to the prostatic sheath. In the female the puboprostatic ligaments are replaced by similar pubovesical ligaments.
- The median umbilical ligament runs between the apex of the bladder to the umbilicus.
- The posterior ligament of the bladder lies between the inferior aspect of the bladder and the lateral wall of the pelvis as a loose sheet of fatty tissue.

Clinically, as has been discussed with respect to the uterus, if there are mechanical tensions within the pelvis, these can create tension on the ligaments supporting the bladder and produce symptoms. As with both bladder and uterine symptoms, we should be mindful not to promise results which we cannot deliver. However, to explain that osteopathy *may* ease ligament tensions supporting the organs is a true statement and therefore an ethical comment. Do ensure that the patient also follows a path of medical investigation where appropriate.

The testes

The male testes are the two hormone and sperm producing organs within the testicular sac. The sperm is sent for ejaculation via the vas deferens to the male penis when appropriate. The hormonal aspect, the function of testosterone, is discussed in Chapter 13: Working with the hormonal system. It is highly professionally unwise to work on these organs, and if there any

possible concerns from you or the patient, refer the patient to their medical practitioner.

Exercise on the pelvis

Figure 9.5 When palpating the pelvic floor, think of the organs as well as the mechanical influences to the spine, sacrum and coccyx.

https://youtu.be/AdhX6bWEouw

REFERENCES

Azzouz, L.L., & Sharma, S., 2022. Physiology, large intestine. In: StatPearls [Internet]. Treasure Island, FL: StatPearls Publishing. Available from: https://www.ncbi.nlm.nih.gov/books/NBK507857/

Bassotti, G., 2021. 1907–2020: more than one century of colonic mass movements in humans. *American Journal of Physiology*. 320(1): G117–G124. Available from: https://doi.org/10.1152/ajpgi.00375.2020.

Britannica.com, 2019. Pancreatic polypeptide. Encyclopaedia Britannica. Available from: https://www.britannica.com/science/pancreatic-polypeptide.

Centers for Disease Control and Prevention, 2019. Alcohol Related Disease Impact (ARDI) Application. Available from: https://nccd.cdc.gov/DPH_ARDI/Default/Default.aspx.

Collins, J., Nguyen, A., & Badireddy, M., 2022. Anatomy, abdomen and pelvis, small intestine. In: StatPearls [Internet]. Treasure Island, FL: StatPearls Publishing.

Available from: https://www.ncbi.nlm.nih.gov/books/NBK459366/

Eaton, D., & Pooler, J., 2013. *Vander's Renal Physiology*. 8th edition. The McGraw-Hill Companies, Inc. Available from: https://accessmedicine.mhmedical.com/content.aspx?bookid=2173§ionid=163663126#1143895696.

GBD 2016 Alcohol Collaborators, 2018. Alcohol use and burden for 195 countries and territories, 1990–2016: a systematic analysis for the Global Burden of Disease Study. *The Lancet*. 392(10152): 1015–1035. Available from: https://www.sciencedirect.com/science/article/pii/S0140673618313102#fn1.

Harvard Health Publishing, 2017. How it's made: cholesterol production in your body. *Harvard Medical School.* Available from: https://www.health.harvard.edu/heart-health/how-its-made-cholesterol-production-in-your-body.

Hoffman, M., 2021. Picture of the kidneys. WebMD. Available from: https://www.webmd.com/kidney-stones/picture-of-the-kidneys.

Holland, K., 2021. Foods to increase your HDL. Healthline. Available from: https://www.healthline.com/health/high-cholesterol/foods-to-increase-hdl.

InformedHealth.org, 2018. 2006. How does the pancreas work? Cologne, Germany: Institute for Quality and Efficiency in Health Care (IQWiG). Available from: https://www.ncbi.nlm.nih.gov/books/NBK279306/

Jones, O., 2020. The diaphragm. Teach me Anatomy. Available from: https://teachmeanatomy.info/thorax/muscles/diaphragm/

Kapila, V., Wehrle, C.J., & Tuma, F., 2022. Physiology, spleen. In: StatPearls [Internet]. Treasure Island, FL: StatPearls Publishing. Available from: https://www.ncbi.nlm.nih.gov/books/NBK537307/

Knipe, H., Hacking, C., El-Feky, M., *et al.*, 2022. Accessory renal artery. Radiopaedia.org. Available from: https://doi.org/10.53347/rID-25835.

Merrell, A. J., & Kardon, G., 2013. Development of the diaphragm: a skeletal muscle essential for mammalian respiration. *The Febs Journal*. 280(17): 4026–4035. Available from: https://doi.org/10.1111/febs.12274.

Monie, T.P., 2017. Monocytes. Available from: https://www.sciencedirect.com/topics/neuroscience/monocyte#:~:text=The%20life%20span%20of%20a,they%20subsequently%20mature%20into%20macrophages.

Newman, T., 2022. What does the liver do? Medical News Today. Available from: https://www.medicalnewstoday.com/articles/305075.

NHS, 2021. Overview: liver transplant. Available from: https://www.nhs.uk/conditions/liver-transplant/

Oertel, M., & Shafritz, D.A., 2008. Stem cells, cell transplantation and liver repopulation. *Biochimica et Biophysica Acta*. 1782(2): 61–74. Available from: https://doi.org/10.1016/j.bbadis.2007.12.004

Office for National Statistics, 2021. Alcohol-specific deaths in the UK: registered in 2020. Available from: https://www.ons.gov.uk/peoplepopulationandcommunity/healthandsocialcare/causesofdeath/bulletins/alcoholrelateddeathsintheunitedkingdom/registeredin2020#:~:text=There%20.

O'Toole, T.J., & Sharma, S., 2022. Physiology, somatostatin.

In: StatPearls [Internet]. Treasure Island, FL: StatPearls Publishing. Available from: https://www.ncbi.nlm.nih.gov/books/NBK538327/

Park, J., & Hirschberg, R., 2011. *Hormones and the Kidney*. Oxford Academic. Available from: https://oxfordmedicine.com/view/10.1093/med/9780199235292.001.1/med-9780199235292-chapter-100201#:~:text=Hormones%20that%20are%20produced%20in,1%20(IGF%2D1).

Rao, M., & Gershon, M.D., 2016. The bowel and beyond: the enteric nervous system in neurological disorders. *Nature Reviews Gastroenterology & Hepatology*. 13(9): 517–528. Available from: https://doi.org/10.1038/nrgastro.2016.107.

Rix, I., Nexøe-Larsen, C., Bergmann, N.C., *et al.*, 2019. Glucagon physiology. In: Feingold, K.R., Anawalt, B., Boyce, A., *et al.*, eds. Endotext [Internet]. South Dartmouth, MA: MDText.com, Inc. Available from: https://www.ncbi.nlm.nih.gov/books/NBK279127/

Science Learning Hub/Pokapū Akoranga Pūtaiao, 2014. Food's journey through the digestive system. Available from: https://www.sciencelearn.org.nz/resources/1849-food-s-journey-through-the-digestive-system.

Seladi-Schulman, J., 2021. Jejunun overview. Healthline. Available from: https://www.healthline.com/human-body-maps/jejunum.

Shaikh, J., 2021. Does it take 30 minutes to digest food? MedicineNet. Available from: https://www.medicinenet.com/does_it_take_30_minutes_to_digest_food/article.htm.

Thau, L., Ghandi, J., & Sharma, S., 2022. Physiology, cortisol. In: StatPearls [Internet].Treasure Island, FL: StatPearls Publishing. Available from: https://www.ncbi.nlm.nih.gov/books/NBK538239/

Valdes, A., Walter, J., Segal, E., & Spector, T., 2018. Role of the gut microbiota in nutrition and health. *BMJ*. 36: k2179. Available from: https://www.bmj.com/content/361/bmj.k2179.

Van Furth, R., & Cohm, Z.A., 1968. The origin and kinetics of mononuclear phagocytes. *J Exp Med*. 128: 415–435.

Van Grunsven, L., 2017. 3D in vitro models of liver fibrosis. *Advanced Drug Delivery Reviews*. 121 (Suppl 2). Doi:10.1016/j.addr.2017.07.004.

Wenzel, V., Idris, A.H., Banner, M.J., *et al.*, 1998. Respiratory system compliance decreases after cardiopulmonary resuscitation and stomach inflation: impact of large and small tidal volumes on calculated peak airway pressure. *Resuscitation*. 38(2): 113–118. Available from: https://doi.org/10.1016/s0300-9572(98)00095-1.

Yazdi, P., 2021. Pancreatic polypeptide: function & associated diseases. SelfDecode. Available from: https://labs.selfdecode.com/blog/pancreatic-polypeptide-function/

Young, R.L., Page, A.J., Cooper, N.J., *et al.*, 2009. Sensory and motor innervation of the crural diaphragm by the vagus nerves. *Gastroenterology*. 138(3): 1091–1101.e1015. Available from: https://doi.org/10.1053/j.gastro.2009.08.053.

Zhang, Y.-J., Li, S., Gan, R.-Y., *et al.*, 2015. Impacts of gut bacteria on human health and diseases. *Int J Mol Sci*. 16: 7493–7519. Available from: https://doi.org/10.3390/ijms16047493.

CHAPTER 10

The Inner Approach to the Thorax

INTRODUCTION

In this chapter we will looking at the thorax from an 'inner' perspective. We will explore this region at a profound level, the deep inner aspects of the anatomy and physiology, and take our awareness as practitioners also to a deeper 'inner' level.

As you have been working through the book, you should have been doing the exercises outlined earlier on centring regularly by this point. Likewise, you should have been practising the hands on, treatment table exercises, perhaps repeating some of them until you felt comfortable and proficient, with each chapter taking you on a progressively more profound inner journey of both anatomy and skill levels. As explained in Chapter 1: Introduction and how best to use this book, it is important not to rush ahead until you feel comfortable with the exercises from all the previous chapters so far. Skipping ahead and finding it tricky or difficult when working at the treatment table will result in 'trying', which may

lead to tissues tightening up in response, leaving your model uncomfortable. This is naturally something we need to avoid, especially as we are now beginning to work with even more significant physiological structures.

In this chapter on the thorax, we will be exploring the physiologically profound aspects of lung function, the pleura, the circulation, the three layers of the pericardium, and the venous and lymphatic return to the heart and the thymus gland – all structures which have a deep and significant effect on the whole physiology. The treatment of the heart itself will not be covered, as that is beyond the scope of this book. It is a highly delicate area both physiologically and emotionally and I would not wish to risk your disturbing its function. I do, however, recommend you take appropriate courses to learn more about the heart and its treatment as the benefits can be quite profound.

ANATOMICAL REVIEW

We will commence with the pulmonary system and then progress to the great vessels of the thoracic inlet, the three layers of the pericardium, and the lymphatic return before finishing with the thymus gland.

The pleura and pleural cavity

The pleura consists of two layers of fascia: the parietal layer, and the visceral layer, with the pleural cavity between the two. The pleura has vitally important functions, without some of which we could not breathe and so would die!

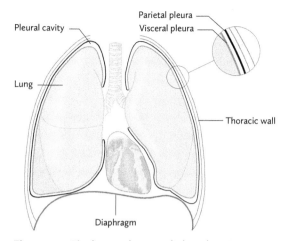

Figure 10.1 The lungs, pleura and pleural cavity.

The outer parietal layer lies immediately underneath the ribs, being adherent to them and the intercostal muscles within the thorax. On the left medial aspect of the thorax, the parietal pleura lies against the fibrous pericardium of the heart and is indented by it. Inferiorly the parietal layer is adjacent to the diaphragm muscle and tendon. It is adherent to the diaphragm muscle. As the right lung is slightly shorter than the left, there is a larger space between the two layers of the pleura on that side, with the costodiaphragmatic recesses at the very inferior aspect at the angles of the dome of the diaphragm. These recesses are only filled by the lungs when a very full inhalation occurs.

The parietal layer should be considered like a fibrous fascial sheath over the visceral pleura, as it is smooth, not following the indentations of the lung fields as does the visceral pleura. The parietal pleura is primarily a protective layer for the more delicate visceral layer and the lungs within. To be highly protective, this parietal layer is highly sensitive to pain, with many sensory nerve endings. The body needs to know if a sharp object is about to penetrate the lungs before it happens, and to get immediately out of the way! These nerves arise from the intercostal nerves at the relative spinal segment levels and also the phrenic nerves which arise from the cervical spine at levels C3, C4 and C5. Compared with the visceral layer, it is much stronger, being more fibrous. The blood supply to the parietal layer comes from the arteries in the intercostal spaces.

The visceral layer, like the pia mater of the meninges, follows all the indentations of the lungs and is much more delicate. It is not adherent to the outer parietal pleura, lying adjacent to it but with a slight gap between them, the pleural cavity. This layer is much more delicate compared with the parietal layer and unlike its stronger sister, it has no nerve supply, making it completely impervious to pain. The visceral pleura is completely adherent to the lung surfaces. At the root of the lungs, the visceral layer reflects on itself, becoming the outer parietal layer. The blood supply to the visceral pleura comes from the bronchial arteries, which also supply the lung tissue.

Between the parietal pericardium and the visceral pericardium (the serous pericardium layers) lies the pericardial fluid. This creates a cushioning effect in protecting the heart and reduces friction from the heart motion (Watson 2018). This film of fluid within the pleural cavity also creates a surface tension between the two layers such that as the parietal layer (adherent to the ribs) moves with inhalation, the inner visceral layer moves with it at the same time. Being adherent to the lung tissue, the visceral layer pulls on the lung tissue, creating expansion with the inhalation process. This expansion of the lungs then reduces the air pressure within the lung fields, resulting in air moving down the bronchial tree to equalise the pressure. It is quite humbling to think that without this tiny volume of surfactant in the pleural cavity we could not survive!

The two pleural layers are kept in their relationship due to physical and ionic factors. The lung tissue naturally likes to recoil, creating an inward pressure on the visceral pleura. Likewise, the parietal layer moves externally towards the rib cage. The two layers of the pleura stay close to each other due to the pleural liquid pressure being less than the recoil pressure. However, they stay very slightly apart, because the phospholipid surface layers within the pleural membranes have the same electrical charge between them, resulting in an electromagnetic repulsion (Miserocchi 2009).

The pleural cavity is vital for lung function and therefore our survival. Luckily (and perhaps it is not luck), the left and right pleural cavities do not communicate with each other. Should one cavity become punctured and exposed to air entering or filling the space causing a pneumothorax, it results in a collapsed lung. The patient in such a scenario is fortunately still able to access oxygen via the other, non-collapsed lung, whilst awaiting medical treatment. Should the cavity fill with body fluids (pleural effusion), this too can cause a partial lung volume reduction. When standing, such an effusion will be at the lower lobes because of gravity, but if supine, it could affect all lobes of the lung. Therefore, such patients need to be raised up when lying in bed whilst awaiting the surgical pleural drainage.

Exercise on the pleura
Centre yourself first then match as appropriate for each separate tissue during the exercise.

https://youtu.be/Pt5vm_vZdzs

The tracheobronchial tree
The trachea is the start of the cartilaginous reinforced tube which becomes the bronchial tree, the internal skeleton of the lungs. The trachea commences at the level of C6, the level of the cricoid cartilage. It continues as a vertical structure before finally dividing (the carinae) into the left and right main bronchi, at the level of T4. However, with respiratory motion, the division of the trachea can move as inferiorly as T6 (when the patient is upright).

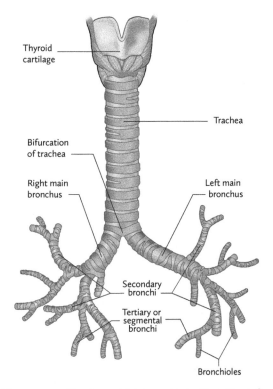

Figure 10.2 The bronchial tree. Note that the left main bronchus is more horizontal and the right main bronchus more vertical. This means that if any food accidently goes into the bronchial tree, it is more likely to get stuck in the right side.

The bronchial tree is not symmetrical on each side, the right being shorter, wider and more vertical than the left. The right lung has three lobes compared with the two lobes on the left (the heart taking up space on the left), resulting in the right lung having a greater volume. (However, do remember that some people (about 1 in 12,000) have their heart on the right side of their body.) The right lung is also influenced embryologically by the descent of the liver, away from the expanding heart. The growth of the liver descends away from the heart, as the whole embryo lengthens, along with the straightening of the whole spine. This creates a slight partial vacuum in the thorax, and the lungs grow into this developing new space. The right lung grows more on the right (because there is no heart and due to the influence of liver growth and descent on that side), and so develops three lobes not two.

Each main bronchus divides and subdivides into the smaller bronchioles which in turn divide and subdivide. At the end of the terminal bronchioles are the functional areas of the lungs, the alveolar sacs.

Exercise on the tracheobronchial tree
Centre yourself deeply first.

https://youtu.be/XHuEoOScC6Y

The lungs

Lung tissue is quite different to the pleura and bronchial tree. All tissues in the physiology which have differing functions will feel different to our osteopathic palpation. Think of one of the main osteopathic tenets: structure and function are interrelated. Consequently, just as with the pleura, the visceral layer feels quite different to the parietal layer, and in the same way, lung tissue feels quite different to the visceral pleura. As you would imagine (because of its function), the lungs feel more sponge-like, yet very, very delicate in comparison to the pleura or bronchial tree. In one of the exercises in this chapter I will guide you on an osteopathic journey to feel the functional point of the lung tissue, the alveolar membrane, where *you will feel the oxygenation process occurring!*

The lungs consist of small alveolar sacs which are described as 'hanging off the bronchioles like a bunch of grapes' (perhaps originally so described by a wine lover!). There are a phenomenal number of alveoli in the two lungs, which for everyday life when both lungs are functional seems a massive over requirement. Ochs *et al.* found that: 'In six adult human lungs, the mean alveolar number was 480 million (range: 274–790 million; coefficient of variation: 37%)' (Ochs *et al.* 2004).

Because the final ending of the terminal bronchioles and the alveolar sacs are so minute (too small for the naked eye), there would be a high risk of the adjacent walls of these tiny structures adhering to each other by surface tension. The alveoli are moist structures to assist with the gaseous interchange, and the surface tension between these moist surfaces would collapse the lumen. Consequently, to prevent this occurring, the terminal bronchioles and alveolar sacs secrete a small amount of surfactant, which eliminates the surface tension and keeps the walls apart. So, this minute volume of fluid enables the lung tissue to breathe and enables oxygenation of the blood to happen.

The pulmonary arteries from the right ventricle, carrying deoxygenated blood, follow the bronchial tree to the alveolar sacs. These sac walls are highly vascular to allow for the essential gaseous exchange occurring there, resulting in lung efficiency. From the capillary beds within the alveolar sac walls, the oxygenated blood flows within the pulmonary veins to the left atrium of the heart.

The extracellular matrix of the alveoli has a supporting role to the capillary bed in the epithelium. As we have already seen in the chapter on the fascia (Chapter 6) the matrix creates links to adjacent cells and has mechanical influences even to the nucleus within. So, a healthy matrix will help to assist the maintenance of healthy alveoli. Osteopathy can help even at this subtle level and thereby help the breathing of our patients – even those whose breathing is compromised.

Why do we need such overcapacity in our lungs?

Although the body can exist with large volumes of lung tissue missing (see Case study 1 below), that does not mean true excellent health can be expressed in such states.

Why do we have such a massive over capacity of our lung potential, if the physiology can manage with just one lung? Perhaps having two lungs gives a safety net should one side get a pneumothorax, but even then, there is still a massive potential available, and we could have two smaller lungs. If under heavy exertion, for example competitive athletic activity, we will use our full lung capacity for a while, so perhaps we needed to evolve such a large lung capacity to run away from danger, with the help of our sympathetic nervous system. However, during normal day-to-day activities we use only a percentage of our full capacity.

Interestingly, advanced meditators have been studied whilst in deep meditation, and it has been shown that their breath rate and volume is extremely low, and at times even stops. Equally their metabolism at such times reflects this low imperceptible breathing:

> We observed, over four independent experiments, 565 criterion-meeting episodes of breath suspension in 40 subjects practicing the Transcendental Meditation technique (TM), a simple mental technique involving no breath control procedures. The frequency and length of these breath suspension episodes were substantially and significantly greater for TM subjects than for control subjects relaxing with eyes closed. (Farrow and Hebert 1982)

As practitioners of the cranial approach, we know that we have an involuntary mechanism, a primary respiration causing a subtle motion within all our (healthy) tissues. Could it be that under the refined 'non-'activity of deep meditation/ mindfulness approaches, all that our physiology requires is the level of oxygenation gained by our primary respiratory motion of the lungs, working with the full lung volume, and not requiring rib movement-based breathing? We are very unlikely to see such persons in our practices whilst engaged in such mindfulness approaches, so this is just my personal conjecture and food for thought!

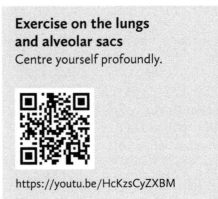

Exercise on the lungs and alveolar sacs
Centre yourself profoundly.

https://youtu.be/HcKzsCyZXBM

The great vessels

The great vessels (aorta, pulmonary trunk, brachiocephalic artery, subclavian arteries and veins, common carotid arteries, pulmonary veins, and brachiocephalic veins along with the superior and inferior vena cava) are all major components of the thorax and thoracic inlet. Many are close to or just underneath the manubrium and sternum. The large veins are under low pressure and so any pressure from the bones above will especially result in poor fluid dynamics within these highly significant vessels.

What are the consequences to disturbed blood flow?

When a pipe becomes distorted, the fluid dynamic within becomes turbulent. Turbulent fluid flow is less efficient and is maintained for a significant distance downstream. A turbulent flow (more easily expressed in the low-pressure veins) will have an influence on the efficiency of the blood flowing to the atria of the heart.

When the blood within the heart is turbulent, the myocardial activity will be less efficient in transmitting the blood through the organ, being a disorganised fluid.

Remember our osteopathic principles are universal throughout the physiology: structure influences function. This even applies to fluid dynamics. If you watch a small river or a stream, and the fluid flow is disturbed by a fixed branch lying in the water, it creates whirls and turbulence which are contrary to the main flow. In addition, turbulent water flow creates nearby areas of stagnant or poor flow. This turbulent water flows more slowly and does not combine well with the main current. Tension in the thorax or the diaphragm (a finding which we frequently see in patients) will negatively affect the fluid dynamics of the vessels passing through it. At areas of poorer flow, there is an increased risk of deposition from the blood occurring on the vessel walls, this possibly leading to atheroma and its pathological sequelae.

Exercise on the great vessels

Centre yourself first and match the tissues, the vessels, involved.

https://youtu.be/q5ZsSrM5nZI

The pericardium

From an osteopathic perspective, the pericardium is a tissue which is often overlooked, yet it plays an important role within the thorax both in assisting the heart and as a mechanical structure, affecting its neighbours. The pericardium is the structure surrounding the heart. This consists of the fibrous pericardium, the parietal pericardium and the visceral pericardium. The parietal and visceral pericardium layers are both called the serous pericardium as they are continuous with each other, the parietal layer reflecting back at the exit and entrance of the great vessels to become the visceral layer (Liverpool University n.d.).

Some sources just refer to two layers, but I shall keep to the above Liverpool University definition as on palpation there are three different qualities, one for each layer (we will be exploring these in the practical session). These layers protect the heart from the surrounding tissues and reduce the friction against adjacent structures caused by the motion of the myocardium.

The fibrous pericardium

The fibrous pericardium is the most external layer. As its name implies, it is very fibrous, giving it great strength. It has two areas of ligamentous attachment. These are more like thickenings of fascia rather than neat distinct ligaments. To quote Dr Frank Willard, the head of anatomy at New England University:

> Visceral ligaments generally are nowhere near as strong as somatic ligaments, nor are they as clearly defined on dissection. Unlike ligaments in somatic tissue, visceral ligaments typically function to carry blood supply and innervation to an organ system or to loosely anchor an organ in the body cavity. (Willard 2012)

The two ligaments to the fibrous pericardium are:
- the sternopericardial ligaments, which attach to the posterior of the sternum
- the pericardiophrenic ligaments, which blend with the central tendon of the diaphragm below the heart.

The function of these ligaments is to stabilise the heart within the thorax and thereby stop it from dancing around under the influence of the heart's beating action. This fibrous layer is continuous with the central tendon of the diaphragm, the fibres blending with each other. Therefore, from a true anatomical perspective it is diaphragm tissue, and the diaphragm is the fibrous pericardium tissue – the fibres are one and the same.

The fibrous pericardium is also adherent to the medial aspects of the fibrous layer of the pleura in the mediastinum, except for those areas separated by the phrenic nerves travelling inferiorly to the diaphragm muscle. Any tension within the fibrous pleura or fibrous pericardium will transfer to its thoracic neighbours (and vice versa).

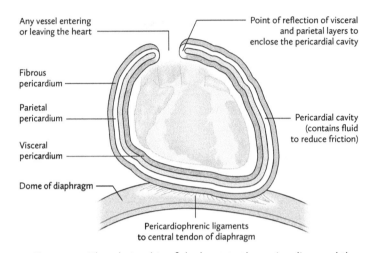

Figure 10.3 The relationship of the heart to the pericardium and the fibrous tendon of the diaphragm (not to scale).

The parietal pericardium (outer layer of the serous pericardium)

The middle layer or parietal pericardium, as has been shown in the above diagram, lies against the internal surface of the fibrous layer and is considered inseparable from it. This layer is not as strong and fibrous as its external neighbour, giving it a quite different quality to our palpation (which we will experience in the exercise on the pericardium).

Visceral pericardium (inner layer of the serous pericardium)

N.B. Some authorities name the visceral pericardium as the epicardium of the heart. This innermost layer is adjacent to the myocardium, not separable from it. Where the visceral pericardium passes from the myocardium to the origins of the great vessels entering/leaving the heart, the visceral pericardium then reflects on itself to fuse with the parietal layer, thus enclosing the pericardial space (see Figure 10.3).

Pericardial space

This is a small, enclosed space between the parietal layer and the visceral layer, containing a minute amount of fluid. This fluid acts as a lubricant to reduce friction between the visceral layer and parietal layers which would otherwise happen from the motion caused by the heart muscle. If the friction were to occur, it would cause inflammation of the pericardium and put the heart itself at risk, a medical emergency.

Pericardial function

Being strong in nature (as composed of both dense and loose connective tissue), and unable to be stretched, the fibrous pericardium creates a restrictive force against the risk of the heart being over filled with blood. If the heart did over fill, it would have serious consequences for the myocardium and heart valves as they would then need to work against an increased resistance from the raised blood volume.

In addition to the prevention of over filling, as has been mentioned, the fibrous pericardium prevents the heart dancing around within the thorax. The beating of the myocardium is of a spiral nature due to the internal arrangement of the myocardial fibres. Unless stabilised, this motion would cause the heart structure to twist and rotate within the thorax, putting pressure on the lungs and tension on the great vessels entering and leaving the heart (including the important cardiac arteries and veins).

Exercise on the pericardium

Centre yourself profoundly first and match with your elbow fulcrum, forearm tone and correct level of third hand intention, with each tissue you are palpating during this practical.

https://youtu.be/w1f6C_Sho8Q

Lymphatic return

The lymphatic system makes its final journey back to the heart within the thorax. It is vital for the body immunity and when it is less than efficient, it affects the whole physiology. All the returning lymph from the lower extremities, pelvis and abdomen flows into the cisterna chyli (on the right side of the aorta and in front of the right medial arcuate ligament of the abdomen), at the level of L1/2. This is a sac about 5–7 cm (2–2.75 inches) long running vertically adjacent to the spine. From the cisterna chyli, the lymph passes into the lymphatic trunk on the left of the dorsal vertebral bodies.

At some point it may then split into the left and right thoracic ducts, however the thoracic duct(s) are highly variable and sometimes the right duct is even absent. The left thoracic duct (not variable) then runs adjacent to the spine until it curves and always proceeds to the junction of the left jugular vein and the left subclavian vein. The lymph in this main left duct drains at this junction into the venous system. Here it has valves preventing back flow of venous blood into the lymphatic duct. The right duct (if present, or it can be several smaller vessels) drains somewhere in the region of the right jugular vein and the right subclavian vein, again with a one-way valve at its exit. Unlike the left side, the right drainage point into the venous system can be variable, but if not at the same location, then nearby.

The left lymphatic duct receives lymph from the whole of the left side of the body along with the right lower extremity, whereas the right upper quadrant of the body drains into the right subclavian vein. The lymphatics of the left side of the heart pass under the aorta to reach to the right lymph duct and the right subclavian vein, whereas the right side of the heart drains into the left thoracic duct and left subclavian vein. This arrangement occurs due to a rotation of the heart during its embryological development.

Like the venous system, the lymphatics flow under very low pressure, and similarly have valves at regular intervals along the vessels. Because of the low pressure within the vessels, they can be strongly influenced by compressive forces, damaging the quality of the spiral fluid flow. Fluids in a pipe naturally take up a spiral motion. If you observe a household tap (without an aeration gauze fitted), which is almost turned off but not quite dripping, you will observe the water flowing from the tap in a spiral fashion.

At the junction of the lymphatic ducts and the venous system, the flow of the strong venous current across the opening valve between the two creates suction on the lymphatic outflow into the streaming venous blood. Hence the final drainage of the lymph into the venous system is a suction-led system. Mechanical restrictions to the clavicle or first ribs could have a distorting effect on the venous flow along the subclavian artery, thus reducing the suction at the lymphatic opening.

Exercise on lymphatic return
Centre yourself first. Match the tissues you are palpating.

https://youtu.be/wOdng9txhY8

The thymus
The thymus is a gland often overlooked in the thorax. It lies immediately behind the manubrium and sternum and is an important part of the immune system. On palpation it has a vastly different quality to the manubrium as it has a delicate glandular quality. Only the lung tissues in the thorax feel this delicate.

The thymus changes in size throughout life, growing from birth to puberty, from which time it then slowly decreases in size with age. It consists of two lobes each subdivided into lobules.

The main function of the thymus gland is the maturation of T cells (lymphocytes). Precursors (stem cells) continually migrate to the thymus from the bone marrow throughout life, and are then known as thymocytes. These thymocytes then mature, gaining the ability to react against a specific antigen, which involves a double selection method. A double selection process occurs in this process. Firstly, to react against an invading antigen in the body, known as positive selection, and secondly, making sure they do not react against normal body tissue, known as negative selection. When the cells have gained full maturity and acquired these selection processes, they leave the thymus as active T cells (lymphocytes). Whilst in the whole-body circulation, the T cells undergo a further maturation process, partly induced by hormones and cytokines secreted by the thymus.

Exercise on the thymus gland
Be very centred and match (delicately) the thymus tissue when palpating it.

https://youtu.be/lmio-TfuhSo

COMMON CLINICAL CONDITIONS

Presented below are a few common medical conditions which we are likely to see at times in our osteopathic practice and the medical treatment approach. This is not intended to be a complete list nor a detailed reference regarding these conditions. If you have a patient with a case history relevant to this chapter, you should read up further on their condition.

Conditions of the pulmonary system
Asthma
We will all see patients in our practice who suffer from asthma. According to research in 2016, 5.4 million people in the UK were receiving treatment for asthma, equating to 1.1 million children (1 in 11) and 4.3 million adults (1 in 12) (Pharmaceutical Services Negotiating Committee 2016).

Asthma is an inflammatory condition of the bronchial tree causing coughing, difficulty in breathing and wheezing. The aetiology is from one or more asthmatic triggers which result in inflammation within the bronchial tree. These triggers can vary from person to person, but common physical triggers include pet fur/pet mites, household cleaning agents, air pollution, tobacco smoke and mouldy surfaces. However, physiological aspects such as exercise, hormonal cycles, chest infections and viral infections can be aetiological factors. Psychological states are now also acknowledged to bring on asthmatic attacks, including emotional stress and anxiety.

As the condition progresses so an increase in bronchial mucus occurs, leading to a reduced bronchial space and further breathing difficulties. The medical treatment for asthma will depend on each individual and may be to avoid the trigger (if known), preventative measures via inhalers or, if more severe, then the use of inhalers alongside steroid medication.

Bronchitis

This is a common condition of the bronchial tree causing it to become inflamed and congested. The UK National Health Service (NHS) estimates that around 2 million people in the UK are affected by chronic bronchitis, with most being adults over the age of 50 (NHS Inform 2021).

The main common symptom is a chronic cough which may be productive, having a yellow mucus. Other symptoms can present like the common cold, resulting in headaches, sore throat and general aches and pains. In long-term sufferers, chronic obstructive pulmonary disease (COPD) may occur. In these cases, the symptoms progress to wheezing, difficulty breathing on exertion, productive cough and frequent chest infections.

Medical treatment in the acute phase is to drink more (not alcoholic) fluids, give the body plenty of rest, take mild anti-inflammatory medication (weak, not prescribed by the GP) and

avoidance of a dry domestic atmosphere. However, if the condition becomes more serious, and depending on the nature of symptoms, cough inhibitors, bronchodilators, antibiotics and/or inhalers may be prescribed to treat the bronchitis or to reduce the risk of secondary conditions occurring in the lungs.

The pleura
Pleurisy

This is a condition where the pleural coverings of the lungs become inflamed. It is characterised by a sharp pain in the thorax which is aggravated with breathing (because of the demanded motion of the pleura). With pleurisy, the swelling from the inflammation of the two layers causes them to rub against each other, creating painful friction when breathing, as the pleural cavity becomes occluded.

Symptoms other than the sharp pain include a shortness of breath as the patient minimises their breathing to avoid pain. Equally the patient will avoid coughing and sneezing at all costs for the same reason. All movements of the thoracic spine or the shoulder girdle also cause pain, as they demand motion of the whole thorax including the pleura.

The medical treatment of pleurisy is to ease the pain with the necessary level of analgesia, along with medication for the underlying cause of the damage to the pleura. There can be a variety of aetiological factors to pleurisy, including bacterial, viral, or fungal infections, as well as autoimmune conditions, lung cancer near the pleura, pulmonary embolism, tuberculosis and fractures to the rib cage.

Conditions of the lungs

I will briefly discuss two well-known conditions of lung tissue which we may see in our practices: pneumonia and lung cancer. If you see such patients, it is important that you should do further reading as to the pathophysiology of the patient's condition. Likely, the patient will have already been to their general practitioner (GP), and will still be on current medical care. If the condition was in the past and no longer requiring medical treatment, the patient may simply require check-ups to ensure all is well from a medical standpoint or they may be medically dismissed altogether.

Pneumonia

This is an inflammatory condition caused by infection of the lung tissues. When the condition is active it can give a variety of symptoms: the air sacs in one or both lungs may fill with fluid or pus, causing cough with phlegm or pus, fever, chills and difficulty breathing. A variety of organisms, including bacteria, viruses and fungi, can cause pneumonia (Mayo Clinic 2022). Unless there are medical complications, the medical treatment is resting at home with a prescription of antibiotics.

Lung cancer

Lung cancer has a high incidence in society and is the most common cause of fatality among cancerous conditions. There are many types of lung cancer, and therefore there are a variety of types of medical or surgical treatments required. Consequently, I recommend (with your patient's permission) liaising with their GP regarding their ongoing treatment regimen and explaining that you will be offering a *very gentle* (emphasise the very gentle) supportive role to the thorax (the GP would not want to think you will be manipulating such patients, especially as lung cancers can in advanced cases create secondary tumours, including to the spine).

According to Cancer Research UK, the estimated lifetime risk of being diagnosed with lung cancer is 1 in 13 (8%) for males and 1 in 15 (7%) for females born after 1960 in the UK (Cancer Research UK 2016). Consequently, we will see cancer patients or those who no longer have the condition coming to our practices at some point in our careers.

The pericardium
Pericarditis

This is a condition where the pericardium becomes inflamed. The symptoms are like pleurisy, that of a sharp stabbing pain in the thorax which is aggravated with a deep inhalation. The condition may be more of a dull ache and can have a gradual onset. Other symptoms can include fever, nausea and feeling lightheaded or just feeling unwell. Pericarditis can also be aggravated when lying supine. This is a condition which needs immediate medical diagnosis and treatment.

OSTEOPATHIC INSIGHTS

The pulmonary system

This is the only way air from the outside world can enter the lungs. Therefore, it is vital that the bronchial tube is kept open and as free from fluids as possible. The cartilaginous rings are formed to reinforce the tube structure and ensure as much as possible that the tube is permanently open. The bronchial tree, like any other firm structure in the body, can be affected by mechanical tensions. If this occurs, then because it is the skeleton of the lungs, the lungs will also be affected. The whole internal tube surface is covered in mucous membrane which secretes mucus as part of the immune system, reducing infection risk from the incoming viruses and bacteria within the air. If, however, the immune system in the bronchial tree becomes overactive, then the mucus production becomes excessive and leads to breathing difficulties.

The working part of the lungs are the alveoli. Like the rest of the physiology, although miniscule, they still follow the same osteopathic mechanical principles of structure affecting function. Any tension within the matrix of the alveoli will affect the adjacent alveoli epithelial cells, whose function is the gaseous exchange of O_2 and CO_2.

Like all other tissues, lung tissue will be affected by life events. Mechanical injuries to the thorax will influence the internal structures to varying degrees. Perhaps such influences may not be in a manner to threaten life, perhaps not even be symptomatic, but their influences will still affect their pulmonary efficiency to some degree. As osteopaths we all see asymptomatic mechanical tensions and lesions in many areas of the physiology where they do affect function in a detrimental manner, but only on a subtle, subclinical level. The lungs, bronchial tree and pleural tissues are no different.

The great vessels

Most of the great vessels are, as stated earlier, close to the clavicle, sternum and manubrium. Many of our patients have a compressed manubrium. If you place your forefinger and middle finger on the flat surface of the bone, in health is should 'spring' up and down under fingertip pressure. There should be a sense of 'give'. However, frequently you will find that it is restricted, particularly at the manubriosternal angle. Many patients develop mechanical tension in this area from trauma or from chronic tension and anxiety, when then leads to problems in the cervicodorsal region. When we get apprehensive, the body develops upper rib breathing, locking up the thoracic inlet and manubrium, the manubriosternal angle. If this becomes chronic, it can pressurise the great vessels lying just underneath.

The heart strings

When we consider arteries, our thinking immediately moves to their role of transporting blood away from the heart. However, we should also consider that arteries are powerful muscular and fascial tubes. Consequently, they can convey mechanical forces along their length, just as any other fascial structure can, especially as they are reinforced with a muscular coat.

The great vessels are large! For example, the ascending aorta is on average 3.3 cm in diameter (this increases with age), and 2.5 cm in diameter at the diaphragm junction. We should also consider that the thoracic arteries are full of arterial blood. From physics, we know that fluids do not compress. Therefore the aorta in both the thorax and abdomen (lying directly in front of the spine, except for the aortic arch) acts as a support to the vertebral column as far down as L4 (where it divides into the common iliac arteries). In the same way, the brachiocephalic and left subclavian arteries, along with the pulmonary arteries (venous blood from right ventricle), help to open out laterally our chest and shoulder girdle.

We should also bear in mind that many of these important structures are just underneath the clavicle, manubrium, sternum and first ribs. Any restriction of the skeleton in this region will cause internal turbulence to the fluid flow and poorer efficiency in supplying their destination with blood. Such turbulence will be even more expressed in veins as they are at a lower pressure.

Emotions and the great vessels

In the UK we have a phrase: 'He/she is pulling on my heart strings.' This is used when we are under emotional distress from someone we care strongly about. I would imagine the same or similar phrase exists for many other languages and cultures across the world. Quite literally the blood vessels (especially the arteries) are our 'heart strings', which when pulled by the emotional tensions within the heart, create mechanical pulls to the rest of the body.

Try this simple exercise.

- Stand comfortably.
- Place one hand over your upper heart

and the other over the mid-pelvis at the front (the level of L4). Your two hands will now be at each end of the aorta.

- Imagine the distance between your two hands is shrinking. Do not move your hand position, but let your body adjust to the new position, of a shorter aorta.
- Notice what has happened: your spine has curved forwards and your neck has become more extended (if you kept looking in the same direction).
- Now imagine the same shortening is happening to the pulmonary arteries, brachiocephalic artery and left subclavian artery. This will further pull your shoulders into a 'hunched' position and further pull (due to the tug on the carotid arteries and carotid sheath) the neck into a deeper, shortening extension, with a deeper strain now occurring at the cervicodorsal area.
- We call this a degenerative posture! Notice how it feels to be in this position, created just by imagining a shortening of the main arteries leaving the heart.
- Now have a good stretch to loosen up this 'heart string pull' posture.

Clearly this exercise demonstrates that chronic/ongoing emotional stress changes our posture, as the changes to our musculoskeletal system then occur as secondary effects from the pull on the heart strings. Giving osteopathic treatment just on the spinal mechanics will create an easing, but unless we address the underlying cause, including the emotional tension pulling on the arteries, the condition will likely return.

It is perhaps important at this stage to drop a physiological 'bombshell'.

The heart is not a pump!

The standard medical model is that the heart pumps the blood around the body. However, this has been refuted and the history of the heart being a pump has, by some, been strongly questioned.

The arch of the aorta is known to become more curved during systole when viewed during open heart surgery: 'During the systolic ejection (period when blood is ejected from ventricle), the aorta's curvature is seen to increase, signifying that the aorta is not undergoing a positive pressure, but rather is undergoing a negative pressure' (Marinelli *et al.* 1995).

As anyone who has a garden hose will know, when you turn on the tap, the hosepipe unwinds under the increased internal pressure of the water. The arch of the aorta should flatten out, not increase its curvature under the increased pressure of systole, but that is not the case. Therefore, another mechanism of force must be occurring, creating a negative pressure on the aortic arch.

However, this negative pressure theory fits in with what happens embryologically. Fluid is 'sucked' by hungry cells in the days before the heart exists. The extracellular fluids around the early embryo flow by osmotic gradient towards the cells where rapid growth is occurring. The growth demand creates a depletion of growth nutriments and sets up the osmotic gradient by the nutritional need of the cells. The 'hungry' cells demand, or quite literally 'suck' the high nutrient fluids towards them.

This means the heart was being formed whilst this suction (demand)-led fluid dynamics was already in existence. Suction (demand) by the cells throughout the whole body for nutrient rich blood would cause a negative pressure state in the aorta hence the curvature increasing, not straightening out, during systole. (I recommend a full read of the 'Heart is not a pump' paper quoted above, as it makes fascinating reading and changes how we should look at our circulation).

Now consider that the myocardium has no antagonist and it beats an amazing amount of times every day: 'The heart beats (expands and contracts) 100,000 times per day, pumping five or six quarts of blood each minute, or about 2,000 gallons [7,570 litres] per day' (WebMD 2018). Therefore, if a person lives 80 years and does not suffer a heart attack, the number of beats is 100,000 x 365 x 80: a total of 2.92 billion heart beats without rest. That does not include the foetal heart beating during its time inside the uterus. The heart tube commences contraction around 15 days after conception, giving a possible extra 27,370,000 extra beats before birth. So the final total based on an average 100,000 per day = nearly 3,000,000,000 beats over 80 years without rest!

According to the Franklin Institute:

The smallest blood vessels measure only five micrometres. To give you some perspective, a strand of human hair measures about 17 micrometres. But if you took all the blood vessels out of an average child and laid them out in one line, the line would stretch over 60,000 miles. An adult's would be closer to 100,000 miles long. (Franklin Institute 2022)

So, if this length is correct (it can only be a very rough estimate), then over a lifetime, the heart beats nearly 3 billion times, pushing blood against the resistance of the circulation, which is about 100,000 miles long, without rest. This simply does not make sense. We would get heart failure in our 20s (or earlier), if the myocardium had to act like any other muscle of the body working against such resistance and over such long distances.

If, however, we now consider that the cells (when in a healthy state) of the body are 'sucking' the nutriment-rich blood towards them as the primary driver, then the beating of the myocardium would be just a relaxed gentle motion, as if going along with the ride, not being the primary engine of blood motion. Only when there was significant added demand – as when running away from danger that required a high level of athleticism – would there be the need for the myocardium to *really work* above its gentle beating state. The heart would also have to 'work' hard when the health of the body deteriorates, resulting in a reduced suction force on aortic outflow. If poor health persists for long periods (years), then the heart is forced to work hard, instead of sustaining a restful beat, resulting in heart disease and hypertension. The heart suffers because it is not designed to work hard as a pump, outside of emergency situations.

The right side of the heart requires venous blood to replenish that which has just been shunted out of the right ventricle, to the lungs. Therefore, there is effectively a suction action on the superior and inferior vena cava pulling blood into the right atrium. So do look at the circulation of the body as a suction/demand-led system, not a heart-pushed system. Healthy demand by healthy cells results in a reduced demand on the myocardium and the heartbeat is just 'going with the flow', not really working at all.

OSTEOPATHIC TREATMENT OF THE THORAX

Osteopathic assistance can be helpful to patients who are undergoing medical treatment or have had a history of conditions in the thorax (or anywhere else in the physiology). Always make sure you gain the patient's understanding that your aim is not to cure their condition but to allow them to cope/live more easily with their condition. However, with some conditions and some patients, you may find that osteopathic help does reduce symptoms. Wisely use your knowledge of the anatomy and physiology of the different systems before you palpate this special area of the physiology. If your patient has an active or recently active medical condition, do always ensure that they are receiving the appropriate medical care, in addition to osteopathic treatment.

If the patient has a past condition to the thoracic cavity that no longer requires medical intervention, the condition may have left the involved tissues with varying degrees of scarring or reduced function. Skilled and gentle osteopathic care can be beneficial and assist such tissues to an improved physiological function.

Questions to consider

- When palpating, do any of these tissues specifically call to your awareness requesting help? N.B. You need to be highly centred within yourself to assess this properly.
- If so, can you refine your palpation and assess exactly where anatomically within that tissue you need to give osteopathic help? Exactly which part(s) of the thorax needs your help?

Do remember, the more accurate your awareness both of tissue type and of anatomical location, the more effective your treatment becomes. The internal therapeutic wisdom of the body seems to respond more effectively to our treatments when we become more specific with our understanding of tissue types and location (and as we will see in Chapter 15, also with the dimension of time).

Pulmonary conditions

If you see a patient with a pulmonary condition (who may have come to see you for a different,

perhaps musculoskeletal concern), osteopathic care for such patients can be highly beneficial. Working on the rib cage, pleura, bronchial tree, lungs and the autonomic system (both the sympathetic and vagal systems) as deemed appropriate can help the patient gain an easier breathing pattern. Also, such patients can commonly be afraid or worry about their breathing (quite understandably), especially if they are not chronic sufferers or who are unfamiliar with the symptomatic process. For these patients we can also help reduce their fear and stress levels by working with the nervous system and diaphragm along with working more directly to assist the pulmonary system.

When treating the tissues with which you are working, when they are at a point close to stillness, invite them to treat themselves *if they want to*. If the patient is in a highly active phase, or has very low vitality, they may say, 'No thank you, not today', or they may take up your (without ego) suggestion and proceed to self-treat to a greater or lesser extent. You are not the boss: the tissues, not you, decide how much they will treat themselves.

If the patient is receiving treatment for an active condition, please use extreme wisdom as to how much osteopathy is applied to the relevant tissues. If in doubt about your skill level (remove your ego before considering this), or about the patient's condition, *do not treat those specific tissues* (you do not want to risk aggravating the condition). However, you can help the patient by working with other supportive areas, to give some ease to their physiology.

OSTEOPATHIC TREATMENT OF THE PERICARDIUM, GREAT VESSELS AND LYMPHATIC SYSTEM

In this book I will not be discussing osteopathic treatment of the heart itself. This requires an

exceedingly high level of skill and should not be undertaken lightly, and it is beyond the scope of this book. Not only could mistreatment of the myocardium and internal structures affect the role of the heart organ in its relation to the circulation, being a key organ associated with our deepest 'heartfelt' emotions, psychological disturbance could also result.

As I hope has become clear, you need to consider the pericardium and circulation with a high level of respect. If the health level of the physiology is not good, then there is the strong possibility that the myocardium is having to *work*, rather than just 'going along with the flow'. Here are some pointers to consider when taking an inner look at the thorax:

- How can you raise the health level of the physiology to bring about a greater 'sucking action' by the tissues and lower the demand on the heart muscle?
- What areas of the body feel sluggish? Sluggish tissues frequently have poor venous return.
- Areas of strong mechanical tension will 'kink the garden hoses', reducing fluid flow quality. Take your hands to these areas, and visualise how the blood vessels could be kinked by the mechanical forces there. Then allow your treatment focus to include these vessels, increasing the flow quality within them.
- Work with the thoracic inlet, as very frequently with our patients it is a quite restricted area. Think about the great vessels underneath it and of the physiological consequences if the flow is being compromised.
- Treat the diaphragm. Remember, it is

the outer layer of the pericardium. Also, the inferior vena cava passes through the diaphragm and aorta under the median arcuate ligament. Make sure they are not being restricted by the diaphragm tone.
- Work directly on the layers of the pericardium. Can you ascertain if one specific layer of the three requires your osteopathic care more than the other two?
- If there are areas of oedema in the body, work to assist the lymphatic return – think cysterna chyli, think lymph glands and certainly think drainage into the subclavian veins.
- Remember the jugular veins and vertebral veins draining the head. Ensure they are not being mechanically compromised at the thoracic inlet, resulting in poorer drainage of the head and brain.
- What advice can you give to the patients about their work–life balance, and how to reduce stress levels?
- Do they need some nutritional advice?

Remember when wishing to treat the tissues of the body, invite the tissues *to treat themselves*.

In the practical exercises below, I will take you through the treatment approach to the thoracic organs and tissues. I have not discussed the treatment of musculoskeletal conditions as I am sure you have much knowledge of such conditions already. The skills you will be developing in this chapter will, however, significantly enhance your palpatory and diagnostic awareness to treat these conditions too.

CASE STUDIES

These case studies are not to indicate my own level of skill, but to inspire you to appreciate how osteopathy can help a wide variety of patients.

CASE STUDY 1
A woman in her mid-70s came to see me who had had all of one lung removed and a quarter

of the other lung removed, because of lung cancer. She had spinal secondary tumours. Her breathing was significantly laboured, and her voice was thin, slow and strained. Taking her case history took much longer than normal. She was still under regular medical care as she was still at risk of the disease. On examination, her thorax was very tight and compressed from the scarring where her lung tissue used to be, yet at the same time very delicate. Her central nervous system was compressed. She spoke of her worries of death (understandably), in addition to the stress of not being able to communicate because of difficulty speaking in anything other than a whisper. Her circulation and autonomic systems were also struggling.

At the initial visit, I just put my hands on the mediastinum and acknowledged the damage to the bronchial tree and lung tissue. By carefully and delicately matching the quality of her remaining lung and the scar tissue on the side of the removed lung (the right side), the lungs, bronchial tree and the space no longer occupied by the right lung were invited to treat themselves. There was no expectation of the outcome nor of how her body might treat itself.

Very slowly and gently, there was a slight motion and changes occurring in her lung fields. When the tissues in the thorax finally returned to a gentle flexion and extension (she had low vitality, so the involuntary expression was still weak), I decided that this was enough treatment for her as I did not think she could handle much change at any one time.

(N.B. Extremely sick tissues cannot handle much change, so always under treat such patients.)

As the treatment finished, I removed my hands, and lowered the table so she could stand up. Much to my total amazement, she carefully stood up from the treatment table,

and in a much louder and more strident voice, said: 'That feels much more comfortable!'

The treatment continued for four months at fortnightly intervals, each time just to support the pulmonary system, pericardium, nervous system, larynx and her spinal mechanics. The treatment process was to simply invite the specific tissue I was working with to treat itself if it wanted to (no fluid drives, no CV4/lateral fluctuation). During that time, she gained greater vitality and better life quality. Sadly, a few weeks after her eighth session, she had a bad fall and could no longer travel (she lived over an hour's drive away). Regrettably, she did not attend again. Perhaps the outcome of the fall had a fatal influence regarding her tumours; I do not know.

Even though it was made clear at the outset that I was not attempting to help her cancer, which she fully acknowledged, she was delighted at my being able to help her quality of life, through easier breathing and speech during those months.

Some of the most significant osteopathic treatments I have ever given to patients have been in circumstances where a better quality of life was gained, up to and until their soul left the body. I do sincerely believe that osteopathy can be beneficially used to help the quality of death, just as it can to help the quality of life!

CASE STUDY 2

A man in his late 80s came to see me who was complaining of heart tension and an unstable heart rate. His voice was a bit thin and his breathing did not appear comfortable. He was under medical investigation at his local hospital, but he had had many osteopathic treatments for a variety of conditions throughout his life and asked if I could assist his health. My response was that I would not be treating his condition, but I would help his whole-body physiology, which would work alongside the medical care he was having.

The osteopathic evaluation showed several significant degenerative findings. The cranial base was rather locked especially on the left occipitomastoid region. The spinal joints reflected those of a person his age and he had a general compression through his thoracic spine. When I evaluated the thoracic viscera, I noted that the parietal and visceral layers of the pericardium specifically were feeling irritated, the outer fibrous layer being a little tight but the most comfortable of the three layers. The lungs felt as if a little congested, but the pleura seemed OK.

Treatment was to the cranial base and to free the occipitomastoid sutures, then moving to the thorax. I mentally asked his physiology if it would be better to focus on his lungs first or the pericardium. The response being that it was best to initially assist his pericardium, I then attuned my awareness to the middle parietal layer and acknowledged its irritability. I recentred myself (to ensure my ego was not involved) and invited the parietal pericardium to treat itself *if it wanted to.* If the body had said it did not want to treat the parietal pericardium at that time, I would have honoured that and moved away (sometimes the body does say no to this invitation).

Then a very subtle change took place initially in the quality of that tissue, before some motion occurred. When this motion settled into a gentle flexion and extension, it was time to move away from the parietal layer, and I then gently took my awareness to the visceral pericardium. Extreme care must be taken when working on this innermost layer of the pericardium as it is inseparable from the myocardium, so at this point I again recentred myself to maintain a deep level of inner stillness. Again, acknowledging the feeling of irritability within this visceral layer, I followed by delicately inviting it to treat itself *if it wanted to.* After a while of nothing happening, the tissues showed a subtle change in tissue quality.

The irritability reduced followed by a return of flexion and extension. After gently removing my hands, he stood up when he was ready.

At the next visit and after further hospital tests, he said he had been given a diagnosis of atrial fibrillation. This is a condition where the heart rate is unstable, often rapid, which results in the heart atria not contracting properly. This results in a slowing of the blood flow or even stagnation, which will then have consequences for the ventricles and especially the lungs. He said that after his initial visit, his heart rate had been more stable than the previous week and his breathing easier. I again worked on the cranial base, the brain stem (thinking about the vagal nuclei, which are discussed more fully in Chapter 11 on the cranial nerves). I also worked with the pericardium (much easier this visit) and in addition, worked with the lungs.

My approach to working on his lungs was to follow the bronchial tree from the trachea all the way to a terminal bronchiole, and into the alveolar wall (the functional site of the lungs). Remember that the bronchial tree is an air tube. When you take your awareness to the functional site of the alveolar wall, there is a significant difference in quality from that of the bronchial tree. The gaseous interchange gives it a definite 'fizzy' active quality to your palpatory awareness (you do need to be highly centred otherwise you will miss this quality). In my experience of teaching, the distance you need to travel along the bronchial tree to arrive at the alveolus is much further than most people realise (see the practical exercise on the lungs earlier in the chapter).

On inviting the alveolar wall to treat itself, a significant sensation of energy increase occurred, and I then finished his treatment. When he came off the treatment table, he said his whole chest felt lighter, more open.

At the time of writing, he is still attending for treatment.

CASE STUDY 3

A male patient in his early 60s had leukaemia. He was fatigued more than his normal state and was under medical care. On examination, his involuntary system was sluggish, the spleen felt slightly enlarged, and his lymphatic system was also sluggish. His venous system felt congested, and on evaluation, the thymus felt hot.

My initial focus was to treat his pelvis to help the venous congestion and then the lungs. The lungs receive greater blood flow when the venous return to the heart is increased, so it is important that the lungs can handle that increased flow. Remember, blood flows in a circle, that is why it is named the circulation, so always consider what happens downstream!

I then moved my awareness to his hot thymus. Clearly the thymus and T cell production were working overtime (probably to compensate for the poorer lymphatic system). The thymus decided to treat itself after my invitation and the organ cooled down significantly. The treatment finished with working on the lymphatic drainage into the subclavian veins.

Afterwards he felt that he had more energy and was mentally stronger. Not living nearby, I was not able to offer follow-up sessions, but he continued receiving treatment from a local colleague.

REFERENCES

Cancer Research UK, 2016. Lung cancer risk. Available from: https://www.cancerresearchuk.org/health-professional/cancer-statistics/statistics-by-cancer-type/lung-cancer/risk-factors.

Farrow, J.T., & Hebert, J.R., 1982. Breath suspension during the transcendental meditation technique. *Psychosom Med.* 44(2): 133–153. Doi: 10.1097/00006842-198205000-00001.

Franklin Institute, 2022. Blood vessels. Available from: https://www.fi.edu/heart/blood-vessels#:~:text=But%20if%20you%20took%20all,arteries%2C%20veins%2C%20and%20capillaries.

Liverpool University, n.d. The pericardium. Available from: https://www.liverpool.ac.uk/~trh/local_html/heart disease/pericardium.htm.

Marinelli, R., Fuerst, B., van der Zee, H., *et al.*, 1995. The heart is not a pump. Available from: http://www.trigunamedia.com/The%20heart%20is%20not%20a%20pump.pdf .

Mayo Clinic, 2022. Pneumonia. Available from: https://www.mayoclinic.org/diseases-conditions/pneumonia/symptoms-causes/syc-20354204.

Miserocchi, G., 2009. Mechanisms controlling the volume of pleural fluid and extravascular lung water. *European Respiratory Review*. Available from: https://err.ersjournals.com/content/18/114/244.

NHS Inform, 2021. Bronchitis. Available from: https://www.nhsinform.scot/illnesses-and-conditions/lungs-and-airways/bronchitis#:~:text=Acute%20bronchitis%20can%20affect%20people,UK%20affected%20by%20chronic%20bronchitis.

Ochs, M., Nyengaard, J., Jung, A., *et al.*, 2004. The number of alveoli in the human lung. *Am J Respir Crit Care Med.* 169(1): 120–124.

Pharmaceutical Services Negotiating Committee, 2016. Essential facts, stats and quotes relating to asthma. Available from: https://psnc.org.uk/services-commissioning/essential-facts-stats-and-quotes-relating-to-asthma/#:~:text=5.4%20million%20people%20in%20the,a%20day%20die%20from%20asthma.

Watson, S., 2018. Pericardium. Healthline. Available from: https://www.healthline.com/health/pericardium.

WebMD, 2018. How the heart works. Available from: https://www.webmd.com/heart-disease/qa/how-many-times-does-your-heart-beat-each-day.

Willard, F., 2012. Visceral fascia. In: Schleip, R., Findley, T.W., Chaitow, L., & Huijing, P., eds. *Fascia: The Tensional Network of the Human Body*. Edinburgh, UK: Elsevier, pp. 55–56.

CHAPTER 11

The Cranial Nerves: An Inner Approach to Treatment

In this chapter we will be looking at the cranial nerves, taking each in succession associated with their anatomical numerical order, with practical exercises following each section. Working with individual nerves can, where diagnostically appropriate, help the clinical outcome more than just working on the cranial base, and where relevant, the foramina of the skull. Each section will revise the anatomical pathway and discuss its function in preparation for the practical session for that nerve.

NERVUS TERMINALIS (CN 0)

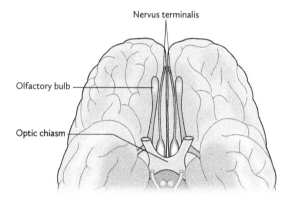

Figure 11.1 Cranial nerve 0 and its relationship to the olfactory nerve, CN I.

Most medical practitioners and osteopaths only think of the 12 cranial nerves when considering this topic. However, when researching the cranial nerves several years ago, I discovered much to my amazement a 13 nerve! This exits the brain stem in the most rostral position, before the olfactory (first cranial nerve), so it was named cranial nerve zero.

Cranial nerve zero (also termed the nervus terminalis) is a bundle of nerve fibres which run either side of the midline in the subarachnoid space just inferior to the frontal lobes of the brain. The fibres pass through the cribriform plate into the basal septum. The fibres pass posteriorly in the subarachnoid space towards lamina terminalis.

Although the nervus terminalis is not mentioned in many anatomy text books, its function is embryologically involved with the migration route of luteinising hormone releasing hormone (LHRH) cells, and is consequently being considered in the pathology of Kallmann syndrome. This is a condition which causes a reduced sense of smell along with a hormonal imbalance which causes the delay or prevention of puberty (Kang 2021).

Czernichowska and Rea at the Glasgow Neuro Conference in 2018 questioned the presence of the nervus terminalis in humans:

We examined 11 formalin-fixed cadaveric brains using gross and histological techniques to try to identify the nervus terminalis… We found that fibre-like structures were identified on visual examination using a surgical microscope. In addition, approximately 830 Masson's trichrome stained sections were examined, taken from the base of the frontal lobes, adjacent and separate to the olfactory nerve. We found fibres adjacent to the olfactory nerve which, although not definitive of the presence of a nervus terminalis, could suggest an anastomosis between the olfactory nerve and a possible nervus terminalis. (Czernichowska and Rea 2018)

However, Sonne *et al.* agree as to its presence in humans:

The CN 0 has been located on the ventral surface of the human brain. Its plexiform fibres appear to run in proximity to CN I, the olfactory nerve. CN 0 rests on the anterior surface of the brain in the region of the olfactory trigone and courses anteriorly on the medial surface of the olfactory tract and bulb. Medially, it forms a plexus of fibres closely associated with the olfactory stria (medial to the anterior perforated space) from where it enters the brain independently… Its structural composition consists of numerous smaller strands that branch and anastomose, elaborating an elongated plexus (plexiform). Its bilateral bundle of unmyelinated nerve fibres is most evident in human foetal stages. However, it is also seen in adult brains. Its fascicles can be seen within the subarachnoid space covering the gyri recti surface of the frontal lobe. (Sonne *et al.* 2022)

Vilenski further describes this nerve passing through the cribriform plate of the ethmoid:

The fibres pass through the cribriform plate medial to those of the olfactory nerve fila. The fibres end in the nasal mucosa and probably arise from autonomic/neuromodulatory as well as sensory neurons… The nerve is referred to as the nervus terminalis because in species initially examined its fibres were seen entering the brain in the region of the lamina terminalis. (Vilenski 2014)

When I first read these conflicting papers on this intriguing nerve, I became fascinated as to why it is neglected in most medical textbooks, especially as some authors indicate that it is a vital nerve in terms of its function. I then wondered whether it could be palpated and/or treated.

I initially worked with an osteopathic colleague and friend so as to get his feedback. With a hand contact over the frontal bone, I visualised the pathway from the lamina terminalis where the nerve is said to originate, passing anteriorly into the subarachnoid space either side of the midline, medial to the olfactory nerve and through the cribriform plate. I then matched any tensions in this area, with my elbow fulcrum, forearm tone and third hand, and mentally invited this nervus terminalis to treat itself if it wanted to. His feedback was intriguing (more on that later).

I then decided to discuss this nerve in the postgraduate course I was running on the first six cranial nerves. This was a class of around 30 students. I described the anatomy and function, also indicating that some authors question its existence. At the end of the practical I asked for the experiences of both being the practitioner and being the patient. Over 70 per cent of the students when being the model lying down had similarities of experience.

At the time of writing, I have repeated this exercise on cranial nerve zero on seven other courses, each having between 20 and 30 students. Again about 60–70 per cent of students indicated similar experiences when being the model lying down and being treated. In all cases I did not give any indication of what they may experience, so as not to influence their own experience during the practical sessions. The feedback from over 200 students working with this nerve has proved to me that:

- the nervus terminalis is present in adults
- the nervus terminalis still has a function affecting the physiology.

So as not to influence the experiences of either you as the practitioner or that of the model lying down, when doing the practical session on CN 0, I will reveal the experiences of my students in the audio practical after you have followed the practical with a friend or colleague. This is not to hide my experiences with my students, nor to make you do the practical session, it is only to make your experiences and those of the model lying down at the treatment table more valid.

Initially, I would strongly advise not working with a patient until you have listened to the audio whilst working with a colleague or friend at the treatment table. Clearly more scientific research, other than osteopathic palpation and treatment, needs to be done on this poorly understood nerve.

OLFACTORY NERVE (CN I)

This nerve and CN 0 are the shortest of the cranial nerves. CN I is embryologically derived from the forebrain and so should be considered an aspect of the central nervous system rather than a separate nerve. Its function is that of the sense of smell. In humans the sense of smell is significantly reduced compared with that of many mammals. As we know, dogs can be trained to detect illegal drugs and other substances and have also been trained to detect clinical states of their owners (by detecting chemical changes within the person associated with a medical condition). Clearly this is an ability way beyond even the most acute human sense of smell.

However, smell does come into play in human behaviour, with the global fragrance market estimated to be worth £40.7 billion per annum (Djordjevic 2022). Clearly this nerve has created a phenomenal industry all by itself. We also use this nerve with our meals. Each and every time we eat, we take our food from the plate or bowl and bring it to our mouth. To get to our mouth it has to pass underneath our nose, and we get a smell of the food before it enters our mouth and reaches our taste buds.

I once had a patient who had an injury to the frontal bone region and on palpation had injured the ethmoid bone. His main complaint was that he could not taste his wife's curries, which he very much enjoyed. His nerves supplying the tongue taste buds were not disturbed, only his olfactory nerve. Treating and releasing the first cranial nerve and the surrounding cranial mechanics restored his enjoyment of his wife's cooking. So, we need to be mindful that sometimes when we are considering a particular sense, we need to ensure it is not being confused with another of our five senses.

Anatomically the olfactory nerve starts in the epithelium of the upper regions of the nasal cavity. These neurons then pass superiorly to traverse the cribriform plate, lateral to CN 0 and the subarachnoid space, where they then accumulate to form the olfactory bulb. The olfactory bulb lies directly underneath the frontal lobes of the brain in the midline. It is here in the bulb that smell detection is received. Axons receiving stimulus from specific chemicals or a variety of chemicals with similar composition each get sent to a specific glomerulus. These glomeruli are balls of nerve tissue which have the effect of amplifying the stimulus from a single smell source, even if only a few axons are stimulated by the chemical.

From the olfactory bulb, the signals are then sent to the amygdala at the base of the brain, part of the limbic system. It is in the amygdala that we attach meanings and associations to our sense of smell, and it is a key area where we process strong emotions and fear. For example, when a person wears a particular fragrance on a date with someone, if the date between the two people is successful and the relationship develops, wearing the same scent at a later date, at an unconscious level via the amygdala, brings about the same loving feelings as that first meeting: hence the perfume industry.

It is worth noting at this point that the olfactory system has a unique ability in repair and regeneration, an ability which stays throughout life. Within the nasal cavity are stem cells, located in the olfactory epithelium, and these stem cells form new neurons throughout life. This ability to form new neurons for the whole of life occurs in both the main nasal epithelium and the neuroepithelium at the basal aspect of the nasal septum (Beecher *et al.* 2018).

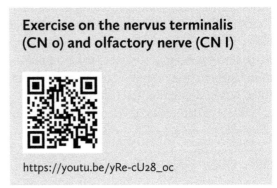

Exercise on the nervus terminalis (CN 0) and olfactory nerve (CN I)

https://youtu.be/yRe-cU28_oc

OPTIC NERVE (CN II)

The optic nerve, like the olfactory nerve, is embryologically an extension of brain tissue, as the eye itself develops from brain tissue. At around day 22 of intrauterine life (IUL) the forebrain develops an extension at each side, the optic vesicle, which is the precursor of the eye. This is covered by surface ectoderm which will evolve to form the lens, the conjunctiva and finally the eyelids. The optic stalk is an outgrowth of the third ventricle which continues to the eye, forming the optic cup with the retina within. The retina being continuous with the brain tissue follows the cup of the eye, and the optic blood vessels supplying nutriment reach the eye via the optic stalk.

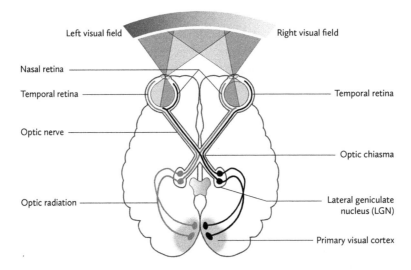

Figure 11.2 Visual pathway from the retina to the visual cortex of the brain.

By three months IUL the eye has eyelids and a fully developed lens, along with the anterior and posterior chambers of the eye. By five months the pupil is developing, and the vitreous humour is expanding to give the eye the fully rounded shape and pressing the retina firmly against the surrounding choroid. The optic stalk invaginates to allow the entry of the optic blood vessels into the centre, and the neural tissue expands around the blood vessels. Eventually the neural tissue fills the space between the outer wall of the stalk and the central artery and vein. Finally, the blood vessels within the posterior chamber get reabsorbed so as not to obstruct vision.

Optic nerve (CN II) function

The optic nerve (CN II) sends visual signals from the retina to the brain. The signals reach the visual cortex of the brain, lying in the occipital lobe, via the optic nerve and tract and the optic radiation.

CN II starts as a disc approximately 1.5 mm in diameter at the posterior aspect of the eye. This disc receives all the axons from the retina and itself has no rods or cones, making it the blind spot of the eye. It then passes posteriorly as the optic nerve through the posterior of the orbit and through the common tendinous ring. Before entering the optic canal, the nerve becomes insulated by glial cells (oligodendrocytes), and then enters the skull through the optical canal of the lesser wing of the sphenoid, adjacent to the ophthalmic artery.

Having entered the skull, the two optic nerves join each other at the optic chiasm. The fibres carrying signals from the lateral aspects of the retina do not cross over, but stay on their respective sides. The fibres conveying signals from the medial aspects of the retina do cross over at the chiasm. After the chiasm, where the fibres from the medial aspect of the retina cross over, some fibres then take a separate journey and instead of going on to reach the visual cortex, have a separate function in sending signals to the reflexes which control pupil size, and the amount of light allowed to enter the eye. This reflex function will be discussed more with CN III.

The vastly greater remaining fibres pass to the lateral geniculate nucleus and then radiate round anteriorly, laterally, posteriorly and then posteromedial, to finally reach their destination in the left and right visual cortices at the posterior aspect of each cerebral hemisphere.

Now, we should remember that the pupil acts like a 'pin hole' in a pin hole camera, causing the light to be reflected upside down and left to right on the retinal surface. Images which are received by the lateral aspects of the retina (i.e., those from the nasal (medial) aspects of our field of vision from each eye) do not cross over at the optic chiasm. Images received by the medial aspect of the retina (i.e., those from the lateral aspects of our field of vision from each eye) do cross over at the optic chiasm (see Figure 11.2). This results in stereoscopic vision and enables us to determine depth and distance, in addition to seeing the image.

Exercise on the optic nerve (CN II)

https://youtu.be/hdS5j5TLM1g

OCULOMOTOR NERVE (CN III)

This nerve, as the name implies, is responsible for most of the muscle movements of the orbit. It also supplies parasympathetic signals which alter the size of the pupil of the eye, in addition to sympathetic fibres which, although not strictly oculomotor fibres, join it to help raise the eyelids.

Eye movement is more complex than at first it may seem. The axes of the orbits are not directed perfectly anteriorly, but the true axes are antero-lateral. Therefore, moving the eye to look at what we want to see may need compensatory muscle actions. Hence the need for muscles working in coordination to take the eyeball to the correct visual position.

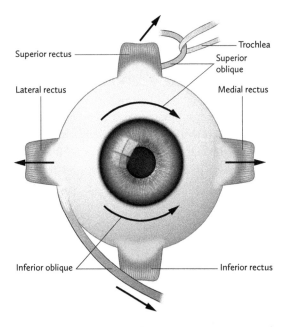

Figure 11.3 The right eye, showing movements created by the different eye muscles.

Control of eye movement

The oculomotor nerve (CN III) controls the following muscles:

- Superior rectus, which elevates the eye from looking straight ahead.

- Medial rectus, which adducts the eye from looking straight ahead.
- Inferior rectus, which moves the eye down from looking straight ahead.
- Inferior oblique, which elevates the eye when the eye is adducted from looking straight ahead.

The trochlear nerve (CN IV) controls the superior oblique muscle, which moves the eye in the inferior and lateral position and intorts it (rotates the eye towards the nose). The abducent nerve (CN VI) controls the lateral rectus muscle, which moves the eye laterally from looking straight ahead.

CN III commences at the Edinger–Westphal nucleus in the midbrain aspect of the brain stem, anterior to the cerebral aqueduct. The nerve then travels anteriorly to leave the brain stem and passes over the petrosphenous ligament. This is the continuation of the dura mater from the tip of the petrous portion of the temporal bone to the posterior clinoid process of the sphenoid bone. From here CN III passes into the superior aspect of the cavernous sinus. Within the cavernous sinus it picks up sympathetic fibres, which hitchhike in its nerve sheath.

The nerve splits into superior and inferior branches close to its passing through the superior orbital fissure of the sphenoid. Once within the orbit the superior branch passes superiorly to the superior rectus muscle and also gives a branch to the levator palpebrae muscle. The inferior branch passes anteriorly and gives branches to the inferior rectus, medial rectus and inferior oblique muscles. It also sends fibres to the ciliary ganglion.

Oculomotor nerve (CN III) function

The superior branch gives motor supply to the superior rectus for elevating the eye and the levator palpebrae superioris for raising the eyelid. The inferior branch supplies the inferior rectus, which moves the eye downwards; the medial rectus, which moves the eye medially; and the inferior oblique. The inferior oblique muscle is the only orbital muscle which does not have its origin in the apex of the orbit but instead arises from the orbital surface of the maxillary bone. Its function is to roll the eyeball in a combination of directions: mainly to roll the vertical meridian of the eye in the direction of the temporal bone (also known as extorsion), secondarily to elevate the eyeball, and lastly to have an abducting effect (see Figure 11.3).

The pupil is controlled by CN III having received information from CN II indicating the brightness of the light entering the eyes. Some of the light signals from the optic nerve (CN II) which do not cross over in the chiasm pass to the posterior part of the brain stem to relay signals in the pretectal area at the most posterior aspect of the brain stem. From there they pass to the Edinger–Westphal nucleus (the origin of CN III) and leave the brain stem anteriorly with CN III and travel back to the ciliary ganglion of the eye to control pupil size.

TROCHLEAR NERVE (CN IV)

This is the smallest cranial nerve in terms of the number of axons and is the only cranial nerve which emerges from the posterior aspect of the brain stem. It also has the longest intracranial journey of all the cranial nerves.

The nerve emerges from the trochlear nucleus at the posterior aspect of the brain stem. At the back of the brain stem, it then crosses over the midline to pass around the sides of the brain stem.

CN IV then passes anteriorly, going immediately underneath the petrosphenous ligament to the cavernous sinus. Here it lies just inferior to CN III on the lateral wall of the sinus, before entering the superior orbital fissure above the superior branch of CN III. The nerve then enters the orbit to enter the belly of the superior oblique

muscle. Unlike the oculomotor nerve, it only supplies this one muscle.

Trochlear nerve (CN IV) function

The role of the trochlear nerve is to innervate the superior oblique muscle of the eye. The superior oblique muscle, which originates at the common tendinous ring at the posterior aspect of the orbit, has its tendon passing through the trochlea (a fibrous sling) to attach to the upper part of the eyeball, but coming from the superior and medial direction, due to the action of the sling. Therefore, the action of the superior oblique muscle is both to pull the eyeball downwards and also to pull the eyeball so that the vertical meridian is pulled in the direction of the nose (also referred to as intorsion, see Figure 11.3).

ABDUCENT (ABDUCENS) NERVE (CN VI)

I hope the reader will excuse me for putting the abducent nerve next, even though the trigeminal nerve (CN V) should come at this point in the list. The reason is quite simple, as CN VI is the last cranial nerve to supply the orbit and eye motion. It is therefore logical to discuss it here, as we are looking at the eye, and so that the

exercise on the eye can then cover cranial nerves II, III, IV and VI.

The abducent nerve arises from its nucleus at the posterior aspect of the pons. The fibres then pass anteriorly though the pons to emerge most medially just below the pons at its junction with the medulla. They emerge just medial to the facial nerve (CN VII). From this point they pass in an anterosuperior direction into the dura and become surrounded in a dural fibrous sheath. The nerve then passes underneath the petrosphenous ligament, more inferior than CN IV, and then to the cavernous sinus.

Within the cavernous sinus it lies towards the lateral wall but just medial to the much larger ophthalmic division of the trigeminal nerve. Passing through the superior orbital fissure of the sphenoid just inferior to the inferior branch of the CN III makes it the most inferior nerve passing though the superior orbital fissure. Once inside the orbit, CN VI then immediately passes through the common tendinous ring as the most inferior nerve, and passes laterally into the belly of the lateral rectus muscle.

Abducent nerve (CN VI) function

Quite simply the CN VI abducts the eye, making that eye look laterally. However, do remember that to look at an object to the right side of our body, for example, the right eye moves laterally, whereas the left eye moves medially and vice versa. Therefore, to look at objects, depending on where they are located relative to our eyes, each eye may be moving in different directions and using a different eye muscle to see them.

N.B. A quick way of remembering which cranial nerve supplies which muscle: CN IV only supplies the superior oblique muscle. CN VI only supplies the lateral rectus and therefore, CN III supplies the other four muscles: superior rectus, inferior rectus, medial rectus and inferior oblique.

Clinical considerations: Treating squints

I have at various times in my career treated patients with squints, a condition where the eyes are not both looking in the same direction. Some patients were children and others were adults. In all cases I was totally honest with the patient (or parent if the patient was a child), explaining that osteopathy may be able to ease the pressure onto the nerves to the eye and reduce the squint; however, if I could not find a clear mechanical reason for the disturbance to the relevant cranial nerve(s), then further medical help would be necessary.

Usually, such patients have already seen a medical specialist and come to see me to ascertain if I can help, whilst awaiting the appointment with the consultant, or if the consultant has recommended waiting a few weeks (or months) to see if it resolves. In such cases it gives me a timescale to see if my osteopathic treatment is helping. Therefore, when you see a patient who has a squint, you need to diagnose whether there may have been a mechanical injury, such as a difficult birth or an accident, which is causing the symptoms.

One such patient was an adult who, following a severe car accident, developed a squint in his right eye, which was looking both inferiorly and laterally when his left eye looked straight ahead. He was told by the specialist to wear a patch over his good eye, to strengthen the muscles of the squinting eye. Having taken a detailed case history, I then made a careful palpatory examination. There was a very strong anterior energetic shift to the right side of his head as if the Sutherland Fulcrum was about 3 metres in front of the right side of his body. This reflected the direction that his car was hit at high speed. The consequence (on my palpatory assessment) was that the temporal bone and sphenoid were sheared strongly in the anterior direction, relative to the left side of his head, putting the dura under immense tension. The dura mater around the petrosphenous ligament region was under a high level of tension. The right orbit was also highly distressed as the lateral aspect was shearing more anteriorly than the left side.

Anatomically, it could easily be evaluated that the cranial nerves supplying the ocular muscles were being disturbed and may be resulting in poor motor supply and the consequent squint. This gave me the ethical justification to accept him as a patient and give a course of treatment. I treated him five times. Over the first two treatments my aim was to bring the Sutherland Fulcrum back within his body and then closer to its home location, the region of the straight venous sinus at the junction of the falx cerebri and tentorium cerebelli. Then once 'he was back inside himself', I worked to release tensions within the orbits, sphenoid and temporal regions. After the five appointments, he was delighted as he was seeing in the same direction with both eyes.

Exercise on the eye: CN III, IV and VI

Here we will be looking at the eye and the role of the above three cranial nerves.

Please be very centred before starting these practical sessions, as you would not wish to disturb the function of these nerves!

https://youtu.be/QuQov5HiojY

Exercise on working with the anterior chamber of the eye and ocular pressure

We will also be looking at the topic of raised intraocular pressure in the anterior chamber and how osteopathy may be able to help reduce the pressure.

https://youtu.be/o3hSJZVWxuU

THE TRIGEMINAL NERVE (CN V)

This is the largest cranial nerve and contains both sensory and motor divisions. The motor division of the nerve arises from its nucleus within the pons and supplies motor signals to the muscles of mastication along with motor signals to tensor tympani, the second smallest muscle of the body after stapedius, located within the middle ear.

The sensory component of CN V arises from the sensory nucleus of the trigeminal nerve (also called the substantia gelatinosa). This is an extensive nucleus which runs from the mid-brain, through the pons, continuing though the medulla and extending into the upper part of the spinal cord. According to Fisch, the nerve nucleus may extend farther into the spinal cord than is often acknowledged:

Within the spinal trigeminal nucleus, pars oralis is the superior-most subnucleus: it spanning from the pons to the mid-medulla; pars interpolaris is the middle subnucleus: lying in the mid-medulla; and pars caudalis is the inferior-most subnucleus, spanning from the lower medulla to the upper cervical spinal cord (variably listed termination is anywhere from C2 to C4). (Fisch 2015)

The sensory nuclei form a sensory nerve root which emerges at the level of the mid-pons. The sensory nerve root passes anteriorly and at the level of the tip of the petrous bone, forms the trigeminal ganglion. This is a very large nerve ganglion, and it even makes a slight depression onto the superior aspect near the apex of the petrous bone. We have to remember that the bones formed much later than the nervous system, which allowed the CN V ganglion to make this impression on the bone because it was there first. This depression along with the surrounding dura is the trigeminal or Meckel's cave.

The trigeminal ganglion is quite variable in size. It is known to be as small as 14 mm and as large as 22 mm in its anterior/posterior distance. This can be deceptive, however, due to its concave shape, which results in an actual ganglion thickness of a mere 1.5–2 mm in the anterior/posterior dimension (Yousry *et al.* 2005).

As can be seen, this is a large ganglion, surrounded by dura in the Meckel's cave and lying directly on top of the petrous tip. The nerve leaves the ganglion as three divisions: the ophthalmic nerve (CN Vi), the maxillary nerve (CN Vii) and the mandibular nerve (CN Viii).

Ophthalmic nerve (CN Vi)

This passes anteriorly to enter the cavernous sinus lying on the lateral wall immediately lateral to the abducent nerve (CN VI). From the cavernous sinus it proceeds to the orbit where it gives off sensory branches, the frontal nerve, nasociliary and lacrimal nerves to:

- the skin above the frontal bone, and scalp, in some cases as far back as the mid-aspect of the parietal bones
- the frontal and ethmoidal sinuses
- the upper eyelid and conjunctiva
- the cornea of the eye
- the skin of the nose except the inferior lateral aspects, which are supplied by the maxillary nerve.

The ophthalmic nerve also carries parasympathetic fibres. These originate from the facial nerve (CN Vii) and then from the pterygopalatine ganglion. They then leave the ganglion with Vii, then pass with Vi to the lacrimal gland. Stimulation of the gland causes creation of tears.

Exercise on the ophthalmic division (CN Vi)
Be very centred.

https://youtu.be/RfRD-JyU6NE

Maxillary nerve (CN Vii)

This leaves the trigeminal ganglion and passes with the ophthalmic nerve into the cavernous sinus where it takes the most inferior lateral position within the sinus. From there it passes through the foramen rotundum of the sphenoid bone to then enter the infraorbital canal. It then continues to the pterygopalatine fossa, where it branches into the pterygopalatine ganglion and distributes parasympathetic fibres along with sensory fibres to the branches to the paranasal sinuses.

The nerve then travels on through the orbit to exit at the infraorbital foramen of the maxillary bone to supply the skin of the mid-face, from the lower eyelid to the level of the upper lip and the inferolateral aspects of the nose. Its dermal supply reach extends posteriorly over the zygomatic bone and continues on to the skin over the pterion area. The branches also supply sensation to the nasal cavity, the upper teeth and gums, and the upper palate.

The maxillary nerve carries parasympathetic fibres from the pterygopalatine ganglion to the lacrimal gland with the aid of CN VI. CN Vii also sends parasympathetic signals to the nasal mucosa, stimulating secretion when necessary.

Exercise on the maxillary division (CN Vii)

https://youtu.be/_bgA-pg6b44

Mandibular nerve (CN Viii)

This is the largest of the three divisions of the trigeminal nerve and is the only division to contain motor nerves.

From the ganglion it passes inferiorly to exit the skull through the foramen ovale of the sphenoid. CN Viii immediately gives off a branch, the auriculotemporal nerve. The nerve is unusual in that it splits and passes around on both sides of the middle meningeal artery before then reuniting. It supplies sensation to the area anterior and superior to the external ear, and also supplies the exterior aspect of the ear and tympanic membrane.

The buccal nerve passes between the two heads of the lateral pterygoid muscle and then passes inferiorly to the cheek, next to the tendon of the temporalis muscle, to supply the skin over the upper lip. It also supplies the upper second and third molar teeth.

The inferior alveolar nerve is both sensory and motor. It soon gives off a branch (the mylohyoid nerve) to supply that muscle and the anterior digastric muscle. The rest of the nerve continues down to enter the mandibular canal in the mandibular bone. During this course through the bone, it gives sensory branches to the roots of the teeth. It finally emerges to the lower face through the mental foramen and continues as the mental nerve to supply the skin to the chin and lower lip.

The lingual branch passes inferiorly under the lateral pterygoid where it is joined by the chorda tympani, a branch of CN Vii. It then goes to the anterior two-thirds of the tongue and submandibular gland, receiving taste and giving parasympathetic supply to the gland.

The motor function is to the muscles of mastication: temporalis, masseter and both the medial and lateral pterygoid muscles. The nerve also gives off motor branches to tensor tympani, which stabilises the malleus bone of the middle ear; tensor veli palatini, which raises the soft palate, preventing food going down into the nasopharynx; and the anterior belly of the digastric and mylohyoid muscles, both of which elevate the hyoid during swallowing.

Exercise on the mandibular division (CN Viii)

https://youtu.be/Z2hN74jn7mg

Clinical considerations: Trigeminal neuralgia

It is a common experience that when the source of a pain gets closer to our head, so it seems to be more severe or more distressing. Frequently people with bad brachial neuritis seem to suffer more than those with similarly bad sciatica. It is as if it becomes more difficult to mentally distance yourself from the pain as it gets closer to the head. Hence trigeminal neuralgia (sciatica in the head) is one of the most distressing conditions, and the patient has to be given high level analgesia to cope with the condition. Can we as osteopaths help? If you diagnose that there is a possibility of mechanical nerve irritation of the sensory aspect of the nerve, then by releasing the offending mechanical forces, osteopathy may be able to help.

Anatomically, consider that the sensory nucleus ranges down into the upper cervical spine, maybe as low as C4. Could the upper cervical spine be causing irritation to the cord? Also, the trigeminal ganglion lies on top of the medial aspect of the petrous bone, being surrounded on all other sides by the dura mater of Meckel's cave. Any tensions to the dura mater or any compressive forces through the temporal bone may be affecting the ganglion.

The three divisions of the nerve pass through the sphenoid: V1 through the superior orbital fissure between the two wings of the sphenoid, V2 through the foramen rotundum and V3 through the foramen ovale, these both being within the greater wing. We all have seen patients where the sphenoid feels tight and compressed. These foramina in the sphenoid could also get compressed and consequently become smaller, resulting in nerve disturbance.

From there you will need to assess the pathway of the trigeminal divisions on leaving the sphenoid bone and the nerve branches, depending on where the symptoms are located.

Always advise patients that you *may* be able to help, in case the treatment response does not ease the highly severe symptoms. However, if you can reduce, even if not eradicate the symptoms, the patient will be delighted.

THE FACIAL NERVE (CN VII)

The main function of the facial nerve is the motor supply to the muscles of the face, the muscles of facial expression. However, it also receives the sensory return from the area around the concha of the external ear, and that of taste from the anterior two-thirds of the tongue. The nerve also carries parasympathetic signals to the submandibular glands, mucous glands of the nose, palate and pharynx, and to the lacrimal gland.

The nerve arises in the pons of the brain as a large motor root and a smaller sensory root. They pass into the internal acoustic meatus on the petrous temporal bone and then enter the facial canal within the bone. This is a 'z' shaped canal within the petrous bone. Within the canal the two roots form a single nerve which then creates the geniculate ganglion (knee bend ganglion) and also gives off the greater petrosal nerve, which carries the parasympathetic fibres to the lacrimal gland and the mucous glands.

Within the canal, the nerve gives off a motor branch to stapedius, the smallest muscle of the body within the middle ear (only 1 mm in length), which stabilises the stapes bone, the smallest bone of the body. Lastly whilst within the facial canal, the nerve gives off the chorda tympani, which receives taste from the anterior two-thirds of the tongue along with sending parasympathetic fibres to the submandibular and sublingual salivary glands.

The nerve then leaves the facial canal at the stylomastoid foramen. This is a small opening between the mastoid and the external ear. (N.B. In babies the mastoid does not exist and is prominent by 2 years of age, continuing to grow until age 6.) This location between the mastoid and external ear gives CN VII protection. Having exited the skull, it gives off branches to the muscles immediately near the ear as the posterior auricular nerve. It then gives branches to the posterior belly of digastric and to the stylohyoid muscles. The remainder of the nerve descends to pass through the parotid gland, without innervating it, to supply the muscles of facial expression:

- The temporal branch supplies frontalis, orbicularis oculi and corrugator supercilii.
- The zygomatic branch supplies orbicularis oculi.
- The buccal branch supplies orbicularis oris, buccinator and zygomaticus.

- The marginal mandibular branch supplies depressor labii inferioris and depressor anguli oris.
- The cervical branch supplies the platysma.

The chorda tympani nerve receives taste from the anterior two-thirds of the tongue. It leaves from within the facial canal and passes across the bones of the middle ear, and exits the skull at the petrotympanic fissure to enter the infratemporal fossa. It then hitchhikes with the lingual nerve of CN VIII to reach the tongue.

Parasympathetic fibres of CN VII leave at the geniculate ganglion within the facial canal, passing anteromedially to enter the middle cranial fossa. It then passes over the foramen lacerum to become the nerve of the pterygoid canal. Having passed through this canal, it enters the pterygopalatine fossa and synapses in the pterygopalatine ganglion. Fibres leave the ganglion to supply the nasal mucosa oral cavity, nasal cavity, pharynx and lacrimal gland.

Clinical considerations: Bell's palsy

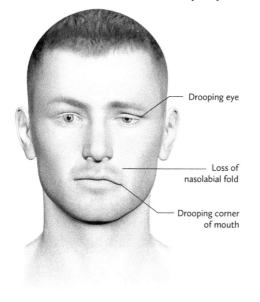

Drooping eye

Loss of nasolabial fold

Drooping corner of mouth

Figure 11.4 Example of a left-sided, lower motor neuron facial palsy.

Bell's palsy is a condition where the patient loses some or all of the control of the muscles of facial expression on one side of the head. This is a highly distressing condition because they look 'odd'. They cannot control their lips on one side, resulting in dribbling of saliva. They cannot show expression on that side of their face, and the affected side looks more 'blank' and will be slightly drooped downwards. The patient will be highly aware of these changes in their facial appearance and may avoid people and choose not to socialise.

As osteopaths we may be able to help such patients as long as we can find a mechanical aetiology. So, we need to consider the facial nerve pathway. Are there any mechanical tensions within the petrous temporal bone on the side of the symptoms? From the entry into the internal acoustic meatus to the exit through the stylomastoid foramen, CN VII is at risk of compression if a trauma were to occur affecting the temporal bone. According to research by Vianna and her colleagues, in non-Bell's palsy patients the facial canal in the labyrinthine segment was 1.83 mm in diameter, with the diameter of the nerve 1.21 mm diameter; in Bell's palsy patients the diameter for the same part of the canal was 1.67 mm, and 1.34 mm for the nerve diameter, a difference of only 0.33 mm (Vianna *et al.* 2014).

As we know when we palpate the temporal bone, it is not rare to palpate a compressive force which could result in a narrowing of the canal by less than 0.33–0.62 mm. So, if a patient with Bell's palsy comes to your practice, do evaluate the anatomy carefully and maybe you can bring about some much-needed help.

CASE STUDY: PETER

Many years ago, I saw a patient with Bell's palsy to the right side of his face, whose work included the use of a pneumatic drill for digging up roads. He had a previous history of pains in his neck on the right side and right shoulder pains. When I examined him, he had a strong mechanical shock and a sense of reverberation to his right temporal bone with compression to the right petrous temporal bone. He also had a chronic tension within his neck especially on the right side, even though that was currently asymptomatic, and similar asymptomatic tension to the right glenohumeral joint and scapula.

This made good diagnostic sense to his Bell's palsy. The strong reverberation forces from the pneumatic drill were travelling up his arms to his neck and head. However, because of the pre-existing tensions to the right side of his neck and shoulder girdle, the shockwaves from the drill would have been travelling to the head without any damping of the shock by the shoulder and neck regions. Hence on the right side of his skull the shockwaves would have been greater and affecting the right temporal bone more than the left, and probably affecting the facial nerve within the facial canal or its exit through the stylomastoid foramen. This working diagnosis gave me confidence to proceed with a course of treatment which proved to be completely successful after four treatments.

Therefore, before you say that you can help a Bell's palsy patient, ask yourself whether you can find a mechanical reason why the facial nerve could be disturbed, interrupting the nerve signals to the muscles of facial expression. If yes, then you *may* be able to help the patient. Even in this situation, do not guarantee to the patient 100 per cent success, just give a guideline statement that there are reasons why you may be successful. Nothing is worse than saying to such a patient that you can certainly help them, and then failing to do so. However, if you can help them, they will be highly delighted.

Exercise on the facial nerve (CN VII)

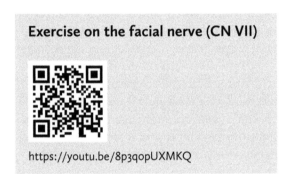

https://youtu.be/8p3qopUXMKQ

THE VESTIBULOCOCHLEAR NERVE (CN VIII)

This nerve comprises two parts, the cochlear nerve to receive hearing signals from the cochlea and the vestibular nerve conveying position in space and motion. In reality they are two totally separate nerves, but they become one nerve before leaving the brain. The vestibular nerve arises from the vestibular nuclei within the pons and medulla of the brain; and the cochlear nerve arises from the ventral and dorsal cochlear nuclei in the cerebellar peduncles between the brain stem and cerebellum. Within the pons they form the vestibulocochlear nerve. The nerve exits the brain anterolaterally and after a short distance, enters the temporal petrous bone via the internal acoustic meatus. Once within the petrous bone it enters the auditory canal (also called the internal acoustic meatus) where the nerve splits into the cochlear nerve and vestibular nerve to reach their differing destinations of the inner ear, the vestibular canals and the cochlea.

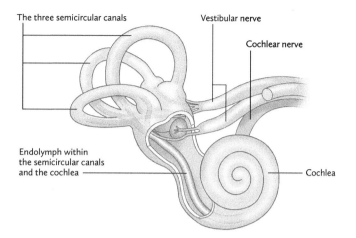

Figure 11.5 The inner ear, showing both the vestibular system and cochlea. Notice the endolymph within the vestibular system and cochlea are continuous. The endolymphatic sac is within the dura mater, subject to tensions of the dura. The cochlear aqueduct is continuous with the CSF.

The vestibular system

The vestibular system comprises three semicircular canals: the anterior canal, posterior canal and horizontal canal, each being in one of the three planes of movement. At the base of the canals are chambers called the utricle and the saccules. The canals and the chambers are full of endolymphatic fluid which is continuous with the fluid within the cochlea.

The utricle and saccules: The static labyrinth

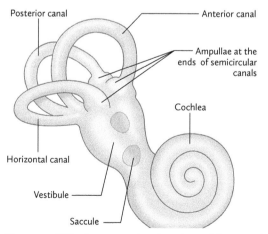

Figure 11.6 The inner ear, showing the utricle, saccule and vestibule along with the ampulla for each semicircular canal.

Both the utricle and saccules detect the position of the head relative to gravity, giving us a sense of up and down. They have a patch of ciliated hair cells in an area called the macula. At the end of each hair, there is a calcium carbonate crystal. Gravity affects these crystals, and such movements then stimulate the vestibular nerve receptors to give the gravity relationship information to the brain.

The semicircular canals: The kinetic labyrinth

These are each angled at 90° to each other. They each have a swelling at the end of the canal which, like the utricle and saccules, contain hair cells similar to those in the static labyrinth. The canals are filled with endolymphatic fluid which moves along the respective canals depending on the direction of head movement. Movement of the fluid causes motion of the cilia of the hair cells to bend and creates an electrical signal. These signals are then sent to the vestibular nerve detectors and back to the brain.

It is worth noting that the brain needs to know if the position of the body relative to gravity is changing, so that it can adjust our posture at an unconscious level, to avoid injury. Consequently, the vestibular signals are sent to the cerebellum, which controls the unconscious postural muscles and prevents us from having falls.

Cochlear nerve (acoustic nerve)

This receives the signals from the cochlea and sends the auditory signals to the brain. The sound waves enter the ear complex via the external ear catching the sounds, which then vibrate the tympanic membrane. This then initially vibrates the malleus, then the incus and subsequently stapes, the three smallest bones in the body. The stapes then vibrates the oval window which is attached to the foot of the cochlea. The stapes bone is stabilised by the stapedius muscle, which prevents excessive vibration of the cochlea. The oval window sets up a vibration in the perilymph which surrounds the endolymph within the cochlea. Being adjacent to the perilymph, the endolymph is then vibrated.

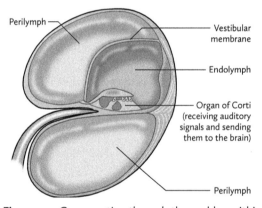

Perilymph
Vestibular membrane
Endolymph
Organ of Corti (receiving auditory signals and sending them to the brain)
Perilymph

Figure 11.7 Cross-section through the cochlea within the petrous bone.

The cochlea, as the name implies, is a spiral shaped organ with the termination narrower than the foot. Consequently, the different frequencies of vibration, due to the varying pitch of sound, vibrate the hairs within the organ of Corti in varying places. The higher pitch sounds activate the hairs towards the apex and lower sounds activate those hairs nearer the foot of the cochlea. The cochlear or auditory nerve then transmits these signals from the organ of Corti to the brain stem. The round window at the foot of the cochlea but just inferior to the oval window, dissipates the 'acknowledged' vibrations in the cochlea back to the air in the middle ear to prevent confusion with the next incoming signals.

Clinical study 1: Vestibular neuritis

Loss of balance and/or dizziness is a distressing condition which may in some cases lead to the patient falling over, with resultant risk of injury. When evaluating the patient, we need to consider if there could be any interference to the vestibular system including the pathway of the vestibular nerve. So be aware of the anatomy of the vestibular nerve pathway through the petrous bone and the auditory canal, where it may be most at risk of nerve interference.

The semi-circular canals (SCC) are very thin: 'The inner diameter measurements of the anterior SCC, lateral SCC, and posterior SCC were 0.101 ± 0.016, 0.135 ± 0.033, and 0.124 ± 0.021 cm, respectively' (Daocai *et al.* 2014).

If you find evidence of mechanical tensions to the vestibular nerve pathway and/or the petrous bone on either side (the organs of balance acting as a balanced pair), then you may be able to reduce the dizziness.

I have helped a number of patients with vestibular imbalance, but not all cases, so do give a cautioned response when a patient asks if you can help. If you do remove or reduce the vestibular condition, your patient will be extremely grateful.

Clinical study 2: Auditory disturbances

Disturbance of hearing (as opposed to loss of hearing) such as tinnitus affects quite a large percentage of the population: 'Around

13% of adults in the UK (7.1 million people) experience prolonged tinnitus' (NICE 2022).

It is worth remembering that sound and smell are the only senses that you cannot consciously turn off. Even touch may be turned off during sleep. We can close our eyes and mouth but not our ears and nose. Hence to have frequent or constant ringing, whistling or other sounds in your ear that do not seem to come or go for any logical reason is very distressing to the patient, as their brain is continually having to ignore the sounds.

Again, with such patients give a response without promises when asked if you can help. Diagnostically, can you ascertain any mechanical reason why the auditory pathway from tympanic membrane to brain stem could be disturbed in some way? If yes, then by reducing such mechanical forces, you may help reduce the symptoms.

Exercise on the ear and CN VIII

https://youtu.be/OFG9QYmOF9o

GLOSSOPHARYNGEAL NERVE (CN IX)

Figure 11.8 The glossopharyngeal nerve (CN IX).

Labels: Foramen ovale; Pons; Hiatus of the lesser petrosal nerve; Otic ganglion; Medulla; Lesser petrosal nerve; Tympanic plexus; Jugular foramen; Superior jugular ganglion; Inferior petrous ganglion; Tympanic nerve; Nerve to stylopharyngeus; Pharyngeal branch; Tonsillar branch; Lingual nerve; Carotid body/sinus branch

As with a number of cranial nerves, CN IX is a mixed nerve. It has motor fibres, special sensory fibres, parasympathetic fibres and sympathetic fibres. CN IX arises from the brain stem at the lateral aspect of the medulla, just anterior to the vagal nerve. It then passes laterally to the jugular foramen.

The glossopharyngeal nerve (CN IX) lying within the jugular foramen, along with the vagus (CN X) and accessory nerves (CN XI), is separated from X and XI by a slip of dura mater which is always present (Colacicco 2021). At the level of the jugular foramen (though some anatomists indicate it is just inferior to the foramen), the nerve has superior and inferior ganglia. Passing inferiorly from the foramen, the nerve has its own individual sheath of dura mater.

The glossopharyngeal nerve leaves the medulla oblongata aspect of the brain stem and then passes laterally and exits the skull through the jugular foramen (the pars nervosa aspect), which is a separate sheath of dura mater (Hacking 2022). The nerve then passes inferiorly beneath the styloid process of the temporal bone and the associated styloid muscles, lying between the internal jugular vein and the internal carotid artery. At the level of the stylopharyngeus muscle, it passes anteriorly to finally reach the palatine tonsil, the mucous membrane of the fauces (the opening at the back of the mouth into the throat), the base of the tongue, and the mucous glands of the mouth.

Branchial motor component
As CN IX passes adjacent to the stylopharyngeus muscle, it gives the muscle its motor supply.

Visceromotor fibres (parasympathetic)
These fibres pass through both the superior and inferior ganglia within the jugular foramen without synapsing, and continue under the new name of the tympanic nerve.

Just before leaving the jugular foramen, the tympanic nerve enters into the petrous bone along the inferior tympanic canaliculus, which lies just anterior to the jugular foramen. The nerve then enters the tympanic cavity (middle ear) where it forms a plexus to provide general sensation. The visceromotor fibres then travel through this plexus to become the lesser petrosal nerve (LPN). The LPN re-enters the temporal bone to the middle cranial fossa.

From here it leaves the skull through the foramen ovale (with CN VIII). As it exits the skull, the LPN synapses on the otic ganglion which lies just inferior to the foramen ovale. From the otic ganglion these visceromotor fibres from CN IX then hitchhike with the auriculotemporal nerve (CN VIII) to enter the parotid gland and secrete saliva when stimulated by these fibres.

Somatic sensory fibres (pain, temperature and touch)
These fibres which arise from the skin of the external ear then hitchhike with the auricular branch of CN X, whereas the fibres from the middle ear travel with the tympanic nerve (CN IX visceromotor). Somatic sensory information from the upper pharynx and posterior one-third of the tongue travel via the pharyngeal branches of CN IX.

The somatic sensory fibres have their cell bodies within either the superior or inferior ganglia within the jugular foramen.

Special sensory fibres (taste from the posterior third of the tongue)
The lingual branch of CN IX leaves the tongue and passes back to the pharynx where it travels with the main nerve superiorly back to the jugular foramen and the brain stem.

Special sensory fibres from the carotid sinus (carotid sinus nerve, Hering's nerve)
This nerve innervates the baroreceptors of the carotid sinus and the chemoreceptors of the carotid body. The feedback from this nerve informs the brain stem if the blood pressure requires adjustment and, if so, will reset the physiology where possible, to rebalance the system. Equally the chemoreceptors which detect both O_2 and CO_2 levels inform the brain stem if the pulmonary breath rate or level of breath volume needs to be adjusted to bring about a normalisation of blood chemistry.

Clinical study 3: Glossopharyngeal neuralgia
Glossopharyngeal neuralgia is described as a sharp stabbing pain in the pharynx, the back of the tongue and also the middle ear, and can be associated with a low heart rate and fainting episodes. Luckily it is considered to be very rare. According to the Weill Institute for Neurosciences (2022), the incidence of this condition is 2–7 people per million population.

Should you ever see a patient with this type of neuralgia (I have not), you would need to consider the anatomical pathway and where it may be at risk. Remember that the nerve has its own dural sheath, in and after the jugular foramen. The sensory cells are within the superior and inferior ganglia. These are often located within the jugular foramen but may be inferior to it.

If the patient had dural tensions around the jugular foramen (as many do), could this be infringing on CN IX? Clearly with such a distressing condition, if you do see such a clinical condition, give a guarded response when asked if you can help. Possibly yes, possibly no.

Exercise on the glossopharyngeal nerve (CN IX)

Please centre yourself before commencing this practical.

https://youtu.be/wdGGLbFN4Cw

THE VAGUS (WANDERING) NERVE (CN X)

This is by far the longest cranial nerve, extending to the distal third of the transverse colon (though the exact end point is variable). It is a mixed nerve having, like CN IX, a variety of functions: motor, sensory, special sensory and parasympathetic.

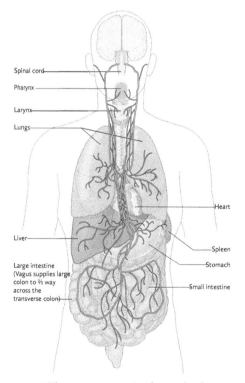

Spinal cord
Pharynx
Larynx
Lungs
Liver
Large intestine
(Vagus supplies large colon to ⅔ way across the transverse colon)
Heart
Spleen
Stomach
Small intestine

Figure 11.9 The vagus nerve in the neck, thorax and abdomen.

The vagus nerve has four nuclei within the medulla of the brain stem: the dorsal motor nucleus, the nucleus ambiguus, the solitary nucleus and the spinal trigeminal, a nucleus which receives a small input from the trigeminal. The dorsal motor nucleus sends parasympathetic fibres to the heart and lungs, and also innervates the smooth muscle of the gut wall and the secretory glands within the gut. The nucleus ambiguus lies within the reticular formation and gives off the fibres for controlling swallowing and also the production of vocal sounds and speech.

The solitary nucleus lies within the dorsomedial aspect of the medulla. This nucleus receives signals with information arising in the carotid sinus and carotid body, which as has been said above, are innervated by CN IX, and also the aortic bodies and sinoatrial node, which are supplied by CN X. The tractus solitarius also receives sensations of taste from the whole tongue. The anterior two-thirds of the tongue are innervated by the facial nerve (CN VII) and the posterior one-third by the glossopharyngeal nerve (CN IX). It is the tractus solitarius (solitary nucleus) which causes us to vomit, produces the gag reflex, carotid sinus reflex and cough reflex. The spinal trigeminal nucleus receives sensory signals from the pinna of the ear, with respect to pain, touch and temperature, in addition to receiving sensory signals from the dura mater within the posterior cranial fossa and the mucosa of the larynx.

The nerve leaves the brain stem and immediately passes laterally to exit via the jugular foramen in the posterior section alongside the accessory nerve (CN XI), CN IX being within its own compartment of the jugular foramen. The small auricular branch of the vagus arises from the superior vagal ganglion, and passes posterior to the internal jugular vein to enter the mastoid canaliculus, which lies on the lateral aspect of the jugular fossa. The auricular nerve of the vagus then passes over the facial canal a few millimetres above the stylomastoid foramen. Finally, the branch reaches its destination by passing through the fissure between the mastoid and the tympanic part of the temporal bone. It receives sensory input from the central area of the pinna and the posterior aspect of the external auditory canal. (N.B. If you ever use a cotton bud to remove ear wax from your ears, you will at the same time be directly stimulating the vagus nerve!)

After descending into the upper neck, the vagus nerve enters the carotid sheath, lying protected between the common carotid artery and jugular vein. At the inferior aspect of the neck, the nerve leaves the carotid sheath. Within the neck, the nerve gives off branches to supply the pharynx and larynx, and also gives off the cervical (superior) cardiac nerve. The upper branches which come from the upper region of the neck are small and communicate with the sympathetic nerves to the heart, in the inner part of the cardiac plexus. The lower branches come from the base of the neck near the first rib.

The branch on the right side of the body passes close to the brachiocephalic artery and goes to the deeper aspect of the cardiac plexus. The thoracic (inferior) cardiac nerve goes to the deep aspect of the cardiac plexus, the right branch coming off the vagal trunk, arriving via the side of the trachea. The left branch comes off the recurrent laryngeal nerve and then passes medially to join the right branch at the cardiac plexus to supply the heart.

The lungs are also supplied by the vagus nerve, via the anterior and posterior pulmonary branches (sometimes called the A & P bronchial branches). There are two or three small anterior branches which pass to the root of the lung where they meet with sympathetic fibres to form the anterior pulmonary plexus. The posterior branches are in greater numbers and larger than the anterior branches. They go to the posterior aspect of the root of the lung where they are also joined by sympathetic nerves. From the pulmonary plexus, the nerves spread throughout the lungs alongside the bronchi. After entering the thorax, the main vagal trunk differs on the left and right sides.

The left vagus passes anteriorly to the subclavian artery to enter the thorax between the subclavian artery and the left common carotid artery. Once within the thorax the nerve passes inferiorly on the left side of the arch of the aorta, separating it from the left pleura. It continues posterior to the phrenic nerve and the root of the left lung. It then passes inferiorly and medially to reach the oesophagus where it combines with the right vagus to form the oesophageal plexus.

The right vagus passes anterior to the right subclavian artery and enters the thorax to the right side of the trachea, separating it from pleura. The nerve then passes posterior to the root (hilum) of the right lung, then passes inferiorly and medially to join the left vagus in the oesophageal plexus.

From the oesophageal plexus the vagus nerve descends into the abdomen. The right vagus forms the posterior gastric plexus on the posteroinferior surface of the stomach, and the left vagus forms the anterior gastric plexus on the anterosuperior aspect. CN X then gives off the coeliac branches, which arise mainly from the right vagus, forming the coeliac plexus of nerves which supplies the pancreas, spleen, kidneys and adrenal glands, and the intestine. The liver is supplied by the left vagus, which joins the hepatic plexus, and the branches are then distributed throughout the whole liver.

Clinical considerations: The vagus nerve

As is very clear, the vagus nerve has a phenomenal consequence to the whole body. I personally think it should be renamed the 'keep me alive' nerve, as it supplies the heart, lungs, liver, pancreas, digestive system, and adrenals and kidneys!

We may see a patient who has a vagal imbalance to a particular organ or tissue. Can we help as osteopaths? As we know this will depend on your diagnostic findings and (if we are honest) the accuracy of your diagnosis. Can you ascertain a mechanical tension in the anatomical region, or even better, the exact location of the vagal nerve pathway from the brain stem to that organ? If yes, then by reducing the offending mechanical forces, then perhaps you can help. However, you may also need to check whether there may be a poor venous return from the organ, creating venous congestion around the tissues. By helping both the nerve supply and the circulation of the tissue/organ, your chances of helping the physiological imbalance will increase.

Frequently the relationship between the sympathetic and parasympathetic nervous systems can get out of balance. This is particularly true in states of anxiety and in the face of the 'fight or flight' stress response. The vagus being the main nerve of the parasympathetic system, it naturally gets involved in such an imbalance. This topic will be further discussed in Chapter 16: The inner relationship of mind, body and emotions.

At this point I will comment briefly on the polyvagal theory and its possible clinical relevance. The theory investigates the shift from reptilian vagal control to mammalian vagal control and the consequent rearrangement of vagal nuclei, giving the nucleus ambiguus a role quite different from the other, more posterior vagal nuclei:

Its specific focus is on the phylogenetic shift between reptiles and mammals that resulted in specific changes to the vagal pathways regulating the heart. As the source nuclei of the primary vagal efferent pathways regulating the heart shifted from the dorsal motor nucleus of the vagus in reptiles to the nucleus ambiguus in mammals, a face–heart connection evolved with emergent properties of a social engagement system that would enable social interactions to regulate visceral state.

In this way, the theory provides a plausible explanation for the reported covariation between atypical autonomic regulation (e.g., reduced vagal and increased sympathetic influences to the heart) and psychiatric and behavioural disorders that involve difficulties in regulating appropriate social, emotional, and communication behaviours. (Porges 2009)

Some scientists question the validity of this theory and others praise it. I have no further comment on this theory as I work with all vagal nuclei, where the palpation indicates it being necessary, without reference to polyvagal theory. However, I felt it should be mentioned at this point in the text as some osteopaths have found it very beneficial when working with patients.

Exercise on the vagus nerve (CN X)

Because of the length and complexity of the vagus, the practical exercise for this nerve will be split into three sections. The first practical will be on the brain stem, the jugular foramen, and its journey through the neck. The second practical session will be on the vagus in the thorax, and the third practical will be on the vagus in the abdomen.

Do have a break between doing the three practical sessions, so as not to tire yourself and to not over treat your friend/colleague on the treatment table.

As always, do centre yourself well before starting the practical sessions.

Exercise on the vagus 1: The head and neck

https://youtu.be/Y22LDXNaNTs

Exercise on the vagus 3: The abdomen

https://youtu.be/u2orbv4BlhM

Exercise on the vagus 2: The thorax

https://youtu.be/TdsDThbyhN8

THE ACCESSORY NERVE (CN XI)

The accessory nerve has both a spinal nerve, the spinal accessory nerve, and also an aspect which arises from within the skull. The origins of the spinal accessory nerve arise in the neurons within the spinal cord at the levels of C1–C5 and sometimes also C6. The fibres then pass superiorly adjacent to the spinal cord to enter the foramen magnum. Once inside the cranium they cross laterally over the posterior cranial fossa to reach the jugular foramen.

The cranial component arises from the lower motor neurons of the nucleus ambiguus lying to the lateral aspect of the medulla. These fibres pass within the medulla to reach the jugular foramen where they meet and combine with the spinal component of CN XI, lying next to the vagus in the same posterior aspect of the jugular foramen. Immediately after leaving the jugular foramen, the cranial fibres which originated in the brain stem combine with the vagus nerve to travel with the pharyngeal and laryngeal branches of the vagus to the soft palate. Because of its anatomical pathway, the cranial component of the accessory nerve is considered part of the vagus nerve.

After exiting the jugular foramen, the spinal accessory fibres pass inferiorly next to the internal carotid artery to reach the sternocleidomastoid muscle to which it gives the motor supply. The nerve then traverses the posterior triangle of the neck to reach the trapezius muscle, again giving it the motor supply.

Clinical considerations: Accessory nerve

The accessory nerve having left the jugular foramen basically lies between the investing and prevertebral layers of fascia of the neck. Consequently, it is at potential risk from mechanical injury to the side of the neck. As will be discussed further in Chapter 16, the trapezius muscle is very much affected by emotions – imagine the stressed person who is described as having their shoulder girdle up around their ears! Could this then create a vicious circle of increasing tension in the trapezius and sternocleidomastoid muscles, which then affects CN XI lying in the cervical fascial system?

Exercise on the accessory nerve (CN XI)
Centre yourself first.

https://youtu.be/VaORc3n350Y

THE HYPOGLOSSAL NERVE (CN XII)

CN XII arises from the hypoglossal nucleus in the most inferior aspect of the medulla oblongata. It passes across the posterior cranial fossa and then into its own canal, the hypoglossal canal, which lies lateral to the jugular foramen. I personally own a skull specimen where the hypoglossal canal is absent on the right side. Presumably, the hypoglossal nerve travelled through the foramen magnum on that side instead.

Having left the skull, the nerve receives fibres from C1 and C2 nerve roots which do not combine with the nerve but just lie within its sheath. These cervical fibres then hitchhike on CN XII to innervate the geniohyoid and thyrohyoid muscles. CN XII then travels inferiorly to the angle of the mandible, passing over both the internal and external carotid arteries to proceed anteriorly into the tongue muscle.

Within the tongue, the nerve gives motor innervation to all aspects of the tongue except palatoglossus, which is supplied by the vagus. CN XII supplies two sets of muscles in the tongue. The extrinsic muscles originate outside of the tongue, and the intrinsic originate and insert within the tongue. The extrinsic muscles supplied by CN XII are genioglossus, hyoglossus and styloglossus, and the intrinsic muscles are the superior longitudinal, inferior longitudinal, transverse and vertical.

Clinical considerations: Hypoglossal nerve

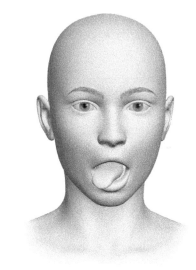

Figure 11.10 Hypoglossal nerve (CN XII) palsy, showing the deviation of the tongue to the affected side when protruded.

Clearly this nerve is highly used for speech and swallowing. As such the tongue is one of the most important muscles of the body. The hypoglossal canal is within the occiput and so may be at risk from compressive forces to the bone. We work with our hands under the occiput on many of our patients, yet we tend to forget this important canal just above our fingers. Do give it some thought when seeing patients.

Hypoglossal nerve palsy is an uncommon condition where the tongue deviates to one side when protruded. The side of the deviation indicates the side of the nerve interference. The cause can be from a tumour, but it can also arise from trauma to the head or neck. If the latter aetiology, then there is the possibility that osteopathy could help.

It is the combination of having both extrinsic and intrinsic muscles which gives the tongue its extraordinary motion ability. Having this amazing motion potential adds to the variety of sounds the mouth can create and can be used within differing languages, and for singing.

Exercise on the hypoglossal nerve (CN XII)

Be centred first.

https://youtu.be/lM5NSTh-eqw

In conclusion, I recommend that you do not take part in too many of the practical sessions at any one time. Working with the cranial nerves can be a very rewarding aspect of our work.

REFERENCES

Beecher, K., St John, J.A., & Chehrehasa, F., 2018. Factors that modulate olfactory dysfunction. *Neural Regeneration Research*. 13(7): 1151-1155. https://doi.org/10.4103/1673-5374.235018.

Colacicco, G., 2021. Conversation with Timothy Marris. Zurich University Anatomy Department, 7 September.

Czernichowska, E., & Rea, P., 2018. The cranial nerve 0 (nervus terminalis) in adult humans. Available from: https://eprints.gla.ac.uk/174138/

Daocai, W., Qing, W., Ximing, W., *et al.*, 2014. Size of the semi-circular canals measured by multidetector computed tomography in different age groups. *Journal of Computer Assisted Tomography*. 38(2): 196-199. https://doi.org/10.1097/RCT.0b013e3182aaf21c.

Djordjevic, M., 2022. 23 perfume industry statistics to catch a whiff of right now. Available from: https://fashiondiscounts.uk/perfume-industry-statistics/#:~:text=The%20global%20fragrance%20market%20is%20worth%20%C2%A340.7%20billion.

Fisch, A., 2015. Clinical examination of the cranial nerves. In: Tubbs, R.S., Shoja, M.M., Barbaro, N., *et al.*, eds. *Nerves and Nerve Injuries*. Elsevier. Available from: https://www.sciencedirect.com/topics/neuroscience/spinal-trigeminal-nucleus.

Hacking, C., 2022. Glossopharyngeal nerve. Radiopaedia.org. Available from: https://doi.org/10.53347/rID-7173.

Kang, O., 2021. Nervus terminalis. Radiopaedia.org. Available from: https://doi.org/10.53347/rID-34852.

NICE, 2022. Tinnitus: how common is it? Available from: https://cks.nice.org.uk/topics/tinnitus/background-information/prevalence/#:~:text=Tinnitus%20is%20a%20relatively%20common,British%20Tinnitus%20Association%2C%202017%5D.

Porges, S.W., 2009. The polyvagal theory: new insights into adaptive reactions of the autonomic nervous system. *Cleveland Clinic Journal of Medicine*. 76 (Suppl 2): S86-S90. Available from: https://doi.org/10.3949/ccjm.76.s2.17.

Sonne, J., Reddy, V., & Lopez-Ojeda, W., 2022. Neuroanatomy, cranial nerve 0 (terminal nerve). In: StatPearls [Internet]. Treasure Island, FL: StatPearls Publishing. Available from: https://www.ncbi.nlm.nih.gov/books/NBK459159/

Vianna, M., Adams, M., Schachern, P., *et al.*, 2014. Differences in the diameter of facial nerve and facial canal in Bell's palsy: a 3-dimensional temporal bone study. *Otology & Neurotology*. 35(3): 514-518. Available from: https://doi.org/10.1097/MAO.0000000000000240.

Vilenski, J., 2014. The neglected cranial nerve: nervus terminalis (cranial nerve N). *Clinical Anatomy*. 27(1): 46-53. Available from: https://onlinelibrary.wiley.com/doi/pdf/10.1002/ca.22130.

Weill Institute for Neurosciences, 2022. Glossopharyngeal neuralgia FAQ. Available from: https://neurosurgery.ucsf.edu/glossopharyngeal-neuralgia-faq.

Yousry, I., Moriggl, B., Schmid, U.D., *et al.*, 2005. Trigeminal ganglion and its divisions: detailed anatomic MR imaging with contrast-enhanced 3D constructive interference in the steady state sequences. *American Journal of Neuroradiology*. 26(5): 1128-1135. Available from: https://www.ncbi.nlm.nih.gov/pmc/articles/PMC8158638/

CHAPTER 12

The Inner Approach to the Brain

For reasons of its great complexity, this section of the book will only offer an overview of neuroanatomy and physiology of the brain and its differing regions, which in itself is a vast topic. However, I hope it will whet your appetite for further study. There are three separate practical sessions for this chapter, relating to the cerebral hemispheres, brain stem and cerebellum of the brain. These will be found at the end of each relevant section.

The central nervous system (CNS), the brain and spinal cord, along with the heart, must be considered the key areas for life. We can survive, though not healthily, on less than one fully functioning lung, we can survive with large parts of our digestive system missing (as patients who have had cancers removed from these tissues can validate), but the CNS is exceptional. Medical science cannot replace the brain with one from a donor. Even if it were medically possible, would you want to receive someone else's brain?

Some interesting facts about the human brain (Lewis and Taylor 2021; Sachdeva 2019):

- The brain makes up about 2 per cent of a human's body weight.
- The cerebrum makes up 85 per cent of the brain's weight. It contains about 86 billion nerve cells (neurons), the grey matter.
- It contains billions of nerve fibres (axons and dendrites), the white matter.
- These neurons are connected by trillions of connections, or synapses.
- Sixty per cent of the human brain is made of fat. Not only does that make it the fattiest organ in the human body, but these fatty acids are crucial for the brain's performance.
- The brain isn't fully formed until age 25.
- The human brain can generate about 23 watts of power (enough to power a lightbulb). All that power calls for some much-needed rest.

OSTEOPATHIC CONSIDERATIONS

The brain is a highly conscious tissue! The brain as a tissue, and perhaps the patient too, will be aware when you are working on it. Therefore, we as practitioners need to be extremely centred when palpating to diagnose or engage therapeutically with the brain. In Chapter 7 on the meninges, I discussed how we need to work with the arachnoid and pia mater with great respect. The same degree of respect must be given when working with brain tissue.

The brain tissue has a specific gravity only slightly greater than the cerebrospinal fluid surrounding it and within it. Back in 1901, Gompertz calculated the brain specific gravity of males and females who had died from a variety of causes. He found in males an average specific gravity of 1.0361 and only a slightly different average in females of 1.0364 (Gompertz 1901). In 1991, a study of the brain specific gravity of rats was done, which found it to be within the range of 1.03–1.26 (DiResta *et al.* 1991). This latter calculation by DiResta was only slightly different from Gompertz's work, 90 years before. It is worth noting that the specific gravity of cerebrospinal fluid was found by Etherington-Wilson (1943) to be between 1.004 and 1.010, just slightly heavier than pure water.

In the days before the Creutzfeldt-Jakob disease (CJD) outbreak in the UK of 1994–1996, it was possible to purchase animal brains from the local butcher. From personal experience before that outbreak, bovine brain tissue had the tactile consistency of cold custard. This tactile quality is in keeping with the specific gravity of brain tissue. Consequently, this cold custard brain floats in the cerebrospinal fluid (CSF). This also gives the brain significant protection (see Ernest's Plum in Chapter 7).

The dural meninges have a mechanical fulcrum in the region of the junction of the falx and tentorium at the straight sinus, the Sutherland Fulcrum (Magoun 1951). The nervous system also has a mechanical fulcrum at the lamina terminalis (LT), which lies at the anterior wall of the third ventricle immediately above the optic chiasm. It is where embryologically the developing brain could no longer grow in the same cephalic direction (due to the restrictions of the membranes surrounding the growing embryo). Instead, it had to branch out laterally and develop into the two cerebral hemispheres.

Involuntary motion of the brain

In the flexion phase of the involuntary mechanism, the whole nervous system recedes towards the LT, which lies at the anterior aspect of the third ventricle. The spinal cord and brain stem shorten towards the LT and the cerebral hemispheres unravel (slightly), retreating the way they developed, towards the LT.

Conversely in the extension phase, the whole CNS lengthens away from the LT. So, it can be considered that the LT is the still point or fulcrum of motion of the whole nervous system. It is easier to follow this if we look at the CNS with the cerebral hemispheres unravelled so that the CNS resembles a tuning fork.

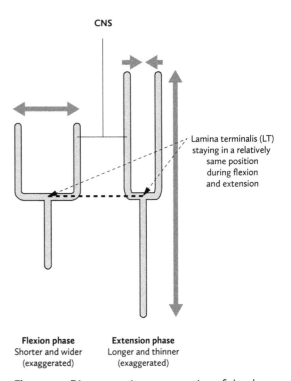

Flexion phase
Shorter and wider
(exaggerated)

Extension phase
Longer and thinner
(exaggerated)

Figure 12.1 Diagrammatic representation of the shape changes of the CNS if unravelled, during flexion and extension.

The functional fulcrum of the CNS

The lamina terminalis is the point to which the CNS recedes (shortening) during the flexion phase, widening at the same time, and lengthening in the extension phase whilst narrowing. Therefore, we can consider this anatomical point the fulcrum of the whole CNS. Knowing this can be of use clinically when the CNS feels as if it is out of balance.

The brain, like any other tissue of the body, is subject to mechanical strains and stresses. Hence patterns of the cranial base and meninges will be reflected in the brain tissues. However, the brain is highly influenced by psychological stresses (as are many other tissues in the body, see Chapter 16). With a physical trauma, the brain tissue will express the force vectors, the direction from where the forces originated. With psychological stresses, the force may be from a variety of psychological and emotional sources.

In such cases there is no directional force vector expressed in the tissues because there has not been any physical trauma. These psychological stresses express themselves in the brain tissue as 'implosions', the brain compressing or contracting in on itself to retreat, or as if to hide away, as does a child when scarred from psychological stress. Consequently, psychological stress-based compressive states of the CNS feel quite different from those of a physical traumatic nature.

We will be discussing ways to help emotional states with osteopathy in greater detail in Chapter 16. I recommend you progress through this book before knowingly taking on a patient with emotional issues unless you already have significant experience.

REGIONS OF THE BRAIN

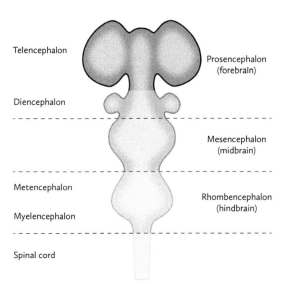

Telencephalon

Diencephalon

Metencephalon

Myelencephalon

Spinal cord

Prosencephalon
(forebrain)

Mesencephalon
(midbrain)

Rhombencephalon
(hindbrain)

Figure 12.2 Embryological regions of the brain, showing the forebrain, midbrain and hindbrain.

The brain is simply described as having three major sections: the forebrain (derived from the prosencephalon) the midbrain, and the hindbrain.

THE PROSENCEPHALON (FOREBRAIN)

This is the largest area of the brain and includes the telencephalon, which becomes the cerebral hemispheres, and the diencephalon, which becomes the thalamus, the hypothalamus, the pineal gland and the limbic system.

The cerebral hemispheres

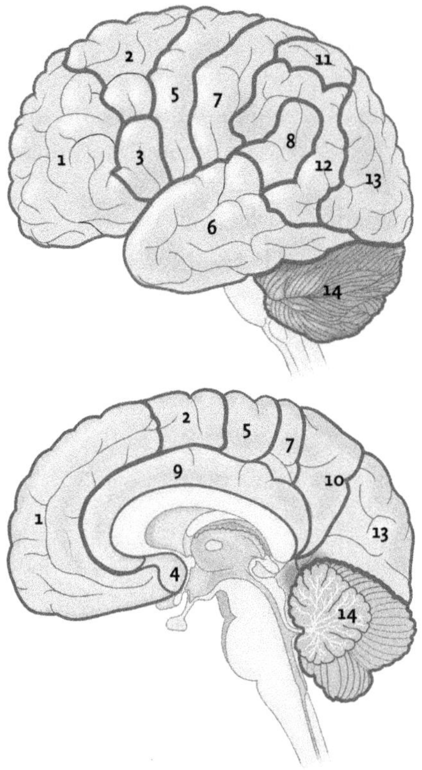

Figure 12.3 The cerebral cortex showing the differing areas of function. Regions 1,2, 3 and 4 are all part of the frontal lobe. Regions 9, 10 and 11 form the parietal lobe, and region 13 is the occipital lobe.

Figure 12.3 shows the anatomical regions of function within the cerebral hemispheres, however there are also functional differences between the two sides. Rush and Burgess (2018) describe these differences very clearly:

- Emotions: this is the domain of the right brain.
- Language and sign language: the left brain is more active in speech production than the right as Broca's area and Wernicke's area are found in the left hemisphere.
- Handedness: left- and right-handed people use the left and right brain differently. For example, a left-handed person uses their right brain for manual tasks and vice versa.
- Attention: the two brain hemispheres also differ in what they pay attention to. The left side of the brain is more involved with attention to the internal world. The right side is more interested in attending to the external world.

Interestingly, our left- or right-handedness can be detected as early as 15 weeks in utero, as revealed by which hand the embryo uses to suck its thumb.

Our language skills, logical and critical analysis, number ability and/or reasoning skills are all left-brain functions, whereas the right side of the brain is where we recognise the faces of other people, and is also involved in creating emotional expression. The right side of the brain is further acknowledged as being involved in our creativity such as in creating music, or the appreciation of colour. It is also considered to be the intuitive side of our brain (Cherry 2020).

Quite clearly there are functional differences between the two sides, however can a person be left- or right-brain dominant as was once previously considered? Scientific evidence now indicates that such conjecture of left- and right-brained people may need to be reconsidered. A 2013 study looked at 3D pictures of over 1,000 human brains, and measured the activity of the left and right hemispheres using an MRI scanner:

Despite the need for further study of the relationship between behaviour and lateralised connectivity, we demonstrate that left- and right-lateralised networks are homogeneously stronger among a constellation of hubs in the left and right hemispheres, but that such connections do not result in a subject-specific global brain lateralisation difference that favours one network over the other (i.e., left-brained, or right-brained). (Nielsen *et al.* 2013)

In other words, neuroscientists are now considering that the so-called left-brained or right-brained people do not exist. We all use both sides of the brain, but differing sections at different times.

The cerebral hemispheres are often referred to as the higher centres, and are associated with our conscious thinking which leads to conscious activity. 'Doing' without 'knowingly thinking' is unconscious activity. In other words, all we consciously think and do happens because of cerebral function. However, the cerebral cortex also processes unconscious thinking.

It is worth noting that we can think we are doing things or saying things as conscious actions, but commonly these are significantly unconscious. We often talk or do things without being conscious of their effects on others, frequently leading to negative unintended consequences. A lecturer when teaching is, or should be, choosing their words selectively, using the correct word for the best educational understanding. That same lecturer could then step down from the stage and have a chat with a friend, no longer in professional mode, and say things without being fully conscious of the consequences. We all do this to a greater or lesser extent.

I recommend that you pause for a moment and consider how this relates to you and your life. When in osteopath mode, we are conscious of how we talk to our patients, but what about at other times? Be natural, but be more aware of what you are saying, even during chatty times. Others will then find what you say much clearer and more understandable, thereby responding more appropriately to what you say. Needless to say, when we are tired or fatigued, we are more unconscious in our interactions even though still awake.

The cerebral hemispheres contain the frontal lobes, parietal lobes, occipital lobes and the temporal lobes. Let us look at each area in turn.

The frontal lobes

This region includes the areas for higher mental functions, the motor function area for the eyes, Broca's area for speech, the olfactory area for smell, and the motor cortex for our voluntary muscles.

The area for higher mental functions such as concentration, planning and judgement are all located in what is called the prefrontal cortex (PFC). This is located within the most anterior aspect of the anterior cranial fossa. One of the functions of the PFC is that it facilitates our decision making by allowing us to anticipate the consequences of our actions. When the PFC is functioning normally it acts like a brake on our impulsive behaviour (Dixon 2016). From my self-observations, this brake does not always function at 100 per cent capacity!

Creativity is a topic which is becoming of increasing interest to the scientific community. It is vital to us all, not just those with an artistic flair. It was a creative impulse in my brain which led to the idea of writing this book, and another separate creative idea which led to the thought of including 'live' practical exercises for you to do at the treatment table. According to Beaty et al.:

> Creative thinking is central to the arts, sciences, and everyday life. How does the brain produce creative thought? A series of recently published papers has begun to provide insight into this question, reporting a strikingly similar pattern of brain activity and connectivity across a range of creative tasks and domains, from divergent thinking to poetry composition to musical improvisation. This research suggests that creative thought involves dynamic interactions of large-scale brain systems, with the most compelling finding being that the default and executive control networks, which can show an antagonistic relation, tend to cooperate during creative cognition and artistic performance. These findings have implications for understanding how brain networks interact to support complex cognitive processes, particularly

those involving goal-directed, self-generated thought. (Beaty *et al.* 2016)

Benedek and colleagues studied the role of cognitive inhibition in increasing creativity. They found that the brain needs to stop following (inhibiting) a well-used train of thought, in order to develop a new creative thought process instead:

We generally found a positive correlation of inhibition and creativity measures. Moreover, latent variable analyses indicate that inhibition may primarily promote the fluency of ideas, whereas intelligence specifically promotes the originality of ideas. These findings support the notion that creative thought involves executive processes and may help to better understand the differential role of inhibition and intelligence in creativity. (Benedek *et al.* 2012)

This implies that the brain, under creative thinking processes, will inhibit previous thinking pathways and link antagonistic relationships to create new and more holistic ideas with a deeper comprehension of possibilities, in other words, thinking outside the box results in creative new solutions. The more our creative faculties become activated, the more that new thoughts, ideas and ways forwards in differing areas in our life will occur.

People with depressive tendencies lose that flair for finding new ways forwards in many aspects of their life and become stuck. This then affects another function of the PFC, that of our emotional expression. From our own experience, there are times when our emotions can be less than positive, or negatively expressed, as seen by ourselves or usually, in the eyes of other people. The consequences of this may lead to negative interactions with others and lead to a lessening of our life quality. Emotions are positively affected by states of mindfulness and states of the prefrontal cortex:

Mindfulness involves non-judgmental attention to present-moment experience. In its therapeutic forms, mindfulness interventions promote increased tolerance of negative affect and improved wellbeing. However, the neural mechanisms underlying mindful mood regulation are poorly understood. Mindfulness training appears to enhance focused attention, supported by the anterior cingulate cortex and the lateral prefrontal cortex. (Farb *et al.* 2012)

Clinical considerations: Prefrontal cortex

The frontal area of the brain is the region most at risk of injury. Injuries to this area can lead to a variety of symptoms, for example, loss of speech, movement, or alterations of social behaviour (Villines 2022a).

Quite often we may experience in our patients a sense of tension or even sometimes a sense of 'buzzing' in the region of the prefrontal cortex, when palpating the anterior cranial fossa. Such findings indicate that the tissue is less than happy. When palpating the CNS, we cannot determine the nature of their thoughts and nor should we attempt to do so, as that would be unethical. However, as osteopaths we are fully entitled to evaluate tissue quality. Depending on the patient and how well I know them, I may ask whether they have a lot on their plate at the moment, or if there is a lot going on in their life. I then rapidly tell them that I do not need to know any details, it's just that their head feels rather buzzy. The patient usually replies and says that yes, they do have a lot going on (or something similar).

We know that centring ourselves is an excellent way of calming our mind and emotions so that we can become neutral and objective when palpating our patients. Centring is one of a number of mindfulness approaches among others such as breathing exercises, meditation, or going for a walk in the countryside (although the latter two are difficult in the middle of a consultation!).

Palpating a tension or a buzzing in the PFC is not a full diagnosis in itself, but it may lead you to consider treating this finding and to see if you can settle the neurological state in this area. In my experience patients do appreciate this benefit and may say such things as: 'It feels as if a big weight has just lifted in my mind.'

A word of caution: *do be cautious to not over treat*. It is very easy to be tempted to help such patients to a greater level than their psychophysiology can tolerate during one treatment session, and consequently over treat them. This caution is especially appropriate if treating a family member.

Non-family members leave after treatment and we do not see them until their next appointment, if necessary. Should they feel a little unsettled due to an over treatment, they will have settled and be feeling OK before you next see them. With family members, you may see them just a few minutes after the treatment, and consequently, you may be highly aware of possible negative emotions from over treating. Also, at an unconscious level, we want to get our family members better even more than other patients because they are our loved ones. So do under treat rather than risk over treating such findings. We do not clean the dust in a room with a stick of dynamite!

Broca's area

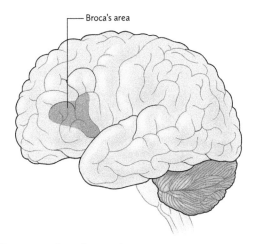

Figure 12.4 Broca's speech area.

This area lying (usually) just in the left hemisphere, is the area for the creation of speech production. Moini and Piran describe this area as regulating breathing patterns while speaking, and the vocalisations required for normal speech. It also coordinates the activities of the muscles of respiration, the larynx and the pharynx, as well as those of the cheeks, lips, jaws and tongue. If a person has damage to Broca's area, sounds can be made, but words cannot be formed (Moini and Piran 2020).

Another region of the brain, called Wernicke's area (see section later in this chapter), is also involved in speech and talking, however there are functional differences between these two areas:

> People with damage to [Broca's] area are considered to have Broca's aphasia, whereby they have difficulties producing speech. A few years after Broca, Carl Wernicke, who was said to be heavily inspired by Broca, found a similar problem with speech in some of his patients. However, the issues with these patients differed from Broca's patients as they were able to produce speech but were unable to comprehend language. These individuals would speak fluently, but with disordered speech, impaired understanding of speech, and impaired silent reading. (Guy-Evans 2021)

Therefore, speaking and conversing are two separate procedures, as with a conversation we need to be able to comprehend the words that the person is saying.

Clinical considerations: Broca's area

Clinically this area is significant if seeing a child with delayed speech development. Speech normally starts around 12 months, near the time of walking commencing. As any parent will know, the child's first words are usually 'Mama' or 'Dada'. If, however, there is a speech delay of a few months (or in the case of some children I helped, over two years), and the parent asks if you can help, you would need to evaluate if Broca's area (and/or Wernicke's area) has been compromised.

The location of Broca's area is close to the left pterion, the junction of the frontal, sphenoid, temporal and parietal bones. It is also close to the area where forceps may be applied to assist a tricky or difficult birth. Easing and releasing possible compressive forces from a forceps delivery may help Broca's area to function better and help the onset of speech.

Delayed speech does not necessarily mean that the child is not still gaining an understanding of sentence construction and understanding, as Wernicke's area may be functioning quite normally. One of my patients was still not talking by the age of three. After a few treatments he started talking, but much to the amazement of his parents, he soon spoke long complex sentences, to a level much in advance of his years when compared with his peers in playschool. (An overview of treating babies and children is presented in Chapter 14.)

Olfactory area
Much of this topic has been discussed in the section on the first cranial nerve (CN I) in Chapter 11. According to Vanderah:

The primary olfactory cortex consists of the cortex adjacent to the lateral olfactory tract (piriform cortex), an area of cortex covering part of the amygdala (peri-amygdaloid cortex), and a small anterior region of the para-hippocampal gyrus... The primary receiving sites for olfactory information project in turn to the hypothalamus, to limbic structures such as the hippocampus and the rest of the amygdala, and to the thalamus. (Vanderah 2021)

As discussed in Chapter 11, these aspects of smell going to the hippocampus, amygdala and thalamus are associated with emotional and historical links to the first experience of that smell. Such aromas may then have a positive or negative influence on how the individual acts when they next encounter it. (For clinical considerations of disturbance to the sense of smell, see the section on the olfactory nerve in Chapter 11.)

Motor cortex for the voluntary muscles
The motor cortex lies at the most posterior aspect of the frontal lobe, directly anterior to the central sulcus. It can be divided into two main functions, that of the primary motor cortex and that of the non-primary cortex.

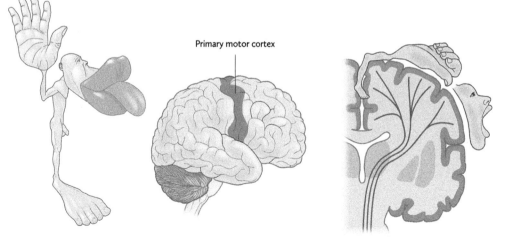

Primary motor cortex

Figure 12.5 Motor homunculus. The size of the image next to the brain indicates the relative number of motor nerves to that area of the body.

The primary cortex is the area that we tend to think of when considering the motor cortex, that of initiating conscious motor movement in our muscles. For example, we choose to raise our arm to get something off a high shelf or we choose to kick a football in a certain direction, and the motor cortex makes those movements happen. The non-primary motor cortex, lying just anterior to the primary motor cortex, contains the pre-motor and supplementary cortex. This aspect of the brain is involved in planning, initiating and selecting the correct movement. In other words, the non-primary cortex decides which is the best way to achieve the muscular action for the desired result.

CLINICAL CONSIDERATIONS: MOTOR CORTEX

The motor cortex gives us conscious control of our musculature, enabling us to interact with life and helping us achieve that which we wish to do. If patients present with a loss of motor function, in addition to checking if there is a nerve interference between the spinal cord and the weakened muscle – a lower motor neuron (LMN) lesion – we must verify that there is no upper motor neuron (UMN) lesion. A reflex test would exhibit very different results between LMN and UMN lesions.

LMN lesions result in one or more of the following: muscle atrophy, fasciculations, decreased reflexes, decreased tone, negative Babinski sign and flaccid paralysis. UMN lesions, however, result in hyper-reflex response, spasticity and a positive Babinski reflex in the foot (hallux flexion to a plantar stroking action and possibly a fanning of the other toes). It should also be remembered that the left motor cortex controls the musculature below the brain stem on the right side of the body and vice versa, due to the decussation of the spinal motor tracts within the medulla.

The temporal lobes

These are the second largest lobes of the brain after the frontal lobe and lie at the distal end of the neural tube, having bifurcated at the lamina terminalis into the two cerebral hemispheres. Their function is that of hearing, short-term memory, equilibrium, emotion, and also understanding spoken and written language (Wernicke's area is in the left cerebral hemisphere).

The auditory cortex region, lying within the posterosuperior aspect of the temporal lobes (number 8 in Figure 12.3), receives the auditory information. Here the data is processed and allows us to experience the sounds we hear, then gives meaning to the sounds and remembers them. For example, the sound signals of music stimulate the cochlea and then pass with the auditory nerve (CN VIII) to reach the auditory cortex. This then processes the sound and remembers the sound from a previous experience – as when a loving couple hear some music and say to one another: 'Darling they're playing our tune!' The auditory cortex then gives a loving meaning to that music based on the emotions felt when the couple heard that music together on a previous occasion. In addition, the temporal lobe has links to the cerebellum, which is then related to the auditory system. If we were to hear an explosion close by, then our body would automatically jump away from the danger, as the temporal lobe recognises the sound as dangerous.

The temporal lobe is also involved with our short-term and long-term visual memories. Here the lobe is communicating with the limbic system, as the temporal lobe is highly important for our conscious memory. When we see an object, the temporal lobe is activated to determine if it recognises the object, based on past experiences – we need to know what we are seeing, recognising it where possible. As with auditory signals, the temporal lobe adds emotions to the sight, based on past experiences. Without this function we would not be able to recognise anyone, even our own family, when we see them.

Wernicke's area is located within the temporal lobe and as has been indicated above, is involved in speech comprehension. When a patient has damage to Wernicke's area, they are able to speak, but have difficulty comprehending words or speech sounds. This is in contrast to damage to Broca's area, where the individual cannot say words, but understands the conversation.

A.T. Still talked to his students of 'being the bone', not 'feeling the bone' (as mentioned in Chapter 3). This requires a shift of spatial awareness by the practitioner, and is a level of working which the less experienced practitioner may find difficult, but one which will come with practice. If there is too much 'noise' going on in the head of the practitioner at these times, then such levels of perception are more difficult to experience. Perhaps the temporal lobes require a certain level of coherence in brain activity before such levels of perception can occur. It is well known that meditative states can calm the state of mind and emotions, with much research having been undertaken on this topic. I am sure that something similar occurs when we become centred and still in our awareness, in readiness to work with our patients.

The parietal lobes

These lie immediately posterior to the frontal lobe and central gyrus. Their role is mainly receiving the sensory signals from the whole body.

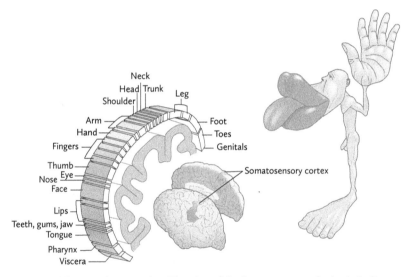

Figure 12.6 Sensory homunculus. The size of the image next to the brain indicates the relative number of sensory nerves to that area of the body.

Having received the sensory signals from the body, the parietal lobe then allows recognition and sensory comprehension, to give meaning to the sensory input. The parietal lobe also allows us to assess the size and shape of objects along with a sense of distance and direction, the latter being essential for giving us a sense of being able to get from A to B. Our ability to differentiate symbols, including written or typed letters, to negotiate mathematical problems, and decipher codes and puzzles are also skills embedded within the parietal lobe. Such deciphering demands memory, and the parietal lobe is involved in both memory and the sensory perception of hearing and sight.

Occipital lobes

As has been discussed with respect to the optic nerve, the occipital lobes process the visual information received by the eyes. The optic lobe, having received the visual signals from the retina, then interprets that information and determines if it recognises anything within the field of vision. To do this it needs to determine the distance from the objects, as well as determining the colour and also what aspects are moving.

Looking at something and seeing something are not quite the same. Only when the signals become conscious do we then realise that we are seeing something, and then, what we are seeing. As we are highly visual creatures (unless severely visually impaired or blind), our visual input has a powerful impact on our emotions, which are created in the visual cortex, based on our memory of past visual input.

The corpus callosum

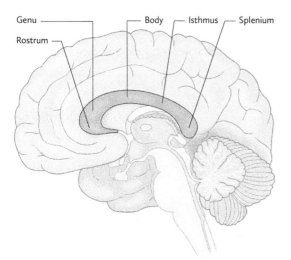

Genu — Body — Isthmus — Splenium
Rostrum

Figure 12.7 The corpus callosum.

The two cerebral hemispheres are connected by the corpus callosum ('tough body' in Latin). It is a very large bundle of white fibres which allows information to pass between the two sides. It is the largest connective pathway in the brain and is made up of more than 200 million nerve fibres (Seymore 2017). As has been described above, differing lobes and hemispheres, with some overlap, control different aspects of our thinking, actions

and/or behaviour. Therefore, with any thought or action, a whole surge of cerebral neural activity occurs. It is the corpus callosum which allows the various regions within the two lobes to communicate and coordinate any thought or action.

Embryologically, the corpus callosum develops towards the end of the first trimester and continues to develop until around 12 years of age. Some babies develop a condition called agenesis of the corpus callosum (ACC). This is where all or part of this connection between the two cerebral hemispheres is missing. It is considered to be among the most frequent human brain malformations, with an incidence of 0.5–70 in 10,000 (Schell-Apacik *et al.* 2008).

If there are few or no other brain development issues, the symptoms of poor corpus callosum function may not be expressed in the child until later in infancy and childhood. At such times the following main symptoms may occur:

> ACC can cause delays in a child's development of motor skills, such as sitting, walking, or riding a bike. It can potentially cause difficulties with swallowing and feeding. Poor coordination is also common in children with this condition. A child may also experience some speech delays in expressive communication... Although cognitive impairment can occur, many people with ACC have normal intelligence. (Case-Lo 2019)

If you as a practitioner see many children, you may or may not see patients with ACC. However, if you see a child who expresses the above symptoms, do ensure that they are referred to a paediatrician.

In older age group patients, an infarction involving the corpus callosum is fortunately considered rare. A 2015 study looked at 10 patients with corpus callosum damage from cranial infarction. The main symptoms expressed in these patients (listed in degree of frequency) were: 'Limb weakness (n = 6), dysarthria [motor speech disorder] (n = 5), dizziness (n = 2), memory loss (n = 2), syncope (n = 1), and unsteady gait (n = 1)' (Huang *et al.* 2015).

From an osteopathic perspective the corpus callosum is an intriguing area. We know from our training and hands-on clinical experience, that cranial base patterns are also reflected in the brain, the patterns of function: torsion, side-bending/rotation, vertical strains and lateral strains, all express in many tissues of the whole body. As the corpus callosum is the connection between the two cerebral hemispheres, it could be considered a mechanical fulcrum between them. This should not be confused with the lamina terminalis, which (as has been discussed above) is the fulcrum for the whole nervous system.

Exercise on the lobes and the corpus callosum of the cerebral hemispheres
Be very centred.

https://youtu.be/D-tc6g9z8DQ

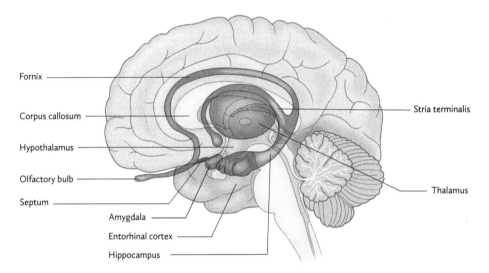

Figure 12.8 The limbic system.

The limbic system
The limbic system is a bilateral neural system located either side of the thalamus immediately inferior to the temporal lobe, located primarily in the forebrain. It is involved in our behavioural and emotional responses, especially when it comes to behaviours we need for survival: feeding, reproduction and caring for our young, and the fight or flight response (University of Queensland n.d.).

The thalamus
Lying between the brain stem and the cerebral hemispheres, the thalamus sends sensory signals from the brain stem to the sensory areas of the cerebral cortices, and equally signals from the motor cortex travel via the thalamus before going to the brain stem, and if appropriate, spinal cord, before continuing to their target muscles.

The thalamus is also considered to be involved in our diurnal rhythms, alertness and levels of wakefulness. Although not carried out in humans for ethical reasons, experiments on rats have shown the involvement of the thalamus in such a role: 'Neurons in the rodent midline thalamic paraventricular nucleus (PVT) receive inputs from brain stem and hypothalamic sites known to participate in sleep-wake and circadian rhythms' (Kolaj *et al.* 2012).

The thalamus has a powerful influence on the whole body by influencing both the endocrine system and the autonomic nervous system. It has a significant connection to the nucleus accumbens, a nucleus anterior to the basal forebrain and anterior to the hypothalamus, which amongst other functions (see cranial nerves X and XI in previous chapter) plays a role in sexual arousal. The limbic system also interacts with the basal ganglia, near to the thalamus and hypothalamus, which direct our conscious movements, as it is the interface between the cortex and the motor centres in the brain stem.

The hypothalamus

The hypothalamus lies immediately inferior to the thalamus, either side of the third ventricle, medial to the two tracts of the optic nerve and superior to the pituitary gland. The hypothalamus is subdivided into three sections: anterior, middle and posterior.

The anterior hypothalamus

This is the area involved in the production of hormones, a significant number of which influence pituitary gland function. It also plays a part in maintaining body temperature by regulating our sweat glands; an increase of sweating results in a lowering of our temperature.

Control of our circadian rhythm, our day and night cycles, is also part of the role of the anterior hypothalamus. This is a role which becomes challenged, for example, in people who have a variable work shift pattern or airline staff who travel long distances and change time zones frequently. When I had a practice close to London Heathrow airport,

I used to treat many of the airport and airline staff. Staff that either worked at the airport on shifts or as long-distance air crew would have sleep problems, since their diurnal rhythms were out of synchrony with the day/night rhythm, with flight staff having to cope with ever-changing time zones as well. Interestingly, many of the female airline staff working on long haul flights had highly irregular menstrual cycles. This would fit in with the anterior hypothalamus being involved with both our hormones and diurnal rhythms.

The middle hypothalamus

The main role of this area is that of determining our appetite and growth. It also produces growth hormone releasing hormone, which then stimulates the pituitary to release growth hormone.

The posterior hypothalamus

This part of the hypothalamus is, like the anterior aspect, involved in maintaining body temperature; it induces shivering and inhibits sweating, resulting in a rise in body temperature. Part of the posterior hypothalamus is also involved in aspects of memory. Seladi-Schulman, in her list of symptoms which may indicate a malfunction of the hypothalamus, includes:

> Unusually high or low blood pressure, fluctuations in body temperature, unexplained weight gain or weight loss, increased or decreased appetite, insomnia, infertility, short stature, delayed onset of puberty, dehydration and frequent urination. (Seladi-Schulman 2022)

Head trauma can sometimes be an aetiological factor resulting in a disturbance of hypothalamic function, so we should be mindful of this when diagnosing our patients.

The epithalamus

This is in the most cephalic part of the diencephalon, lying at the floor of the third ventricle, with the pineal gland at its posterior border. Its main role is to create a connection between the limbic system and other regions of the brain. This part of the brain also includes the pineal gland, which secretes the hormone melatonin. Melatonin is involved in the circadian rhythms of the body and is involved, along with the thalamus, in sleep regulation and diurnal rhythms. The pineal gland is also involved in bone metabolism, and our mental health and wellbeing. It is also affected by recreational drugs and is even thought to be associated with our ageing process (Villines 2022b).

The subthalamus

This is the most ventral aspect of the diencephalon, lying between the thalamus and midbrain. The functions of the subthalamus are in regard to our sexuality, food and water intake, the maintenance of hydration and our cardiovascular activity (Brain Made Simple 2022). In addition, the subthalamus functions to inhibit movements of the body; this is when the body stops muscles working or over working whilst carrying out a specific motion. If holding a full glass of beer, then it is important that the body does not make muscles quiver within your holding arm, nor cause your postural muscles to twitch, which might cause shaking, and consequent spilling of the beer.

Deep brain stimulation (DBS) with electrodes to the subthalamus, which has been used in the treatment of Parkinson's disease, has revealed side effects of memory disturbance and apathy:

> Many patients who receive DBS experience not only an improvement of their Parkinsonian symptoms, but also develop side effects that include cognitive and emotional changes like memory disturbances and apathy. It has been proposed that disruption of the function of the subthalamic nucleus might be responsible for these side effects of DBS. (Neuroscientifically Challenged 2022)

Studies of patients having DBS therapy have revealed further roles of the subthalamus:

> In the past 20 years, the concepts about the functional role of the subthalamic nucleus have changed dramatically: from being an inhibitory nucleus to a potent excitatory nucleus, and from being involved in hyperkinesias to hypokinesias. (Temel *et al.* 2005)

Clearly this is an area of the brain physiology where neurologists are still uncovering its full role.

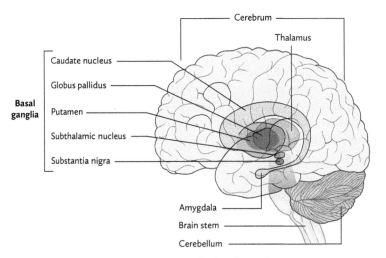

Figure 12.9 The basal ganglia.

The basal ganglia

This is a group of nuclei which are described as deeply hidden, inferior to the cerebral cortex. They consist of a group of structures which are the caudate nucleus, putamen and globus pallidus in the cerebrum; the substantia nigra in the midbrain; and the subthalamic nucleus in the diencephalon (see above).

The role of the basal ganglia is mainly to process information relating to movement and to refine brain activity in relation to specific requirements in specific situations. For example, the basal ganglia help understand the best way to kick a football or catch a ball with our hands. The basal ganglia tell the brain how to achieve an outcome by specific movements, which the higher thought processes want to achieve. They are therefore involved in learning movement habits and using existing motor skills in new situations.

One part of the basal ganglia, the substantia nigra, is highly involved in our posture and movement. Should this area be deprived of adequate dopamine, then Parkinson's disease symptoms are likely to develop. Dopamine is formed from tyrosine, an amino acid. Within the brain, the amine is synthesised by the removal of a carboxyl group from a molecule of its precursor, L-DOPA and hence is named 'dop/amine'. Dopamine functions both as a hormone and a neurotransmitter; it is this latter function which is involved in the muscular control of the body.

An osteopathic insight into Parkinson's disease

Parkinson's disease is not so much a disease but a set of symptoms, and so is more a syndrome. These symptoms are tremors, muscle rigidity and slowness of movement. According to the UK National Health Service (NHS):

1 in 500 people are affected by Parkinson's disease. Most people with Parkinson's start to develop symptoms when they're over 50, although around 1 in 20 people with the condition first experience symptoms when they're under 40. Men are slightly more likely to get Parkinson's disease than women. (NHS 2022)

With some patients suffering with Parkinson's, it is possible to detect a degree of compression around the substantia nigra (that part of the basal ganglia affected by Parkinson's). However, before making assumptions as to what can be treated osteopathically, always give a cautioned prognosis as further assessment needs to be undertaken of causes and to determine if osteopathic input may help. If the patient is expressing Parkinson's symptoms and not already under the care of a neurologist, they should be directed to their general practitioner for further referral.

When seeing a patient with Parkinson's (perhaps they have come to see you about another condition) and when taking their case history, if the patient gives a history of significant head trauma, or if the head and neck were whiplashed in the past, and importantly, you can still feel the force vectors of such events being expressed in the cranium, then you might be able to reduce their symptoms. It is important not to raise the hopes of such patients when discussing the osteopathic viewpoint. I have worked with some patients with head trauma history and Parkinson's who have benefitted from my treatment, but also some who didn't. It is important to explain in simple terms how, if they still have effects of an injury present in their physiology (which may be at an underlying level), osteopathy may be able to reduce these underlying mechanical forces. Then explain how you may therefore be able to improve the function of those areas of the brain so affected.

A 2020 study looked at the relationship between traumatic brain injury with loss of consciousness and increased risk of developing Parkinson's disease. The authors found that:

Traumatic brain injury (TBI) is a significant

non-genetic risk factor for developing Parkinson's disease (PD) later in life. While TBI has been implicated in several neurodegenerative disorders the strongest emerging evidence is for a causative relationship with late onset PD. Accumulating evidence suggests that inflammation may play a significant role in PD pathogenesis following TBI. (Delic *et al.* 2020)

This study by Delic and his team verifies that significant brain trauma can and does result in some patients developing Parkinson's disease after a period of time, possibly years later. As osteopaths, especially those of us who work with the involuntary mechanism, we are experts at palpating and reducing mechanical forces within the head. Following a severe head trauma, in all likelihood the patient will already have been under medical care. However, such patients may come to see us a few weeks or months later complaining of headaches or head pains after being discharged, or only requiring occasional medical check-ups. Reducing the latent mechanical strains in such patients may (we don't know for certain) have a preventive effect on reducing the risk of future Parkinson's disease.

THE MESENCEPHALON (MIDBRAIN)

The midbrain consists of two regions, the tectum and tegmentum. It is located in the brain stem between the prosencephalon (forebrain) and rhombencephalon (hindbrain). It is involved with muscular movement relating to our special senses, especially that of eye movement, but is also involved in visual and auditory processes.

The tectum
The tectum (Latin for 'roof') is a small area on the posterior aspect of the (mid)brain stem. It consists of two rounded areas, the superior and inferior colliculi.

Superior colliculus
This small region of the brain receives signals from both the retina and visual cortex. It consequently is involved in a number of visual reflexes, especially that of tracking objects in our visual field, e.g., watching a specific person walking across a street or watching the ball when playing or watching live sports.

The inferior colliculus (IC)
This is highly associated with our sense of hearing, receiving fibres from the brain stem which receive signals from the auditory nerve. The IC processes this auditory information from both ears. It also has the important role of filtering out unnecessary sounds. For example, filtering out such sounds as our breathing, eating and heartbeat, perhaps the sounds of other people talking in a room, so that these do not interfere with a conversation or listening to music.

The tegmentum
The tegmentum (Latin for 'covering') is inferior to the tectum, forming the floor of the midbrain. It is made up of fibre tracts and three regions, each distinguished by their respective colours: the red nucleus, the periaqueductal grey and the substantia nigra.

The red nucleus
This is an area which appears to need further neurological research as currently there is still debate over some aspects of its internal anatomy and function, though some functions are generally agreed:

Its participation in speech production, pain processing, sensory discrimination and completing complex tasks has been demonstrated by functional magnetic resonance imagery studies conducted over the past 20 years. These functionalities have therefore attributed the red nucleus with execution of learnt behaviour. (Crumbie 2020)

Periaqueductal grey (PAG, central grey)

This area surrounds the cerebral aqueduct (hence the name). The functions of the PAG include having a significant role in the autonomic system and also in how we respond to threatening situations. Recent evidence has also revealed the PAG's potential involvement in the perception of breathlessness (Faull *et al.* 2019).

Responding to danger can be a lifesaving response, ensuring that we are on high alert, and where appropriate, that we move away from the threat. The PAG is also involved with the body pain response. A good example of PAG interaction is being in danger from excess heat from being too near a fire. This will excite the danger response, eliciting the motor cortex to move away. It also creates changes within the autonomic system to cool the overheated body, and also to elicit pain so that we remember not to go too close to a fire in the future.

When stimulated, the PAG can inhibit pain signals if necessary: 'The PAG is also a major component of a descending pain inhibitory system. Activation of this system inhibits nociceptive neurons in the dorsal horn of the spinal cord' (Behbehani 1995). There will be times when it is important to ignore pain for a higher cause. If injured, it may be painful to move away from a seriously threatening situation, however the need to move is perhaps vitally important. In such a situation the pain stimuli will be switched off to allow movement to a safer place, after which the pain levels then return.

There was a famous case of a football (soccer) goal-keeper who, during the English FA Cup Final in 1956, collided with another player, severely hitting his head and neck. He continued playing for the rest of the match. Only after the final whistle did he feel any pain, which soon became severe. On examination, he was found to have fractured several cervical vertebrae! Clearly his periaqueductal grey region was inhibiting the pain signals until he had completed the vitally important (to him) football match.

Substantia nigra

This is named from the Latin for 'black substance'. This area of the brain contains significant amounts of neuromelanin in its dopaminergic neurons. This results in its darker pigment and hence its name. Although located in the midbrain, it is functionally part of the basal ganglia.

The dopamine released by the substantia nigra affects motor control (see pars compacta below). However, dopamine also has a significant involvement in the reward, pleasure and addiction regions of the brain. For example, when doing an activity which is highly satisfying, it is the dopamine which makes sure that your brain remembers the satisfaction experience. This makes you desire to do the activity again in order to receive that stimulus/pleasure. Such an activity could be as simple as eating curry, an ice cream, or a cake, or it could be taking in a more harmful substance such as cocaine. All these examples would stimulate the reward centre of our brain due to the release of dopamine, and lead to the desire to eat or take those substances again, just to get that dopamine hit.

Highly sugared foods can lead to relative levels of sugar addiction (much to the profit of some food companies and children's sweets manufacturers). Leyell, in his article for 'The Dopamine Project', discusses how:

In the pursuit of triggering dopamine flow: drug addicts ingest, imbibe, inhale, inject. Food addicts gorge. Safety addicts flock. Power addicts prey. Acceptance addicts pledge. Esteem addicts flaunt. Religion addicts judge. Money addicts work, cheat, connive, steal. (Leyell 2013)

This is quite an impressive list of common major personality faults. Clearly we need to ensure our substantia nigra and dopamine levels are kept in a healthy balance and do not get out of control.

The substantia nigra has two aspects: the pars compacta and the pars reticulata. The pars compacta supplies the basal ganglia with dopamine, and hence is involved with Parkinson's disease (see section on the basal ganglia above). Its main (although indirect) role is with motor function. 'Pars compacta-lesioned rats exhibited deficits in fine motor functions as previously described in animal models of Parkinson's disease, (Pioli *et al.* 2008).

The pars reticulata receives the finally processed signals from the basal ganglia and passes these to the thalamus and superior colliculus. It is an aspect of the motor control systems within the brain. However, it is also involved with the control of seizures and aspects of epilepsy. Velísková and Moshé looked at the role of the pars reticulata and seizures from epilepsy: 'The substantia nigra pars reticulata represents an endogenous seizure suppressing system, which may be targeted to develop treatments for generalized or multifocal epilepsies' (Velísková and Moshé 2006).

Clinical considerations: Pars reticulata

Could this area, if hindered by mechanical stresses, develop epilepsy? As has been mentioned above, mechanical trauma can lead to Parkinson's disease, so perhaps such an injury, if affecting the pars reticulata, can increase the potential for epileptic attacks.

This area sends impulses incredibly quickly (68 Hz) compared with the dopamine-activated signals of the pars compacta (lower than 8 Hz). Signals from the pars reticulata go to the frontal and oculomotor cortex and hence are involved with visual orientation, fixation and rapid eye movement. Clearly if the orientation function was reduced, then the individual would feel distressed, perhaps dizzy, and probably quite nauseous.

THE RHOMBENCEPHALON (HINDBRAIN)

The rhombencephalon comprises the lower aspects of the brain stem: the pons, medulla oblongata and also the cerebellum. It comprises two parts: the metencephalon and the myelencephalon.

Metencephalon (pons and cerebellum)

In addition to the pons and cerebellum, the metencephalon also includes the superior aspect of the fourth ventricle along with the nuclei of the trigeminal (V), abducens (VI), facial (VII) and part of the vestibulocochlear (VIII) nerves (see Chapter 11 on the cranial nerves).

The pons

The pons (Latin for 'bridge') is named because it bridges the cerebellum lying immediately anterior to the fourth ventricle and the cerebellum. It contains vital centres for the maintenance of pulmonary respiration. It controls the involuntary breathing process via the apneustic centre (causing sudden deep breaths, followed by a partial release) and the pneumotaxic centre (antagonistic to the apneustic centre) controlling our respiratory volume levels and breath rate.

The pons is the location of the nuclei for cranial nerves V, VI, VII and VIII, which are both sensory and motor in their action. In addition to its association with these cranial nerves, the pons also receives the afferent fibres from the cerebellum via the middle cerebral peduncles, allowing our postural information to be relayed to various cerebral centres. It also passes information to and from the spinal cord as well as from both cerebral hemispheres.

The cerebellum

The cerebellum lies inferior to the tentorium cerebelli in the posterior cranial fossa. 'Although the cerebellum accounts for approximately 10% of the brain's volume, it contains over 50% of the total number of neurons in the brain' (Knierim 2020). Having half of the total brain neurons indicates the vital role of the cerebellum. This is the area generally associated with controlling our coordination, balance, posture and voluntary movements, along with motor learning (trial and error). However, research is now revealing a much wider function of the cerebellum, and it is now shown to exhibit cognitive functions:

Recent anatomical studies demonstrate that the output of the cerebellum targets multiple nonmotor areas in the prefrontal and posterior parietal cortex, as well as the cortical motor areas. The projections to different cortical areas originate from distinct output channels within the cerebellar nuclei. The cerebral cortical area that is the main target of each output channel is a major source of input to the channel. Thus, a closed-loop circuit represents the major architectural unit of cerebro-cerebellar interactions. The outputs of these loops provide the cerebellum with the anatomical substrate to influence the control of movement and cognition. Neuroimaging and neuropsychological data supply compelling support for this view.

The range of tasks associated with cerebellar activation is remarkable and includes tasks designed to assess attention, executive control, language, working memory, learning, pain, emotion, and addiction. These data, along with the revelations about cerebro-cerebellar circuitry, provide a new framework for exploring the contribution of the cerebellum to diverse aspects of behaviour. (Strick *et al.* 2009)

In addition, studies by Koziol have indicated that the cerebellum also has cognitive functions (Koziol *et al.* 2014).

Clinical considerations: Cerebellum

As osteopaths we know that the posterior cranial fossa is a common site for tension and compression with our patients. The above quotation from Strick and colleagues gives much food for thought, as they imply that the cerebellum is involved with many significant functions in addition to its role of coordination.

We see many children with attention deficit issues which lead to degrees of hyperactivity at home and school. We see children with delayed speech and learning development. The bones of the occiput are separate at birth: basiocciput, the condylar parts and the basi/supraocciput. During childbirth these highly cartilaginous cranial base bones move with the forces of labour, which can result in significant tensions within the occiput itself and the rest of the cranium (see Chapter 14). Consequently, this relatively new knowledge about the functions of the cerebellum becomes highly significant as distortions to the four occiput bones at birth will have a profound impact on the cerebellum within the posterior cranial fossa. Therefore, osteopathic treatment and consequent tension resolution or reduction of these forces will have considerable therapeutic benefit.

Almost every patient we see is in some degree of pain; we also have patients who have negative emotional issues, e.g., anxiety and depression, and we see some patients with addictions, such as to alcohol, cigarettes, gambling, computer games and even social media. As with the temporal lobes, when more research is done to increase our knowledge of the full function of the cerebellum, then the true potential of our osteopathic work in these areas will fully unfold.

Exercise on the cerebellum

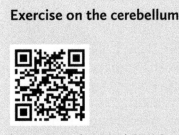

https://youtu.be/DOV1hQWAQww

Myelencephalon

This area lies between the pons and the spinal cord, being the final part of the brain stem, finishing at the foramen magnum. It comprises the medulla oblongata (often just referred to as the medulla) along with the inferior aspect of a portion of the fourth ventricle. It comprises the nuclei of the glossopharyngeal (IX), vagus (X), accessory (XI) and hypoglossal (XII) nerves, and a part of the vestibulocochlear nerve (VIII) (see Chapter 11 on the cranial nerves). Being at the pons/brain stem junction, this region naturally must transmit all signals to and from all regions of the brain.

From an osteopathic perspective it should be noted that the myelencephalon contains what Sutherland referred to as the 'magic inch' (2.54 cm) when describing the CV4 technique at the floor of the fourth ventricle. He did so because it contains all the nuclei that keep us alive, controlling our vital autonomic activities: respiratory lung breathing, heart, digestion, sneezing, swallowing and vomiting. It contains chemoreceptors which cross the blood–brain barrier, allowing detection of toxic substances. The medulla also contains baroreceptors to relax and constrict the blood vessels and so control our blood pressure.

The areas above the brain stem such as the thalamus regulate what we consciously experience such as consciousness, sleep and alertness. We could refer to the thalamus as the regulator, but it is the brain stem which activates that regulation into the body to create the desired result via our basic functions and our basic means of survival.

CONCLUSION

In this chapter, I have attempted to give you an overview of the functions of the differing regions of the brain without going too deeply into the neuroscience. We must remember that even with the amazing topic of brain tissue, A.T. Still's principle of structure affecting function still applies. Science still has much to discover about the brain and its functions and our consciousness as individuals. As that scientific knowledge increases, the role of osteopathy in helping patients will also increase. I hope that you now have a greater hunger to read further into the anatomy and physiology of the brain.

Exercise on the thalamus and brain stem

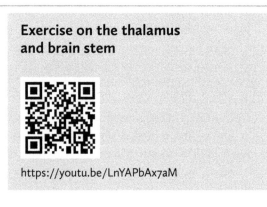

https://youtu.be/LnYAPbAx7aM

REFERENCES

Beaty, R., Benedek, M., Silvia, P., & Schacter, D., 2016. Creative cognition and brain network dynamics. Available from: https://www.sciencedirect.com/science/article/abs/pii/S1364661315002545.

Behbehani, M., 1995. Functional characteristics of the midbrain periaqueductal gray. *Progress in Neurobiology.* 46(6): 575–605. Available from: https://www.sciencedirect.com/science/article/pii/030100829500009K.

Benedek, M., Franz, F., Heene, M., & Neubauer, A.C., 2012. Differential effects of cognitive inhibition and intelligence on creativity. *Personality and Individual Differences.* 53(4): 480–485. Available from: https://doi.org/10.1016/j.paid.2012.04.014.

Brain Made Simple, 2022. Subthalamus. Available from: https://brainmadesimple.com/subthalamus/

Case-Lo, C., 2019. Why does my child have agenesis of the corpus callosum? Healthline. Available from: https://www.healthline.com/health/corpus-callosum-agenesis#:~:text=For%20example%2C%20ACC%20can%20cause,in%20children%20with%20this%20condition.

Cherry, K., 2020. Left brain vs right brain dominance. Available from: https://www.verywellmind.com/left-brain-vs-right-brain-2795005.

Crumbie, L., 2020. Red nucleus. Available from: https://www.kenhub.com/en/library/anatomy/red-nucleus.

Delic, V., Beck, K.D., Pang, K.C.H., *et al.,* 2020. Biological links between traumatic brain injury and Parkinson's disease. *Acta Neuropathol Commun.* 8: 45. Available from https://doi.org/10.1186/s40478-020-00924-7.

DiResta, G., Lee, J., & Arbit, E., 1991. Measurement of brain tissue specific gravity using pycnometry. *Journal Of Neuroscience Methods.* 39(3): 245–251. Available from: https://doi.org/10.1016/0165-0270(91)90103-7.

Dixon, T., 2016. The frontal lobe and the prefrontal cortex. IB Psychology. Available from: https://www.themantic-education.com/ibpsych/2016/10/27/the-frontal-lobe-and-the-prefrontal-cortex/

Etherington-Wilson, W., 1943. Specific gravity of CSF in spinal anaesthesia. *Br Med J.* 2(4309): 165–167. Available from: https://www.ncbi.nlm.nih.gov/pmc/articles/PMC2284692/?page=1.

Farb, N., Anderson, A., & Segal, Z., 2012. The mindful brain and emotion regulation in mood disorders. *Canadian Journal of Psychiatry.* 57(2): 70–77. Available from: https://journals.sagepub.com/doi/abs/10.1177/070674371205700203,

Faull, O.K., Subramanian, H.H., Ezra, M., & Pattinson, K.T.S., 2019. The midbrain periaqueductal gray as an integrative and interoceptive neural structure for breathing. *Neuroscience & Biobehavioural Reviews.* 98: 135–144. Available from: https://www.sciencedirect.com/science/article/pii/S0149763418306067.

Gompertz, R., 1901. Specific gravity of the brain. Available from: https://physoc.onlinelibrary.wiley.com/doi/pdf/10.1113/jphysiol.1902.sp000884.

Guy-Evans, O., 2021. Wernicke's area location and function. Simply Psychology. Available from: https://www.simplypsychology.org/wernickes-area.html#:~:text=Essentially%2C%20Wernicke's%20area%20works%20to,as%20the%20Wernicke%2DGeschwind%20model.

Huang, X., Du, X., Song, H., *et al.,* 2015. Cognitive impairments associated with corpus callosum infarction: a ten cases study. *Int J Clin Exp Med.* 8(11): 21991–21998.

Available from: https://www.ncbi.nlm.nih.gov/pmc/articles/PMC4724017/

Knierim, J., 2020. Chapter 5: Cerebellum. Neuroscience Online. Available from: https://nba.uth.tmc.edu/neuroscience/m/s3/chapter05.html.

Kolaj, M., Zhang, L., Ronnekleiv, O., & Renaud, L., 2012. Midline thalamic paraventricular nucleus neurons display diurnal variation in resting membrane potentials, conductances, and firing patterns in vitro. *Journal of Neurophysiology.* 107(7): 1835–1844. Available from: https://www.ncbi.nlm.nih.gov/pmc/articles/PMC3774578/

Koziol, L.F., Budding, D., Andreasen, N., *et al.* 2014. Consensus paper: the cerebellum's role in movement and cognition. *Cerebellum.* 13(1): 151–177. Available from: https://www.ncbi.nlm.nih.gov/pmc/articles/PMC4089997/

Lewis T., Taylor, A., 2021. Human brain: facts, functions & anatomy. Live Science. Available from: https://www.livescience.com/29365-human-brain.html.

Leyell, C., 2013. Dopamine profile: why power/money/esteem addicts are more dangerous than junkies. The Dopamine Project. Available from: https://dopamineproject.org/2013/01/why-power-money-and-esteem-addicts-are-more-dangerous-than-junkies/

Magoun, H.I., 1951. Mechanics of physiological motion of the sphenobasilar symphysis and sacrum. In: Magoun, H.I, ed. *Osteopathy in the Cranial Field.* Kirksville USA: The Journal Printing Company, p. 38. (Note to reader, this is the only edition of this book which was read and approved by Sutherland).

Moini, J., & Piran, P., 2020. Cerebral cortex. *Functional and Clinical Neuroanatomy.* Available from: https://www.sciencedirect.com/topics/neuroscience/brocas-area#:~:text=Broca's%20area%20is%20also%20known,vocalizations%20required%20for%20normal%20speech.

Neuroscientifically Challenged, 2022. Know your brain: subthalamic nucleus. Available from: https://neuroscientificallychallenged.com/posts/know-your-brain-subthalamic-nucleus.

NHS, 2022. Overview: Parkinson's disease. Available from: https://www.nhs.uk/conditions/parkinsons-disease/

Nielsen, J., Zielinski, B., Ferguson, M., *et al.,* 2013. An evaluation of the left-brain vs right-brain hypothesis with resting state functional connectivity magnetic resonance imaging. *PLoS One.* Available from: https://doi.org/10.1371/journal.pone.0071275.

Pioli, E.Y., Meissner, W., Sohr, R., *et al.,* 2008. Differential behavioral effects of partial bilateral lesions of ventral tegmental area or substantia nigra pars compacta in rats. *Neuroscience.* 153(4): 1213–1224. Available from: https://doi.org/10.1016/j.neuroscience.2008.01.084.

Rush, T., & Burgess, L., 2018. Left brain vs. right brain: fact and fiction. Medical News Today. Available from: https://www.medicalnewstoday.com/articles/321037.

Sachdeva, K., 2019. 11 fun facts about your brain. Available from: https://www.nm.org/healthbeat/healthy-tips/11-fun-facts-about-your-brain

Schell-Apacik, C., Wagner, K., Bihler, M., *et al.,* 2008. Agenesis and dysgenesis of the corpus callosum: clinical, genetic and neuroimaging findings in a series of

41 patients. *American Journal of Medical Genetics Part A.* 146A(19): 2501–2511. Available from: https://doi.org/10.1002/ajmg.a.32476.

Seladi-Schulman, J., 2022. Hypothalamus overview. Healthline. Available from: https://www.healthline.com/human-body-maps/hypothalamus.

Seymore, T., 2017. What does the corpus callosum do? Medical News Today. Available from: https://www.medicalnewstoday.com/articles/318065.

Strick, P., Dunn, R., & Fiez, J., 2009. Cerebellum and nonmotor function. *Annual Review of Neuroscience.* 32(1): 413–434. Available from: https://www.annualreviews.org/doi/10.1146/annurev.neuro.31.060407.125606.

Temel, Y., Blokland, A., Steinbusch, H., & Visser-Vandewalle, V., 2005. The functional role of the subthalamic nucleus in cognitive and limbic circuits. *Progress in Neurobiology.* 76(6): 393–413. Available from: https://www.sciencedirect.com/science/article/pii/S0301008205001048.

University of Queensland, n.d. The limbic system. Available from: https://qbi.uq.edu.au/brain/brain-anatomy/limbic-system.

Vanderah, T., 2021. The chemical senses of taste and smell. Available from: https://www.sciencedirect.com/topics/medicine-and-dentistry/olfactory-cortex/

Velísková, J., & Moshé, S.L., 2006. Update on the role of substantia nigra pars reticulata in the regulation of seizures. *Epilepsy Currents.* 6(3): 83–87. Available from: https://doi.org/10.1111/j.1535-7511.2006.00106.x.

Villines, Z., 2022a. What does the frontal lobe do? Medical News Today. Available from: https://www.medicalnewstoday.com/articles/318139.

Villines, Z., 2022b. What is the pineal function? Medical News Today. Available from: https://www.medicalnewstoday.com/articles/319882.

CHAPTER 13

Working with the Hormonal System

I shall describe the various aspects of the hormonal system, starting at the superior aspect of the physiology and finishing with the most inferior. Please remember that all hormones have a highly beneficial regulatory effect on the physiology and that these are not being described in order of importance, only on the basis of their anatomical location.

THE PINEAL GLAND

This is located at the posterior aspect of the third ventricle in the midline. It is also just inferior to the anterior aspect of the straight venous sinus, the anterior aspect of the junction of the falx cerebri and the tentorium cerebelli. Hence it is located between the two cerebral hemispheres. Its name is derived from it having a pinecone shape.

This gland has a fascinating evolutionary history. Palaeontological findings have shown from reptile skull fossils that millions of years ago, before the dinosaurs, reptiles had a pineal 'eye' located in the midline of their skulls between their true visual eyes. Even today some larger reptiles such as monitor lizards and iguanas still have a pineal 'eye' in the area around the nasion. Benoit, a post-doctoral student in South Africa, discusses how the pineal gland migrated from this position on the anterior aspect of the reptilian skull, covered in scales but still letting light through, to the mammalian position in the middle of the skull:

> It seems that cold-blooded reptiles needed to know exactly when night-time and daytime were changing, presumably to make sure they get the heat back into their body as morning rises, and to be somewhere warm as evening descends. So, this gland moved its position with the advent of warm-blooded mammals sometime between 200 and 300 million years ago. (Benoit 2016)

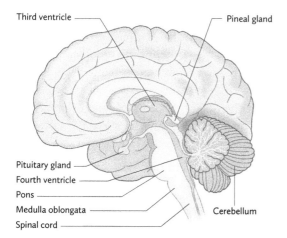

Figure 13.1 Location of the pineal and pituitary glands and the third ventricle.

It is worth considering, even though the pineal is in the midline at the posterior aspect of the third ventricle, whether light could still be affecting the pineal gland directly. If we hold our fingers against a flashlight, we can see the light passing through the soft tissues of the fingers. So, it is not beyond the realms of possibility that light could reach the pineal, especially when we consider the anterior anatomy.

Directly in front of the pineal is the third ventricle, which is full of cerebrospinal fluid. Anterior to that is the lamina terminalis and then the two layers of the falx cerebri. These two layers arise from each separate cerebral hemisphere and so there may be a small or potential space between each side of the falx cerebri. Even if no space exists, the falx is comprised of collagen fibres. These are hollow tubes which will allow light to be transmitted along their structure.

Anterior to the dural falx cerebri is the fontal bone. However, this is also the location of the frontal sinuses, where an air-filled sinus makes the osseous component at this area very thin, compared with the normal vault table. Taking these considerations into account, there is the possibility that the pineal can receive light, even though deep within the brain.

Vigh and his team looked at varying species of mammals:

> In all species examined so far, deep brain photo-receptors play a role in the circadian and circannual regulation of periodic functions. Mainly called pineal 'glands' in the last decades, the pineal organs actually represent a differentiated form of encephalic photoreceptors. Supposed to be intra and extracranially outgrown groups of deep brain photoreceptors, pineal organs also contain neurons and glial element. (Vigh *et al.* 2002)

The total function of the pineal gland is still fully open to question, though it is well known for the production of melatonin. Melatonin has the effect of maintaining our circadian rhythms, having a regulating effect on our sleep patterns by informing the body when to sleep, and when it is time to wake up. Research on melatonin produced by the pineal now also indicates a role in detoxifying the visual eyes: 'The pineal gland – which regulates the cycles of sleep and waking – appears to have evolved as an indirect way to improve vision, by keeping toxic compounds away from the eye' (NIH/National Institute of Child Health and Human Development 2004).

In the anterior hypothalamus (see Chapter 12), there is an area which is described as a pacemaker for our circadian rhythm, the suprachiasmic nucleus (SCN). The SCN receives information about daylight levels and sends that information to the pineal. The pineal gland then produces and releases melatonin during the night and inhibits its production during the day.

Nowadays, people frequently go to bed later than perhaps the pineal would advise, and also, perhaps due to shift work, are sleeping in irregular patterns. Additionally, some people choose to stay in bed longer than the sunrise and the pineal might advise, perhaps due to a late night. I am not being critical of people's life habits, job demands or desires, but one has to wonder if long-term habits such as these dysregulate the pineal function and have a detrimental physiological effect, possibly in ways we have still yet to discover.

Other functions of the pineal have been indicated such as: bone metabolism, mental health, pituitary function, drug metabolism and ageing, although much research needs to be done in this field. Sharan *et al.* looked at the role of melatonin produced in the pineal and noted in rats that bone mass levels changed if melatonin levels decreased:

> Pineal gland-specific deletion of *Tph1*, the enzyme that catalyses the first step in the melatonin biosynthesis, leads to a decrease in melatonin levels and a low bone mass due to an isolated decrease in bone formation while bone

resorption parameters remained unaffected. (Sharan *et al.* 2017)

With respect to mental health and ageing, Ferrari *et al.* did some observational studies on the impairment of melatonin secretions in elderly patients. They found that reduction of melatonin secretion was related to the mental wellbeing or age of the patient, and that melatonin does appear to affect the pituitary:

> A selective impairment of the nocturnal melatonin secretion has been observed in elderly subjects, being significantly related either to the age or to the severity of dementia. A significant increase of serum cortisol levels during evening- and night-times was found in elderly subjects, particularly if demented, when compared to young controls. Besides, both the circadian amplitude of cortisol rhythm and the nocturnal cortisol increase were significantly reduced in relation either to age or to cognitive impairment. (Ferrari *et al.* 2000)

This work indicates that pineal melatonin production does have an influence on the ageing process and its interactions with cortisol metabolism via the adrenal glands. Clearly further work needs to be done in this field of pineal physiology and ageing.

Clinical considerations: Pineal gland

As has been said above, the pineal is located at the posterior aspect of the third ventricle and also just underneath the anterior junction of the falx cerebri (falx) and the tentorium cerebelli (tent). We know from palpating our patients that this area can become disturbed. Being close to the Sutherland Fulcrum, it is close to the *relative* still point of the meninges, but that also means that it is in an area which has to adapt to many body movements. Could tensions in this area influence pineal function? If we follow Still's structure

influencing function principle, then clearly, yes it could.

The pineal gland is known in some patients to calcify and, if so, is clearly shown on an MRI, between the cerebral hemispheres. Ratini comments:

> A research study done in the 1990s found high concentrations of fluoride in the pineal glands of study participants. Fluoride from water and pesticides accumulate in the pineal gland more than in any other part of the body. After accumulation they form crystals, creating a hard shell called calcification.
>
> ... Some research shows that a reduction in the production of melatonin causes older adults to have disruptions in their sleep patterns. For example, they may feel sleepy during the day and stay awake at night. Another study found no relationship between the size of your pineal gland and sleeping problems. The size of the pineal gland usually reduces with age. (Ratini 2021)

Not having X-ray nor MRI facilities in my practice, I have never knowingly palpated a patient with a calcified pineal gland. Theorising for a moment, I would think that such a patient would have a significant chronic disturbance to their involuntary mechanism, such that the arterial blood flow and venous drainage to the pineal was affected.

Exercise on the pineal gland

https://youtu.be/Ri-uSZoqC9Q

THE HYPOTHALAMUS

The hormonal function of the hypothalamus has been described in Chapter 12 on the brain and so will not be repeated here.

THE PITUITARY GLAND

The pituitary, as has been mentioned in Chapter 12, hangs from the hypothalamus by the pituitary stalk. The pituitary lies within the space between the four clinoid processes of the sphenoid bone, under the sella tursica, one of the body's transverse diaphragms. On the lateral aspects of the pituitary are the left and right cavernous sinuses. Thus, the pituitary lies in a very protected space surrounded by the strong fibrous dura mater, and based on its incredible function, it needs that protection.

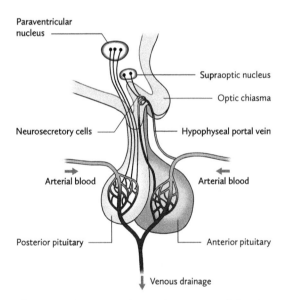

Figure 13.2 Anterior and posterior aspects of the pituitary gland.

The pituitary has two separate functional regions, the anterior and posterior pituitary. These are separate not only in their functions, but also in how they develop. The anterior pituitary is derived from oral ectoderm which evaginates in a superior direction. The posterior pituitary, however, is an extension of the neural brain tissue and descends until it meets with the rising, future anterior pituitary to form the pituitary gland. We must bear in mind that bones form last embryologically, so the pituitary is able to find its resting place, above the future sphenoid body, before the sphenoid bone forms.

Anterior pituitary hormones
Adrenocorticotrophic hormone (ACTH)
ACTH is secreted by the anterior pituitary, which stimulates the adrenal glands to secrete cortisol (see below and also Chapter 9 on the abdomen). This is the main stress hormone enabling the body to run away from 'the tiger'. However, it also has other important functions. It has a regulating effect on our metabolism and how we use carbohydrates, proteins and fats. It reduces or suppresses our inflammatory responses, it has a regulating influence on our blood pressure, and it also regulates our blood sugar levels. Like the pineal, cortisol will affect the sleeping/waking cycle of the physiology. All these functions when put together give the body the energy and requirements to get our muscles working to best effectiveness to escape the danger of 'the tiger', but these functions can also affect the body independently of each other. If the cortisol levels are either too high or too low, then the health of the body could be at serious risk.

Thyroid-stimulating hormone (TSH)
TSH stimulates hormone production in the thyroid. Excessive production leads to

hyperthyroidism, affecting the metabolic rate of the body (see thyroid gland, below).

Luteinising hormone (LH)

Luteinising hormone is a gonadotrophin secreted in the anterior pituitary, but it is the hypothalamus sending a hormone to the pituitary which causes this to happen. LH has a regulating effect on the female and male sexual organs.

In males, it causes the synthesis and secretion of androgens which are produced in the testes, and results in the formation of testosterone, a necessary hormone for the formation of the male sperm. In women, LH is responsible for egg release by the Graafian follicles within the ovaries. In addition, it also maintains the corpus luteum which forms in the ovaries following egg release, and which secretes progesterone.

Follicle-stimulating hormone (FSH)

FSH, as the name implies, results in the ovaries creating the female eggs and releasing them at the appropriate time, into the awaiting fallopian tube. Like LH, FSH formation is stimulated by the hypothalamus, although it is formed in the anterior pituitary. Orlowski and Sarao describe the influence on the male testes:

> In males, FSH stimulates Sertoli cell proliferation, which is the most significant contributor to testicular volume in children. The Sertoli cells produce an anti-Müllerian hormone (AMH), which causes the involution of the Müllerian ducts, preventing the formation of female internal genitalia. (Orlowski and Sarao 2022)

Quite clearly this hormonal influence on the differentiation of the male and female sexual organs is partly responsible for the human race as without it, human reproduction could be called into question.

Prolactin (PRL)

As the name implies, in women during pregnancy, prolactin is secreted which causes the growth of mammary alveoli, the sites of milk production in the breast. After the baby stops breast feeding, the levels of prolactin drop and milk formation ceases.

Contrary to what you may expect, prolactin is also secreted by the pituitary in males. It is now being understood that either low or high levels of prolactin in males create changes affecting sexual function:

> The results showed low prolactin was linked to several signs of poor sexual health, as well psychological health. Men with levels of prolactin that were lower than average, although still within the normal range, were more likely than men with higher levels to say their sexual function was getting worse, particularly their enjoyment of orgasm. They also had more symptoms of depression. (Gholipour 2013)

A high level or excess of PRL in males is associated with low sexual desire and erectile dysfunction:

> In men, high prolactin levels can cause galactorrhoea [inappropriate production of milk], impotence, reduced desire for sex, and infertility. A man with untreated hyperprolactinemia may make less sperm or no sperm at all. (ReproductiveFacts.org 2014)

Thus PRL, once considered strictly a female hormone, is clearly active in males and has an influence on male sexual function.

Growth hormone (GH)

Growth hormone (also known as human growth hormone (HGH) or somatotropin) is generally considered to be responsible for growth regulation during our development, in our childhood years, as Brinkman *et al.* explain:

HGH induces growth in nearly every tissue and organ in the body. However, it is most notorious for its growth-promoting effect on cartilage and bone, especially in the adolescent. Chondrocytes and osteoblasts receive signals to increase replication and thus allow for growth in size via HGH's activation of the mitogen-activated protein (MAP) kinases designated ERKs (extracellular signal-regulated kinases) 1 and 2 cellular signalling pathways. (Brinkman *et al.* 2022)

The same authors continue to clarify how growth hormone affects other tissues:

> In general, cells enter an anabolic protein state with increased amino acid uptake, protein synthesis, and decreased catabolism of proteins. Fats are processed and consumed by stimulating triglyceride breakdown and oxidation in adipocytes. Additionally, HGH suppresses the ability of insulin to stimulate the uptake of glucose in peripheral tissues and causes an increased rate of gluconeogenesis in the liver, leading to an overall hyperglycaemic state. (Brinkman *et al.* 2022)

If there is an excess of growth hormone in children, it can result in acromegaly and gigantism, depending on the level of excess. This is expressed in significant overgrowth of the long bones of the body. Consequently, there would be normal or only a mild increase in the size of the vertebra, so the spine may be the normal length, but the arms and legs would be significantly long and out of proportion compared with the norm.

In adults, the changes are not shown in long bone growth, but in facial features becoming more extreme, such as a larger nose. Also, the tongue can become furrowed and the skin and hair become thicker and coarser. Women also may produce breastmilk even when not breast feeding due to an increased release of prolactin. Men may develop erectile dysfunction.

There is much in the news about athletes defying the athletic federation laws (as also occurs for other sports) with some rogue competitors using growth hormone to enhance their competitive performances. Clearly such actions are unfair in terms of their sport but are also unwise from a health perspective.

Melanocyte-stimulating hormones (MSH)

These are a series of hormones which are produced in the skin, hypothalamus and the anterior pituitary. The hormones respond to ultraviolet light, which increases production in the pituitary and also the skin. The action is to make melanocytes create the darker pigmentation which is present in our skin, hair and eyes.

Contrary to what one might expect, the tanning ability of the individual does not increase if hormone levels are higher than normal:

> ...people with a high blood level of melanocyte-stimulating hormone do not necessarily tan very well or have even skin pigmentation. Very fair-skinned people tend to produce less melanin due to variations in their melanocyte-stimulating hormone receptors, which means they do not respond to melanocyte-stimulating hormone levels in the blood. (You and Your Hormones 2021)

Posterior pituitary hormones
Anti-diuretic hormone (ADH)

Anti-diuretic hormone (also called arginine vasopressin (AVP)) is produced by the posterior pituitary and influences the kidney glands. It regulates water within the physiology by controlling the levels of water reabsorption in the nephrons. With higher levels of ADH, more water reabsorption occurs, conserving body fluid levels. This then increases blood volume, lowers the osmotic levels of the blood, and raises blood pressure. When low body fluid levels are detected, more ADH is secreted. If this does not produce the required rehydration levels, then a thirst experience is produced to make the individual drink more water.

Low ADH levels result in excess water excretion from increased urination, and a consequent feeling of being very thirsty. High levels result in concentrated urine and may have consequences of high blood pressure and chemical imbalances due to the changes within the blood.

Oxytocin

This hormone is actually produced by the hypothalamus but is released into the circulation by the posterior aspect of the pituitary gland. It stimulates the muscles of the uterus to contract, and at the same time, it increases the synthesis of prostaglandins, which further increase uterine contractions at the end of pregnancy, thus initiating the process of childbirth. Following birth, oxytocin stimulates the release of milk to the mother's nipples from the milk glands in the breast and increases bonding between mother and the newborn baby.

Oxytocin is also said to be released at times of (healthy) physical contact or sexual intimacy between people, and when a couple fall in love with each other. Hence it has been called 'the love hormone' or the 'hugging drug'. In this regard it is one of the four 'feel good hormones' of the body, the others being dopamine, serotonin and endorphins.

Exercise on the pituitary gland
N.B. For obvious reasons please ensure you are very centred and only let the body treat itself if it chooses to do so – DO NOT treat it yourself. It is vital that the pituitary is not disturbed in a negative manner.

https://youtu.be/IMxPBaxS5lc

THE THYROID GLAND

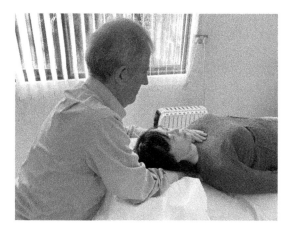

Figure 13.3 Working via the forearm to palpate the fascia, the extracellular matrix, cell membrane and also intracellular palpation.

The thyroid gland lies in the anterior aspect of the neck, inferior to the thyroid cartilage. So do remember that the thyroid cartilage does not protect the thyroid gland but the vocal cords in the larynx. The thyroid is partially protected by the cricoid cartilage, which articulates with the thyroid cartilage at the level of C6, which lies immediately superior to it. The gland lies directly anterior to the trachea and posterior to the sternothyroid muscle, with the pre-tracheal fascia between the two. The gland is made up of two lobes conjoined by a narrow isthmus.

The function of the thyroid
The main function of the thyroid is to take the iodine which we ingest with our foods and utilise

it to synthesise two hormones. The thyroid gland is the only gland in the whole physiology which can absorb iodine. The thyroid combines the iodine with the amino acid tyrosine to form the hormones thyroxine and triiodothyronine (also known as T4 and T3, respectively).

Thyroxine (tetraiodothyronine, T4)

Triiodothyronine (T3) is a hormone synthesised within the thyroid gland; however, when required, T4 can be converted to T3 in other tissues. The normal thyroid gland produces about 80 per cent T4 and 20 per cent T3, but, T3 is around four times as potent as T4 (Sargis 2019).

Thyroxine (T4) regulates the body metabolic rate and thus the levels of energy consumption. Consequently, it is involved with the digestive tract, the cardiac output and even our muscular system. Low thyroxine levels (hypothyroidism) can lead to muscular symptoms, caused by disturbances to the body oxidative metabolism. Symptoms include muscle stiffness, myalgias, cramps and easy fatigability (Sindoni *et al.* 2016).

T4 also has an influence on brain function and even the maintenance of our bones. An excess of T4 results in an increase of osteoclastic activity which osteoblasts may be incapable of compensating for, with subsequent osteoporosis.

Triiodothyronine (T3)

In addition to working alongside T4, T3 has a significant influence on the brain, affecting its development, neural cell differentiation and migration. 'T3 acting through the nuclear receptors, controls the expression of genes involved in myelination, cell differentiation, migration, and signalling' (Bernal 2005).

Calcitonin

Calcitonin, which is secreted by the thyroid gland, works in collaboration with parathyroid hormone (see below). Its action is to regulate the body's levels of calcium by reducing it in the blood. Equally it then increases calcium deposition into bone tissue. It can do this by the inhibition of the osteoclasts within the bone. It also reduces the blood volume of calcium by reducing the kidneys' reabsorption of calcium back into the blood stream. As can be seen, the thyroid hormones are vital to the physiology.

Clinical considerations: Thyroid gland

The thyroid gland is only protected by muscle and fascia anterior to it, and consequently it may be subject to trauma if the front of the neck is injured. I heard of a case many years ago where a patient complained of pains in her neck. She had fallen onto a blunt metal rod with her neck hitting the rod as she fell towards it, some 10 years previously. The patient subsequently developed hypothyroid symptoms and was told it was unlikely she would be able to have children, due to the resulting low thyroid levels. This was confirmed by her and her husband being unable to conceive.

The osteopath treated her neck using the involuntary mechanism to reduce the mechanical forces to the anterior and posterior of the neck, including the thyroid, cricoid cartilages and the thyroid gland itself. After about six sessions the patient was discharged, being free of her neck pain. About a year later, the practitioner received a thank you card from the patient, informing him that she had just given birth to a baby girl! So osteopathic treatment can have a positive influence on the thyroid, but probably only if a mechanical lesion is diagnosed in that area. Again, as has been said in previous chapters, do not promise success to a patient when there is only a possibility of success.

THE PARATHYROID GLAND

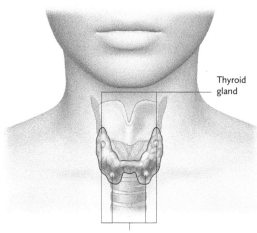

Thyroid gland

Parathyroid glands

Figure 13.4 The parathyroid glands.

The parathyroid glands are four small glands, each lying on the posterior aspect of the superior and inferior ends of the two lobes of the thyroid gland. They are described as being the size of a grain of rice. They produce just one hormone, parathyroid hormone.

Parathyroid hormone (PTH)

As has been mentioned above, parathyroid hormone works in collaboration with calcitonin, which has an antagonistic effect on blood calcium levels. PTH increases blood calcium levels and reduces bone calcium levels.

It is vital that blood calcium is kept at the correct levels at all times, and as such calcium is the most closely regulated mineral in the physiology. Calcium is the only mineral which has its own hormone to regulate it. The three main and vital roles of calcium in the physiology are

to create electrical energy for the function of the nervous system, to provide electrical energy for the muscles of our body, and to give strength to our skeleton.

Research is now finding that calcium plays an important role in the physiology of microtubules within the body, possibly even at the cellular level:

> Microtubules (MTs) are important cytoskeletal superstructures implicated in neuronal morphology and function, which are involved in vesicle trafficking, neurite formation and differentiation and other morphological changes. The structural and functional properties of MTs depend on their high intrinsic charge density and functional regulation by the MT depolymerising properties of changes in $Ca2+$ concentration. (Priel *et al.* 2008)

As can be seen from this brief summary of the parathyroid glands, it is phenomenal how four structures, each only the size of a rice grain, can influence the whole physiology.

Exercise on the thyroid and parathyroid glands

https://youtu.be/YgLZ7wFwFgE

ADRENAL GLANDS AND PANCREAS

The adrenal glands and pancreas have been described along with their hormonal function in

their respective sections in Chapter 9: An inner evaluation of the abdomen and pelvis.

OVARIES AND TESTES

The ovaries

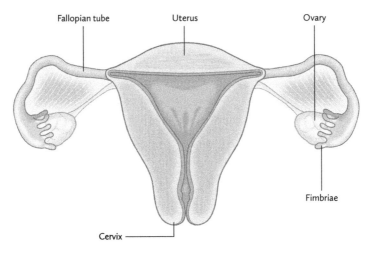

Figure 13.5 The ovaries and uterus.

These are involved in the production of the female egg cells, and they also produce the hormones oestrogen and progesterone.

It has long been considered that a woman is born with all the egg cells she will produce during her fertile life. However, in 2004, a study on mammals, published in *Nature*, showed:

> Their results indicated that female mammals continue to create egg cells after birth, contrary to long-held scientific belief that females are born with all the eggs they will ever have. The researchers became convinced that the traditional picture of ovarian function was wrong after a relatively simple experiment. They counted the number of dead follicles in ovaries of mice (which are thought to have reproductive systems similar to humans). Follicles are tiny sacks within the ovary that hold the egg cells. When the follicle dies, so does the egg. That initial experiment had a startling result, indicating that up to 1,200 follicles, or close to one-third of the mouse's entire egg supply, were dying at any given time in each ovary as the females approached adulthood. (Powell 2004)

Consequently, this study raises many questions about ovarian function.

Ovarian hormones: Oestrogen, progesterone and...testosterone
Testosterone

Contrary to popular opinion, testosterone is not only a male hormone but is also produced in the female adrenal gland, though in much lower levels. Testosterone levels in a woman will vary throughout her life, with respect to her monthly menstrual cycle and even at different times throughout the day. If a woman's level becomes low, the rate of new blood cell production can be reduced, as well as levels of other reproductive hormones, and she may find it difficult to maintain her sex drive. It is considered that women should have 15–70 nanograms of testosterone per decilitre of blood, though there are no accepted guidelines as to what is considered a low female testosterone level (Fletcher 2018).

In females, testosterone is mainly converted into oestrogens due to the actions of aromatase within the ovary, which converts the testosterone into oestradiol (E2), one of the three oestrogens, the other two being oestrone (E1) and oestriol (E3). The remaining testosterone could be directly affecting bone health, although this is an area of conflicting research. Arpaci and his team found that when looking at serum testosterone levels in post-menopausal women:

> There was no correlation between serum testosterone levels and patient age, body-mass index, or any measured bone mass density (BMD) values. Given the findings in our study, which failed to demonstrate a statistically significant relationship between testosterone and BMD, adjustment of other risk factors for osteoporosis might have a more distinctive effect in this setting. (Arpaci *et al.* 2015)

However, Zborowski and his team a few years later looked at osteoblasts and their androgen receptor sites. Their conclusion was:

> Oestrogen replacement in aromatase-deficient males has also been shown to increase bone mass. These observations suggest that oestrogen plays a crucial role in mediating bone mass in both men and women, a theory recently articulated by Riggs and colleagues in the bone literature. However, the presence of androgen receptors on osteoblasts also suggests a potential direct effect of androgens on bone regardless of gender. (Zborowski *et al.* 2000)

What is not in doubt is the role of oestrogen levels in helping to maintain good bone density, with low levels bringing about osteoporosis in post-menopausal women. So, after the conversion of testosterone into oestrogens, it does then have a strong benefit to bone health in women, even if not as testosterone itself.

Oestrogens: A brief outline of function
There are three types of oestrogen: oestrone (E1), oestradiol (E2) and oestriol (E3). However, E3 is produced within the baby in the womb, affecting the mother's physiology via the placenta. I will include it here as it is an oestrogen.

Oestrone (E1) is a weaker type of oestrogen which continues to be produced following menopause. It can be converted into oestradiol (E2) if required, thus acting as a source of E2. The direct role of oestrone is involved with sexual function and the health of the reproductive system.

Oestradiol (E2) triggers the hormonal and the sexual changes to the female physiology during pregnancy. It also stimulates emission of luteinising hormone by the pituitary, causing the release of eggs by the ovary during the menstrual cycle. E2 also causes, in conjunction with progesterone, the uterine wall to thicken in preparation for the arrival of a fertilised egg. Oestradiol levels drop during the menopause.

Oestriol (E3) is not actually formed in the ovary but by a combination of the foetal adrenal glands and the liver of the developing baby within the uterus. E3 is mentioned here due to its effect on the uterus, and whilst discussing E1 and E2. It is the main oestrogen which influences pregnancy via the placenta and then influencing the maternal uterine wall. Around the eighth week of intrauterine life, E3 levels start increasing. These continue increasing for the remainder of the pregnancy with the highest levels found about three weeks prior to the birth. Consequently, some premature deliveries take place when oestriol levels are at their greatest and hence the dominant pregnancy hormone. E3 is the hormone that prepares the mother's physiology for labour, delivery and postnatal breast feeding (Cleveland Clinic 2022).

Progesterone
This is the main female hormone which regulates the menstrual cycle and also pregnancy. Following ovulation, progesterone prepares the uterine wall for implantation of the egg should it become fertilised. If implantation does occur, then progesterone continues to maintain the status of the uterine wall for the duration of the pregnancy.

It is secreted by the corpus luteum within the ovary. This cyst-like structure forms within the ovary following ovulation and produces progesterone. However, it should be noted that some progesterone is secreted by the adrenal cortex in both sexes, and is even synthesised within the male testes. In males, progesterone stimulates spermatogenesis. Should the female egg be fertilised and implanted into the uterine wall, the developing placenta then takes over the role from the corpus luteum for production of progesterone at around week ten of the pregnancy.

During pregnancy one of the main roles of progesterone is to regulate the tone of the blood vessels and muscle contractility within the uterine wall:

> One of the primary responsibilities of progesterone throughout pregnancy is to maintain a decreased level of vascular tone in the myometrium. Progesterone also influences the production of inflammatory mediators, such as human T-cells within the uterine cavity. Thus, a loss of progesterone leads to an increase in myometrial contractility coupled with a decrease in fighting off immunologic threats, ultimately leading to a higher risk of miscarriage and early delivery of the foetus. (Cable and Grider 2022)

Should the female egg not become fertilised, and no uterine implantation occurs, then the progesterone levels drop. This results in shedding within the uterine wall, producing the monthly menstrual bleed.

Exercise on the ovaries

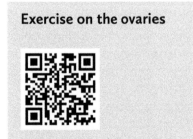

https://youtu.be/lubwoBHO4FA

The testes

The male testes produce the male sex hormone testosterone. It is formed by the Leydig cells, which lie between the seminiferous tubules. However, the testes also secrete other hormones: inhibin B and anti-Müllerian hormone from Sertoli cells, and insulin-like factor 3 and oestradiol from the Leydig cells (You and Your Hormones 2018).

Follicule stimulating hormone (FSH), which is produced by the pituitary, combines with proteins within the testes to form inhibin B:

> FSH stimulates testicular growth and enhances the production of an androgen-binding protein by the Sertoli cells, which are a component of the testicular tubule necessary for sustaining the maturing sperm cell. This androgen-binding protein causes high local concentrations of testosterone near the sperm, an essential factor in the development of normal spermatogenesis. Sertoli cells, under the influence of androgens, also secrete inhibin, a polypeptide, which may help to locally regulate spermatogenesis. (Jabbour 2020)

Anti-Müllerian hormone (AMH)

This is associated with the development in the foetus of the male reproductive tract. It is produced by the Sertoli cells within the testes and is one of the first testicular hormones to be formed. When Müllerian hormone is present in the foetus then the Müllerian ducts develop into the female fallopian tubes, the uterus, the cervix and the vagina. Therefore, when the anti-Müllerian hormone is present, it blocks the action of the Müllerian hormone, and so blocks the development of the female reproductive system, and the foetus develops into a male.

Insulin-like factor 3

This is produced in the Leydig cells of the male testes, and its main role is that of promoting the descent of the testicles and also the development of the male scrotum. It also is involved with bone growth and with male reproductive behaviour. It is said to be present in females where it is thought to act alongside follicle stimulating hormone and luteinising hormone from the pituitary, though this synergistic action in the female physiology is not currently understood.

Oestradiol

This hormone, as has been mentioned above, is one of the oestrogen family of hormones, and normally is considered a female hormone. However, in males it also has a variety of functions. In men whose sex is the same as that assigned at birth (also known as cisgender or cis men) the role of oestradiol is quite widespread:

> In cis men, oestradiol modulates sex drive, supports regular erectile function, and regulates healthy spermatogenesis (the production of sperm). Outside of the reproductive system, oestradiol has numerous applications and functions, including: maintaining bone health, regulating the balance of lean muscle mass and fat mass, supporting regular brain function, metabolising lipids (fats and fatty acids), supporting healthy skin, producing nitric oxide (a molecule that has an important part in vasodilation). (Miller 2021)

Testosterone

Testosterone is formed in the Leydig cells of the testes but is also formed within the female ovaries in much lower quantities than that of the male. It is also produced by the adrenal glands of both males and females. In women the majority of the testosterone is converted within the ovary into the main oestrogen hormone, oestradiol.

Testosterone is responsible for male sexual characteristics and for the development of male sexual organs in the foetus. It also causes the secondary male characteristics of male facial hair growth, a deepening of the voice and the sudden growth spurt during puberty. Following puberty, testosterone maintains these secondary male characteristics throughout the person's life. It is also responsible for stimulating sperm production within the testes.

CLINICAL CONSIDERATIONS: HORMONAL SYSTEM

As has been described with respect to the thyroid hormone, osteopathic treatment on the hormonal system requires great caution when consciously treating these glands. I say 'consciously' because somehow, when we are consciously treating a tissue or an organ then its influence seems more powerful in that part of the body, as opposed to an indirect influence. In all cases, do ensure that the patient is receiving the appropriate medical treatment for their condition. Equally, if the patient is being prescribed hormone replacement therapy by their medical practitioner, we should be careful not to over treat and possibly upset the levels of their prescription which were prescribed based on the lower levels of that hormone in the blood.

In general, ask yourself the key question: 'Are there mechanical forces present, which if reduced, may promote better function of the gland in question?' If yes, then cautiously proceed. I would recommend that you inform their medical practitioner that osteopathic treatment to reduce mechanical strains to that area is taking place, and that it may have a positive influence on the gland for which they are receiving medical therapy.

Now it goes without saying that the hormonal glands are subtle glandular tissues. On palpation they feel very delicate because they are amongst the most delicate organ structures in the physiology. With respect to the pituitary gland, it sits directly above the body of the sphenoid bone and is surrounded by the dura mater and is roofed in by the dura formed by the sella tursica between the four clinoid processes of the sphenoid bone. It is suspended down into the pituitary fossa by the pituitary stalk, which arises from the hypothalamus aspect of the brain. Consequently, dural and neural tensions could, though not necessarily, influence the pituitary gland.

REFERENCES

Arpaci, D., Saglam, F., Cuhaci, F., et al., 2015. Serum testosterone does not affect bone mineral density in postmenopausal women. *Archives of Endocrinology and Metabolism*. Available from: https://www.scielo.br/j/aem/a/6bqTKzBfzgZSmt8YD6r8LsN/?lang=en.

Benoit, J., 2016. What our ancestors' third eye reveals about the evolution of mammals to warm blood. The Conversation. Available from: https://theconversation.com/what-our-ancestors-third-eye-reveals-about-the-evolution-of-mammals-to-warm-blood-68454.

Bernal, J., 2005. Thyroid hormones and brain development. *Vitamins and Hormones*. 71: 95–122. Available from: https://doi.org/10.1016/S0083-6729(05)71004-9.

Brinkman, J.E., Tariq, M.A., Leavitt, L., et al., 2022. Physiology, growth hormone. In: StatPearls [Internet]. Treasure Island (FL): StatPearls Publishing. Available from: https://www.ncbi.nlm.nih.gov/books/NBK482141/

Cable, J.K., & Grider, M.H., 2022. Physiology, progesterone. In: StatPearls [Internet]. Treasure Island (FL): StatPearls Publishing. Available from: https://www.ncbi.nlm.nih.gov/books/NBK558960/

Cleveland Clinic, 2022. Estriol. Available from: https://my.clevelandclinic.org/health/articles/22399-estriol#:~:text=Estriol%20is%20one%20of%20three,body%20for%20labor%20and%20delivery.

Ferrari, E., Arcaini, A., Gornati, R., et al., 2000. Pineal and pituitary-adrenocortical function in physiological aging and in senile dementia. *Experimental Gerontology*. 35(9–10): 1239–1250. Available from: https://doi.org/10.1016/S0531-5565(00)00160-1.

Fletcher, J., 2018. What happens when a woman has low testosterone? Medical News Today. Available from: https://www.medicalnewstoday.com/articles/322663.

Gholipour, B., 2013. Men's sexual problems linked to low prolactin levels. LiveScience. Available from: https://www.livescience.com/41322-low-prolactin-men-sexual-impairment.html.

Jabbour, S.A., 2020. Follicle-stimulating hormone abnormalities. Medscape. Available from: https://emedicine.medscape.com/article/118810-overview.

Miller, N., 2021. What causes high estradiol levels in males? Everlywell. Available from: https://www.everlywell.com/blog/testosterone/what-causes-high-estradiol-levels-in-males/#:~:text=Functions%20of%20Estradiol%20in%20Men&text=In%20cis%20men%2C%20estradiol%20modulates,Maintaining%20bone%20health.

NIH/National Institute of Child Health and Human Development, 2004. Pineal gland evolved to improve vision, according to new theory. ScienceDaily. Available from: www.sciencedaily.com/releases/2004/08/040817082213.htm.

Orlowski, M., & Sarao, M.S., 2022. Physiology, follicle stimulating hormone. In: StatPearls [Internet]. Treasure Island (FL): StatPearls Publishing. Available from: https://www.ncbi.nlm.nih.gov/books/NBK535442/

Powell, A., 2004. Examining cell death, researchers explode belief about life. The Harvard Gazette. Available from: https://news.harvard.edu/gazette/story/2004/03/examining-cell-death-researchers-explode-belief-about-life/

Priel, A., Ramos, A.J., Tuszynski, J.A., & Cantiello, H.F., 2008. Effect of calcium on electrical energy transfer by microtubules. *Journal of Biological Physics*. Available from: https://pubmed.ncbi.nlm.nih.gov/19669507/

Ratini, M., 2021. What to know about calcification of the pineal gland. WebMD. Available from: https://www.webmd.com/sleep-disorders/what-to-know-about-calcification-of-the-pineal-gland.

ReproductiveFacts.org, 2014. Hyperprolactinemia (high prolactin levels). Available from: https://www.reproductivefacts.org/news-and-publications/patient-fact-sheets-and-booklets/documents/fact-sheets-and-info-booklets/hyperprolactinemia-high-prolactin-levels/#:~:text=In%20men%2C%20high%20prolactin%20levels,or%20no%20sperm%20at%20all.

Sargis, R., 2019. How your thyroid works. Endocrineweb. Available from: https://www.endocrineweb.com/conditions/thyroid/how-your-thyroid-works.

Sharan, K., Lewis, K., Furukawa, T., & Yadav, V.K., 2017. Regulation of bone mass through pineal-derived melatonin-MT2 receptor pathway. *Journal of Pineal Research*. 63(2): e12423. https://doi.org/10.1111/jpi.12423.

Sindoni, A., Rodolico, C., Pappalardo, M., et al., 2016. Hypothyroid myopathy: a peculiar clinical presentation of thyroid failure. Review of the literature. *Rev Endocr Metab Disord*. 17: 499–519. Available from: https://doi.org/10.1007/s11154-016-9357-0.

Vigh, B., Manzano, M.J., Zádori, A., et al., 2002. Nonvisual photoreceptors of the deep brain, pineal organs and retina. *Histology and Histopathology*. 17(2): 555–590. Available from: https://doi.org/10.14670/HH-17.555.

You and Your Hormones, 2018. Testes. Available from: https://www.yourhormones.info/glands/testes/#:~:text=What%20hormones%20do%20the%20testes,known%20as%20the%20Leydig%20cells.

You and Your Hormones, 2021. Melanocyte-stimulating hormone. Available from: https://www.yourhormones.info/hormones/melanocyte-stimulating-hormone/

Zborowski, J.V., Cauley, J.A., Talbott, E.O., et al., 2000. Bone mineral density, androgens, and the polycystic ovary: the complex and controversial issue of androgenic influence in female bone. *The Journal of Medical Endocrinology and Metabolism*. 85(10): 3496–3506. Available from: https://academic.oup.com/jcem/article/85/10/3496/2851114.

Part 3

ADVANCED OSTEOPATHIC CONSIDERATIONS

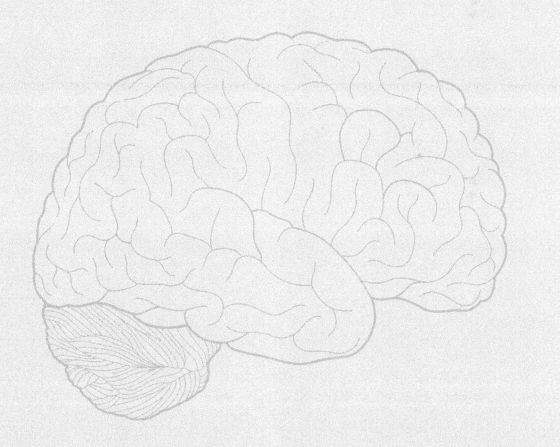

CHAPTER 14

An Overview of Working with Babies and Children

In this chapter I do not intend to train you as a practitioner in paediatric osteopathy. I consider this area to be one which requires a specialised knowledge of embryology, development within the womb, childbirth and its possible complications, along with an understanding of the differences of newborn physiology from that of the adult. Consequently, this requires separate postgraduate osteopathic training, and is beyond the intended purpose of this book. However, many readers may already treat children and so I will just give an overview of my thoughts and just some of my experiences on this topic. For those who have not yet undertaken paediatric osteopathy courses, I hope this chapter will inspire you to do so.

EMBRYOLOGY AND DEVELOPMENT

Working with babies and children is clearly a vital area of study as it helps us to understand the developmental processes of the body and organs during the first eight weeks of life. From that time forwards the developing foetus is maturing and organs undergo organ refinement, not creation.

As well as being a fascinating area of study, embryology is considered to give us an understanding of the blueprint or foundations of our physiology. As has been already quoted in Chapter 4, the late Dr James Jealous regarded embryology as a vital study in order to fully comprehend the self-therapeutic forces of the physiology in adults. I will repeat the quotation again here because of its strong relevance: 'The forces of embryogenesis become the forces of growth and development, healing and repair' (Jealous 1998).

Certainly, a study of embryology helps our learning of anatomy as it gives us a sense of how the structure came to be in the adult form. Should there be any issues with the embryological phase affecting the baby or child, there may possibly be ways that can be helped. This will be discussed in more detail in Chapter 15: Back to the time: an inner approach.

CHILDBIRTH

There is no such thing as a normal birth, only the more common aspects of childbirth. Each and every childbirth is unique for that mother and baby. The nature of the baby's presentation to the maternal pelvic floor, the state of the mother's sacrum and pelvic floor, the length of the labour and the nature of the delivery all create a unique event. Unfortunately, not all of the above are always ideal, which may have less than desirable consequences.

If the baby's head presents to the maternal pelvis in a less than ideal manner, it can result in a greater degree of rotation needing to occur during labour, or a wide part of the baby's head lying in a narrower dimension of the maternal pelvis than would be otherwise expected. In a so-called normal birth, the baby's head descends into the upper pelvis, with the baby's occiput to the left side of the mother's pelvis, i.e., the baby's head facing laterally to the right. As the baby's head descends to the lower pelvis, so it ideally needs to have its head with its face towards the sacrum, so that it can be delivered occiput first, the diameter of the mother's pelvis being greatest in the anterior/posterior direction in the lower pelvis.

Should there be any complication or difficulty with the birth, a forceps or ventouse delivery may be required to help the process. Such interventions will have been decided upon by the medical team at the birth, to ensure a healthy baby is born and that the mother is also healthy afterwards, given the tricky circumstances that prevailed. However, as osteopaths, we can palpate and detect tensions and forces which may not be clinically expressed. Sometimes the baby may have bruising or redness around the point of forceps application to its head. If a ventouse delivery, there may still be nonclinical palpatory signs of the suction forces to the parietal bone area where the ventouse was applied.

At times a baby might be delivered with a brow presentation, sometimes called a 'face to pubes' presentation or even a lateral presentation, where they were not able to turn the baby in time for the delivery. Any such irregularities can result in excessive forces to the baby's cranium which can be palpated and properly assessed by the appropriately trained osteopath.

A premature birth has issues for the baby. I once saw a baby who was born at 28 weeks of intrauterine life and was brought to see me two weeks later. He had a low birth weight of just 3 pounds and 9 ounces (1.61 kg). With a premature birth, there is often no complication with the delivery due to the small size of the baby. However, foetal tissues are not yet ready to experience the birth forces, and the lungs may struggle with breathing and need medical assistance.

In the latter stages of the pregnancy, the lungs and especially the alveolar sacs are still undergoing changes in readiness for breathing air, the digestive tract is undergoing preparation for milk intake, and the brain is still going through maturation. It is the maturation level of the lungs which determines whether a premature baby can still survive: 'By the time you're 24 weeks pregnant, the baby has a chance of survival if they are born. Most babies born before this time cannot live because their lungs and other vital organs are not developed enough' (NHS 2021).

Equally a delayed birth date (after 40 weeks) can lead to other issues, if prolonged. The longer the pregnancy, the larger the baby will become, thus putting greater pressure on the maternal pelvis, and so increasing the chance of a trickier delivery. So, the baby after a long pregnancy is less delicate than with a premature delivery, but the delivery risks increase.

The length of the mother's labour can also be a factor affecting the baby after birth. A precipitous (very quick) labour, is described as: 'the experience of being in labour and then giving birth less than 3 hours after regular contractions start – that is, when a stable pattern of contractions has developed' (Larson 2020).

A fast labour does not give enough time for the baby's head to be moulded by the forces of birth and the rotations required on the journey through the maternal pelvis and birth canal. By contrast, a long labour which can last up to 30 hours or more puts a tremendous amount of pressure on the baby's head, resulting in strong mechanical forces remaining after the birth process.

ANATOMICAL DIFFERENCES WITH BABIES

Babies are not simply small adults. Their brain is at a different stage of development and much neuron and axon development is still occurring, especially in the first five years. However, it should be borne in mind that even in teenagers, although the brain may be done growing in size, it does not finish developing and maturing until the mid- to late 20s. The front part of the brain, the prefrontal cortex, is one of the last brain regions to mature (National Institute of Mental Health 2020).

The baby's gut does not develop its truly effective microbiota until several years after birth: 'Early reports suggested that the infant microbiota would attain an adult-like structure at the age of 3 years, but recent studies have suggested that microbiota development may take longer' (Derrien *et al.* 2019).

The liver in a new baby is proportionally much, much larger in size, relative to that of the adult liver. This reflects the phenomenal volume of chemical processing that is happening in the baby's digestive system. This also reflects the incredible growth and cellular reproduction rates which are happening throughout the body.

SYMPTOMS FROM BIRTH

The symptoms arising from a tricky birth can be quite varied and will depend on the level of mechanical trauma and where it is located.

Sleep patterns can often be poor if the baby is distressed or compromised from the birth. So-called colic is a common baby symptom that frequently distresses parents too, as they also suffer from lack of sleep. According to the UK National Health Service (NHS):

> All babies cry, but your baby may have colic if they cry more than 3 hours a day, 3 days a week for at least 1 week but are otherwise healthy. They may cry more often in the afternoon and evening. It may also be colic if, while they are crying, it's hard to soothe or settle your baby, they clench their fists, they go red in the face, they bring their knees up to their tummy or arch their back, their tummy rumbles or they're very windy. (NHS 2022)

Many babies with colic, in my experience, respond well to cranial osteopathic treatment though it is important that other more serious conditions are ruled out by the paediatrician, if symptoms persist and do not respond to osteopathic help.

Some babies have difficulties with breast feeding, and they may or may not be accurately diagnosed as having a tongue tie. If there is no tongue tie, then if there is a mechanical tension which may be influencing CN XII, osteopathic treatment may help.

Sometimes the baby may be happier breast feeding on one side more than the other. In such cases the mother usually blames herself for not having sufficient milk being produced by one breast. However, if the baby has tensions in the suboccipital area, which are quite common after birth, this may result in the baby finding it more difficult to rotate the head and neck to one side, consequently having difficulty feeding on the affected side.

Squints in babies are not that uncommon, as the ocular muscles are still developing their coordination and strength. However, if the squint persists, then osteopathy may be able to help. Such a positive outcome would depend on there being an accurate diagnosis of mechanical forces to the baby's head such that CN III, IV and VI are being compromised. If, with skilled treatment to the head, the mechanical tensions around the pterion area, affecting the sphenoid, or tensions to the side of the head, affecting the temporal bone and its relationship to CN III, IV and VI, can be reduced, then the possibility of reducing the symptoms significantly increases.

The above symptoms are just some of the more common issues resulting from a difficult or tricky birth. If you already treat babies, you may have already seen many such patients in your practice.

As a child grows, so the influences of their birth develop in ways appropriate for the types of behaviour at their current age group. A 4 to 12 year-old child is unlikely to be a frequently crying child, but they may easily be a hyperactive child, or a child who does not turn their head to one side as much as the other. They may also have learning difficulties at school due to poor concentration, this being from an underlying hyperactive mind.

Some children at primary school (until age 11 in the UK) frequently get aggressive towards other peers in their class. In some cases, I have found this to be associated with the brain tissue being under strain and compressive forces still expressing from their birth, unless perhaps they have had additional injuries to the head after birth. Unless treated, birth stresses can and sometimes do result in negative personality traits or behaviour due to the continual negative pressure and tension on the child's head and brain tissue that 'just won't go away'.

Naturally as a child becomes older, they start pursuing more adventurous activities and sports. They naturally want to engage in horse riding, climbing trees, skiing, cycling and many other pursuits which are more exciting, but potentially injurious activities. Depending on the age of the teenager even motorised sports are pursued such as having a motorbike or learning to drive a car (depending on the age limit in your own country). As we can see, or may have experienced ourselves during our own youthful years, injuries from such pursuits can be quite severe, leaving additional strains and tensions within the physiology, on top of any birth strains and tensions.

CONSIDERATIONS WHEN TREATING BABIES AND YOUNGER CHILDREN

First of all, we have to remember that the parent (usually the mother) who brings their baby or child for treatment is frequently anxious about their condition. So, as you take your case history and evaluation, you need to be very aware of this and choose your words carefully when talking to the parent about your thoughts and findings, so as not to increase their worries unnecessarily. Also always remember that if the patient is a child not a baby, do look directly at the child and ask them some questions and not only the parent. This makes them feel that they are important, and that they are involved in what you are discussing with their mother or father. An important reason why this is necessary is it that the parent may say that the child feels the symptoms in a particular place. However, when asking the child to touch the place that hurts, it may be different from where the parent said. If the child is old enough to explain, then asking the child when and what makes it worse may reveal a view that is different from that of the parent. So always remember the view of the child, as they are the person who has the symptoms.

When treating babies, however, the information you receive verbally is a second-hand version from the parent, the baby not being able to express themselves. This is why the palpatory evaluation with a baby may be even more important than the case history, though both still are very necessary.

As has been mentioned in Chapter 3 on diagnosis, do unobtrusively observe family interactions if more than one child comes to the treatment room, or between child and parent. Depending on the age group of the children, this can give insights as to the level of family harmony. Also notice if there is a degree of attention seeking happening during the case history. This may be from the patient who feels they need attention whilst you talk to the parent, or perhaps a sibling who keeps jumping in and directs everyone's attention to them instead of the patient. If they do this in the consulting room, then probably they do this at home too, much to the frequent annoyance of the patient child.

Where to treat the patient in your consulting room?

This may seem like a strange question, and you may be thinking, 'Well on the treatment table of course.' However, for babies, I personally like to place a large pillow on both my knees and the parent's knees. To achieve this, I ask the parent to sit facing me with their knees almost touching mine, with our thighs closed. I then place the pillow on both our laps. Asking this is very important as having one's own knees almost touching another person's knees could be seen as inappropriate, unless the reason for it is explained.

I then ask the parent to put the baby lying down supine on the pillow between us. Some practitioners like to palpate babies starting from the feet and then working their way up towards the head. However, I personally like to start at the head and work towards the feet. It technically does not matter which way it is done as long as the whole body is assessed. The reason I prefer to work initially on the baby's head is that this means that the baby is initially looking directly towards mum or dad. They do frequently extend their neck to look me directly in the eyes too, an 'eyeball to eyeball experience'!

Being able to see the parents is reassuring to the baby whilst I evaluate the stresses and strains in his/her physiology. Sometimes I move my arms lower down the pillow to evaluate the pelvis and lower extremities, or sometimes I ask

the parent to help me carefully rotate the pillow 180 degrees, so that I have an easier contact to the lower aspect of the baby.

Obviously when the age of the baby increases and the baby outgrows the pillow size, then they 'graduate' to the treatment table.

Do babies cry during treatment?

This is a common question, both from osteopathic students and parents alike. The answer, as is necessary with many specific osteopathic questions, is a 'definite maybe'!

All patients are unique and the same is true for babies. Some are 'good as gold' and just lie there smiling at both me and the parent, but some are not. Some can be happy and calm until I place my contact near the areas of most strong tensions within their physiology. At these times some babies let loose, and howl strongly. If this occurs, I immediately reassure the parent, saying: 'As you can see, I am still touching the baby incredibly delicately, just as I did a moment ago.'

I then explain to the parent how I am now working on an area of strain and tensions caused by their (difficult?) birth, and that my working at this place is making the baby conscious of tensions that have always been there since they were born. I then continue to work on the area of most significant tension, seeking a release to some degree, but always being ready to come off if the parent expresses anxiety or the level of crying increases. Then I let the parent cuddle the baby for a few minutes and then work somewhere else, away from that key area. I then arrange to see the child a few days or a week later and continue at this place. Usually after the first treatment their crying is much less or in some cases they no longer cry when working at the high-tension area.

In some cases, I have treated babies or young children whilst the mother is holding and cuddling them. Depending on how self-conscious the mother may be, I have also on occasions treated the baby whilst the mother is breast feeding, but such times are rare and this is only advisable if the father or other chaperone is present as a witness to safeguard all parties. Again, in such circumstances, do get the mother's full understanding of why this may be a good idea, to settle the baby whilst you treat them, and give her full permission to say: 'No thank you, I do not wish to do that.'

Needless to say, to work when a baby is sometimes crying and/or the parent is anxious does require you as the practitioner to be very highly centred. It is easy for that anxiety energy in the consulting room to throw you off centre and make you lose your objectivity when palpating and treating. Therefore, I would recommend a few minutes to centre yourself in advance of a baby patient entering your consulting room.

THE JOYS OF TREATING BABIES AND CHILDREN

We all know that there is a great level of fulfilment when helping a patient of any age and they walk out of your treatment room in a better way than when they arrived. When treating babies and children, there is also the same joy expressed by the parent, but somehow the level of relief expressed in their faces and body language when a baby or child is happier and expressing no or fewer symptoms is on another level.

From the practitioner perspective, shears, strain and mechanical forces being expressed in the physiology of a very young person are carried forwards in the physiology as they grow and have to be accommodated to in their later years. I have seen patients in their 80s who still have birth issues being expressed, though being significantly compensated for by the rest of the physiology. Would their physiology have been happier if such birth strains had been reduced by good cranial osteopathic treatment soon after, or within a couple of years after birth? This cannot be answered categorically, but it is probably yes.

Throughout life, the physiology is always attempting to modify and reduce the influence of mechanical tensions. It does this by a series of compensations. We call these compensations patterns of health (see Chapter 3). The greater the number of compensations having to occur, whether from birth or from life events following birth, the lower the body's tolerance of postural tensions, psychological tensions, or traumatic tensions becomes. So, treating babies and children on one level is helping the future life of the child. A number of practitioners I know have devoted their latter years in osteopathic practice to only treating such age group patients, for this very reason.

I hope that this short chapter has inspired you, if you do not already treat babies and children, to attend a postgraduate course on paediatric osteopathy, and if you have already done so, that it has given you some added enthusiasm for this field of osteopathic work.

REFERENCES

Derrien, M., Alvarez, A.-S., & de Vos, W., 2019. The gut microbiota in the first decade of life. *Trends in Microbiology.* 27(12): 997–1010. Available from: https://www.science direct.com/science/article/pii/S0966842X19302148.

Jealous, J., 1998. Conversation with Timothy Marris. June.

Larson, C., 2020. Precipitous labour: when labour is fast and furious. Healthline. Available from: https://www.health line.com/health/pregnancy/precipitous-labor-when-labor-is-fast-and-furious.

National Institute of Mental Health, 2020. The teen brain: 7 things to know. Available from: https://www.nimh. nih.gov/health/publications/the-teen-brain-7-things-to-know#:~:text=Though%20the%20brain%20may%20 be,%2C%20prioritizing%2C%20and%20controlling%20 impulses.

NHS, 2021. You and your baby at 24 weeks pregnant. Available from: https://www.nhs.uk/pregnancy/ week-by-week/13-to-27/24-weeks/

NHS, 2022. Colic. Available from: https://www.nhs.uk/ conditions/colic/

CHAPTER 15

Back to the Time: An Inner Approach

As mentioned in Chapter 4, I was introduced to the possibilities of working with osteopathic timelines, by Dr Robert Fulford, one of Dr Sutherland's students, whereby the practitioner could take their attention back in time to a period or even a day, when a specific event happened to the physiology.

Dr Fulford outlined this approach to me when I had only been in practice for about five years. When I heard him talking about it, it was a revolutionary moment in my perception and thinking. In the subsequent years I honed my skills and explored differing applications of the approach with my patients. It was not until 2012 that I created a three-day course on this topic and started teaching it to others. I called the course 'The Other Temporal Factor' as it is about time, not the temporal bone. Interestingly one student who attended one of these courses I taught in Germany informed me that the temporal bone is called that because the hair over the anterior aspect of the temporal squama is the first hair on the body to turn grey!

In this chapter and in the associated practical sessions, I will be presenting the essence of the method so that you as the reader can start developing your own skills in this approach. By now, if you have followed the strong advice to not jump ahead, but work through all the practical sessions of the preceding chapters in sequence, your palpatory skills will have been increasing such that you are probably now ready for working with this aspect of diagnosis and treatment. If you did jump ahead due to enthusiasm or pure inquisitiveness, I politely ask you to go back to where you jumped forwards from and slowly work your way through all the chapters. I hope you understand this request. As you will appreciate, I have written these chapters in sequence, on the basis of the reader's increasing skill set for each successive chapter, and so decided it was appropriate to explore this topic in Chapter 15, not earlier in the book.

In Chapter 3, on the topic of working on your diagnosis, we realised that we primarily palpate with our third hand, that of our attention. Our other two hands are giving us a strong 'helping hand' to allow our perception and attention to link our anatomy and physiology with where we wish to send our awareness. We have been using these 'three-handed' approaches to take our awareness to varying places within the physiology, working with the three anatomical dimensions of: left and right, anterior and posterior, plus superior and inferior. Now with this approach of working we will be working with the fourth dimension, that of time.

THE FOURTH DIMENSION AND SPACE-TIME

According to physics, there are many more levels of dimensions:

> While on the local level we are trained to think of space as having three dimensions, general relativity paints a picture of a four-dimensional universe, and string theory says it has 10 dimensions – or 11 if you take an extended version known as M-Theory. There are variations of the theory in 26 dimensions, and recently pure mathematicians have been electrified by a version describing spaces of 24 dimensions. (Wertheim 2018)

Quite clearly with our limited level of consciousness, we cannot comprehend what more than four dimensions could be, let alone 24 or 26 dimensions. So you will be relieved to know that the scope of this book will remain with just exploring the four easily comprehended dimensions, that of space and time.

The concept of space-time dates back to the early 20th century:

> Space-time, in physical science, a single concept that recognizes the union of space and time, was first proposed by the mathematician Hermann Minkowski in 1908 as a way to reformulate Albert Einstein's special theory of relativity (1905). Common intuition previously supposed no connection between space and time. (Britannica.com 2018)

With space and time having been unarguably linked by Einstein, who is considered by many to be the greatest mind of the 20th century, it is surprising that many osteopaths still do not work with timelines. As a reader, doing cranial work already, I hope this chapter will inspire you to explore this approach with your patients.

Our awareness is amazingly flexible and adaptable and in many cases is only limited by our own beliefs. There are many practitioners within the profession who do not fully believe what cranial practitioners can palpate and treat. Unfortunately, this limits the desire to attend a course and learn new experiences under their own fingers. If, however, you have an open mind and are happy to explore the unknown, then a whole new experience may unfold to your awareness.

CENTRING OUTSIDE OF TIME

To develop the skill set for going back in time within your patient's tissues and working on a past event which affected the physiology as it if happened recently, not many years ago, we have to be highly centred within ourselves, 'outside of time'. This requires a much deeper level of inner stillness and being without practitioner ego. Part of the reason I placed this chapter at this stage in the book is so that not only will your palpation and attention levels have significantly progressed with working your way through each chapter, but your centring skills will also have been significantly improving, even if you are not conscious of that having occurred.

TIME ARROWS AND THE 'PARENT UNIVERSE'

Sean Carroll, an American research professor of physics, describes the nature of The Big Bang (fortunately in easy-to-understand terminology) and how it was not the first event of our universe. Initially he discusses how everything heads towards entropy, a more chaotic state, over time:

> ...the particular aspect of time that I'm interested in is the arrow of time: the fact that the past is different from the future. We remember the past, but we don't remember the future. There are irreversible processes. There are things that happen, like you turn an egg into an omelette, but you can't turn an omelette into an egg... It's not, 'Why did the universe begin with low entropy?' It's, 'Why did part of the universe go through a phase with low entropy?' (Carroll 2010)

He then continues to discuss a parent universe, this being outside of time itself – a state of permanent present – which only occasionally sprouts a daughter universe, then reverts to a non-changing present state, with no past and no future. The occasional daughter universe is then 'in time' and sprouts further generations of universes, one of which is our universe.

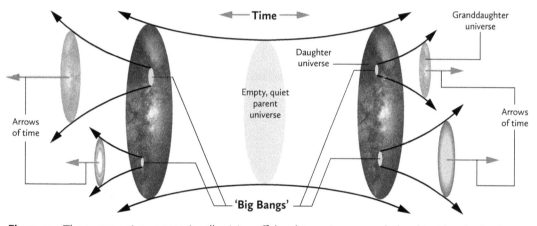

Figure 15.1 The parent universe occasionally giving off daughter universes, each daughter then having its own unique arrow of time. Each daughter subsequently has its own Big Bang to create a granddaughter universe.

If this theory is correct, it would fit in with the current astrophysical understanding that our universe is just one of an almost infinite number of universes within a multiverse. For those of you who are curious, according to MIT, Linde and Vanchurin calculated that the number of universes is 10 to the power 10, to the power 10, to the power 7. In an attempt to explain how big this number is:

> Linde and Vanchurin say that the total amount of information that can be absorbed by one individual during a lifetime is about 10 to the power 16 bits. So, a typical human brain can have 10 to the power 10 to the power 16 configurations, and so could never distinguish more than that number of different universes. (MIT Technology Review 2009)

So, the parent universe (if it exists, as some experts consider) is quite literally beyond our comprehension, and so could be also outside of time itself, as Carroll suggests. Carroll continues to describe the parent universe in terms of two aspects of time:

There are different moments in the history of the universe and time tells you which moment you're talking about. And then there's the arrow of time, which gives us the feeling of progress, the feeling of flowing or moving through time. So that static universe in the middle has time as a coordinate but there's no arrow of time. There's no future versus past, everything is equal to each other. (Carroll 2010)

When I read this statement by Carroll, I immediately thought that this parent universe is probably the ultimate still point!

We can now use this concept of a parent universe outside of time when doing our centring exercise to help our consciousness to be more objective to time. When we centre ourselves, before having read this chapter, we are coming to a still point in three dimensions within ourselves. We can use the notochordal axis, the original positional axis for the early embryo, to find the relative still point of the three dimensions of space within the physiology. By becoming more still within ourselves and so becoming more objective to the three dimensions of space, we become more objective to the three dimensions within our patients' physiology, helping us to be more objective, anatomically aware and accurate.

We may also choose to centre ourselves with subtle aspects of our breathing or combine this with an awareness of our own notochord, to get closer to a physiological still point. Breathing techniques are well known for bringing about a calmness to the psychophysiology, so can therefore be valuable in helping to centre ourselves, especially if we are feeling a little stressed or mentally too busy.

Now we can now progress to a whole new level of centring by using the concept of a parent universe, to become objective to the fourth dimension, that of time.

Exercise on yourself, centring outside of time

https://youtu.be/OiwYsspy1EQ

I suggest you repeat this centring exercise a few times before starting the first treatment table exercise for this chapter. Do give yourself about 30 minutes or so between each time you listen, otherwise you may get a bit too 'spaced out'. By having a few practices, it will give your consciousness a little time to get used to this deeper centring approach before we go to the treatment table and work on a friend or family member.

APPLICATIONS OF WORKING WITH TIME

I will now take you through a series of examples of going back in time to treat various stages of the physiology, beginning at the very beginning, that of the time of conception. Then we will look at the implantation of the egg into the uterus and stages of embryological development. We will progress to look at the birth process, childhood and adulthood. In each scenario, we will be palpating and then treating the physiology as if that event was happening today, not in the past.

I am sure many of you will, like me, have treated members of your own family, perhaps just after an injury. If you treat the physiology immediately after a traumatic injury, it feels very fresh, and there are no long-term tissue compensations needing resolution, as the injury happened only moments ago. If you have ever experienced such a situation, then you will know that it feels very different to treat, compared with an event that happened a few weeks or months, or many years ago.

By going back in time, with our awareness 'centred outside of time', it feels that we are literally palpating a fresh injury. When we proceed to work at the embryological stages of development, then the physiology feels totally different to when palpating the adult body, which we were doing only moments before we used the timeline approach.

CONCEPTUAL TIME UP TO THE THIRD WEEK OF INTRAUTERINE LIFE

Conception is when Mr Sperm meets Ms Egg. This is not about the patient on the treatment table, but the energetic phase of the two biological parents. The patient had no control over this event, they were just the consequence! However, the energetic state of the genetic parents at that moment becomes intertwined at the moment of conception. As we know, in a very high proportion of cases, this is a moment of bliss, happiness, love and tenderness (you can think of other adjectives yourself).

Following ejaculation, the male sperm have to travel about 15–18 cm to reach the female egg. Depending on the circumstances and the readiness of the egg, this can take a varying amount of time. In a normal situation, the sperm can reach the egg within 15 to 45 minutes following ejaculation. However, this time scale could be significantly longer if the woman has not ovulated by the time of the sexual intercourse. In such circumstances, sperm are capable of living within the female reproductive tract for as long as five days whilst waiting for an egg to arrive (Kallen 2022).

From the time of intercourse to the time of sperm implantation into the egg, the mother's feelings and emotions will be very much influenced by her emotions (positive or negative) during the time of intercourse. Also, the feelings of the male partner towards his female sexual partner will be influencing her feelings at this time. Consequently, the energetic state of her vaginal, uterine and fallopian tube tissues within her physiology, where the sperm are swimming and, if present, where the egg is waiting, will be bathed by these feelings and emotions.

Unfortunately, not all intercourse between a man and a woman is a time of loving, tender intimacy between consensual partners. It can simply be a moment of stress release by one or both partners, it can follow times of aggression, or can be a non-consensual act of forceful violence. It is not necessarily the man who is the offensive partner, and can (although far less commonly) occur between a dominant woman and a non-consensual man.

As osteopaths we are not here to speculate what may have happened nor why, whether a good and loving, less good, or bad, intimate event. We are tissue experts, and our role is to feel tissue quality and not delve into inappropriate questioning about such aspects. However, if perhaps a patient knows they were adopted as a baby, then there will have been a reason behind the adoption, and why the mother was unable to bring up the child. Strong negativity, or a lack or absence of love between biological parents may (we don't know for certain) be the reason.

Equally, you can use this approach to see if the energy of the conception time was harmonious and loving for the biological parents, as long as your reason for taking the approach is professionally justified and ethical, and not just out of pure curiosity. Obviously, like all other osteopathic practical learning, using this approach for a learning experience on a colleague, friend or family member is perfectly acceptable, as long as you have permission from the person you will be working on, legally termed informed consent.

From your timeline diagnosis, it may become apparent that the emotional state of the mother at the time of the intercourse was not happy, tender and loving as it should be. Consequently, if 'the act' was very emotionally or physically distressing for the mother, her physiology would have tightened up in response to the highly negative emotional circumstances. This would then have influenced the tissue states of her pelvis around the time of conception. Fortunately, with this timeline osteopathic approach, we can ease and reduce some or all of such energetic negative influences occurring within the mother, affecting the newly conceived individual.

Following intercourse, if fertilised, the egg travels to the uterus, reaching it a few days later. The egg once fertilised rapidly divides and grows. After about three to four days following the fertilisation, the egg starts entering the uterus (Nazario 2020). Whilst still within the fallopian tube, the cells are organising into a ball of cells, the blastocyst. By the time it reaches the uterus it may simply float for an extra two to three days before entering the uterine wall. In other words, it is usually approximately day seven or eight before the actual implantation into the uterine wall occurs.

So not until day seven or eight does the blastocyst gain a direct absorption of rich nutriment from the uterine wall. If the blastocyst does not implant into the uterine wall, then the egg is lost with the removal of the uterine wall during menstruation. The incidence of such loss is relatively high: '...a plausible range for natural human embryo mortality from fertilisation to live birth in normal healthy women is approximately 40–60%' (Jarvis 2016).

Around the second week the ball of cells has differentiated according to which part of the ball was the first area to get a higher level of nutrition, that area which started the implantation process. The region of the ball of cells closest to the uterine wall undergoes differentiation and becomes the trophoblast, the area of cells responsible for the absorption of nutriment and which later becomes the placenta. Against these trophoblast cells is the amniotic cavity and then the newly differentiated epiblast and hypoblast, lying between the amniotic cavity and the primary yolk sac.

The epiblast and hypoblast evolve into the ectoderm and endoderm respectively. The ectoderm within the embryo becomes our nervous system, pituitary gland and skin. However, it also develops into the lens of the eye and epithelial tissues of the sense organs, such as the nasal cavity and mouth. It also creates the lining at the other end of the gut tube, the anus. It could be considered that the ectodermal tissues are those which are involved in contact with the outside world and how we relate to it (Britannica.com 2019a).

The endodermal tissue, on the other hand, develops into the epithelial tissue linings. In the head and neck, these are within the pharynx, tonsils and auditory tube. The endoderm also creates the linings for the thyroid and parathyroid endocrine glands along with the larynx.

At the base of the neck, the endoderm forms the epithelial tissue for the thymus and in the thorax, the lungs. The endoderm has a strong relationship to the gut wall, creating the epithelial lining for the whole tube, except for the mouth and anus. In the pelvis in addition to the rectum, it forms the epithelium of the vagina (in females) and also that of the bladder and urethra (Britannica.com 2019b).

Within the following week, the embryo undergoes a further significant development, the formation of the trilaminar germ disc. Within the bilaminar germ disc, an invagination of the ectoderm occurs, creating the primitive groove, primitive pit and primitive node. This invagination of the ectoderm between itself and the endoderm creates a third layer. This new layer differentiates into what becomes the mesoderm layer.

The mesoderm gives rise to all the other tissues of the body not created by ectoderm and endoderm. These include the somites and the whole of our musculoskeletal system, along with the notochordal axis. Mesoderm is highly extensive in the physiology as it also forms the connective tissues and fascial system throughout the body. The epithelium and the tissues of our blood and lymphatic systems are also of mesodermal origin, creating our circulatory system. Being the most common tissue type in the body, in addition the mesoderm is responsible for the formation of many of our organs (Britannica.com 2012).

The mesoderm also forms the somites, which later become our muscles and bones, fascia and mesenchyme tissue throughout the body. As you can see, the advent of the third layer during the third week of development is a profound embryological shift.

It is probably around the third week following fertilisation that the mother is thinking, 'Oh, my goodness, my period is late.' Whether this is good news or bad news will depend on the readiness of the parents to start having a family, or to have another child. Consequently, this will be a time of great joy, or a time of perhaps negative shock.

Exercise on the timeline for conception, 7 days, 2nd and 3rd week of intra-uterine life

Read these instructions to the practical, before scanning the QR code/accessing the web page which follows.

- Be deeply centred within, referencing to the parent universe above and beyond time!

- Take a comfortable hold anywhere (it does not really matter where, as long as you and your model are comfortable).
- Do not focus on any particular tissue.
- Have in your awareness the moment of conception, the moment of fertilisation.
- Be aware of the energetic state of the fluids surrounding the egg and sperm.
- Bring the physiology of your model to a point of balanced tissue tension.
- Repeat for the significant very early embryological milestones
  - At 7 days: implantation
  - At 2 weeks: bilaminar germ disc
  - At 3 weeks: trilaminar germ disc.

https://youtu.be/4M1F1OK2zQg

Having reached the trilaminar germ disc stage and, if necessary (but not otherwise), treated the varying stages to get to this point, the embryo goes through the embryological development of the varying organs and tissues of the body along with the development and formation of the limbs.

I will give two examples of how to treat such tissues during their formation, those of the eye and the heart. These are just examples to demonstrate the principles; I could have chosen any part of the body. After having learned the method of the principle, you can apply the approach to wherever you feel is clinically appropriate for your patient.

PRINCIPLES FOR TREATING THE EMBRYOLOGICAL DEVELOPMENT OF ASPECTS OF THE PHYSIOLOGY

- You will have needed to read up on the embryological development of the part of the body you wish to work on. This could be from a good physiology book or perhaps online.
- Get an idea of the key times of the stages of development for that organ, i.e., how many days after conception, for each key stage.
- If necessary, print out some images of those key times and stages so you can place those images near you when working at the treatment table. If you choose to do this, explain to your patient that you are going to do some work which requires you to have an exact knowledge of an early stage of their physiology, and that is why you will be at times looking at the images whilst working. The patient will, in my experience, be quite impressed by your doing that.
- Centre yourself with reference to the parent universe, outside and beyond time.
- Mentally, gently think of the start date after conception, for the formation of that organ, e.g., day 22 for the eye. This will, as if 'magically', shift your awareness to that exact day embryologically, and you will feel an immediate dramatic shift in tissue quality from that of the adult to that of an early embryo, it now feeling incredibly fluid.
- Work your way through the key stages you have outlined, but only inviting that key stage to treat itself if you detect some negative tension. If it feels good, then do not treat it, but move on to the next stage, only inviting the physiology to treat itself where necessary, until you reach the time of the formed organ.

- The embryological phase is where the tissues have formed the organ, but there may still be maturation to occur within the organ. Whether you stop at the embryological formation or continue through the time to full completion is your choice.

When teaching this approach, I stop at the end of the embryological formation stage, which is what I will be doing for the practical sessions linked to this chapter.

Embryological development example 1: The eye
Key stages of eye development

1. At around 22 days following conception, the neural ectoderm of the developing brain folds and creates two optic vesicles.
2. At 28 days the surface ectoderm thickens over the optic vesicle as a lens placode.
3. At around 31 days the optic stalk lengthens to form the optic nerve and the optic cup indents to create an early-stage optic cup. The surface ectoderm over the optic cup develops into a lens placode and a lens pit.
4. At 33 days, whilst the optic cup is forming, the optic stalk also invaginates to create the optic blood vessels, and the hyaloid artery and vein within this developing fissure. These will later develop into the blood vessels to supply the future developing retina.
5. Also at 33 days, the lens placode develops into two regions, the true lens itself and also an area anterior to it, which will become the anterior chamber of the eye. The retina at this stage is now covering the inside of the eye surface.

6. By 41 days the retina is enclosing the posterior chamber. This posterior chamber is growing in size to push the retina closer against the back of the eye. The lens at this stage is now detached from the surface aspect of the eye and a cornea is developing from the ectodermal tissue.

7. By 67 days the eye is looking quite similar to the adult eye, although the hyaline artery and vein are now at this stage just dissolving away so as not to obstruct the future light passage from the lens to the retina. The surface ectoderm and mesoderm beneath it are now invaginating to form the cornea and our eyelids. The iris muscle and ciliary body, which creates the fluid of the anterior chamber, have also now formed. The lens is now properly suspended by the suspensory ligament.

8. By 112 days (16 weeks), the eye formation is close to that of how it is at birth. The eyelids remain fused until about week 20 (140 days) and the hyaloid artery and vein are fully disintegrated around the 16-week stage, just leaving the gel-like vitreous humour of the posterior chamber of the eye.

Exercise on treating the embryological development of the eye

Before starting the practical you will need to centre yourself using the concept of the parent universe to bring your awareness closer to being outside of time and space.

Having just gained an insight into the key stages of eye development, we can now progress to the hands on practical. However, you may wish to clarify the embryology of the eye further, on your own from books or online, before proceeding to the practical.

https://youtu.be/J3gU4vtpepA

It is worth noting that the eye is formed to adult size by the age of seven years, and so a child's eyes are much larger proportionally to the size of the face than in adults.

Embryological development example 2: The heart
Key stages of cardiac development

It is fascinating that the start date of the initial beating of the heart tube is around that of another momentous occasion:

> The initiation of the first heart beat via the primitive heart tube begins at gestational day 22, followed by active foetal blood circulation by the end of week 4. The start of early heart development involves several types of progenitor cells that are derived from the mesoderm, proepicardium, and neural crest. (Tan and Lewandowski 2020)

This beating of the primordial heart tube is just after the trilaminar germ disc stage of development. However, this is also likely around the time when the mother (if she has a regular menstrual cycle) is thinking: 'My period is a bit late, could I be pregnant?' We know that this can either be a time of great joy to the mother, or not. So, the fact that this time of (hopefully) joyful celebration and wonder to the mother occurs around the time that the heart tube starts beating, is certainly a strange coincidence.

We must also bear in mind that the mother will be feeling this emotion as a heartfelt feeling, quite literally in her heart tissues, the heart being a key emotional tissue (see Chapter 16 for more on this topic). Did the cosmic laws of nature make these two events coincide on purpose? We will never know, but we cannot deny the fascinating fact that both happen at a similar time!

1. The primitive blood vessels start to coalesce in the area of greatest embryological activity, that of the brain, their then being in a cephalic position, relative to the developing brain.
2. By day 18, the primitive blood vessels which initially are cephalic to the brain are growing to form along the growing sides of the brain.
3. As the brain then undergoes phenomenal growth and development, it has to grow into the space available which is then cephalic to the heart tube, making the heart tube now below the brain. It is not the heart that moves down into the thorax, but its position is the consequence of the brain growing: the heart actually stays in the same place.
4. By day 20, as the brain grows into what becomes a cephalic position relative to the future heart, the two blood vessels start coming towards each other from the left and right sides.
5. By day 21 these two tubes meet in the midline at the area which will become the thorax, and fuse to form the early heart tube.
6. By day 22 the fusion of the two endocardial tubes has completed with the two arterial trunks (the future aorta and pulmonary artery) most superior, and what will become the atria of the heart, most inferior.
7. Due to there now being a lack of space in the thorax, the heart tube has to start twisting and turning on itself, creating the helical ventricular band.
8. Between day 24 and day 35 the heart has developed its adult shape with the two ventricles inferior and the two atria now being superior. The atria have to fold posteriorly as the ventricles are expanding and twisting more anteriorly in front of the atria.
9. From day 35 to the 20th week of intrauterine life, the heart completes its internal maturation of the muscle walls and the formation of internal valves and is simply growing in size between week 20 and birth.

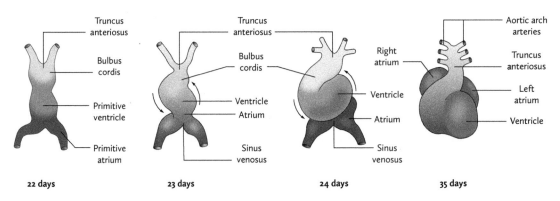

Figure 15.2 Stages of development of the heart.

A research team at Leeds University discovered that the heart continues to mature internally until week 20. This is some ten weeks later than was previously thought. Their research was from human studies and not mammalian studies as done previously:

A University of Leeds-led team developing the first comprehensive model of human heart development using observations of living foetal hearts found surprising differences from existing animal models. Although they saw four clearly defined chambers in the foetal heart from the eighth week of pregnancy, they did not find organised muscle tissue until the 20th week, much later than expected (Leeds University 2013)

The helical ventricular band mentioned above is one muscular structure that becomes both the left and right ventricles. It was discovered by Torrent-Guasp, and revolutionises the way we think about heart contractions: 'The helical ventricular myocardial band of Torrent-Guasp is a revolutionary new concept in understanding global, 3-dimensional, functional architecture of the ventricular myocardium' (Kocica *et al.* 2007). I strongly recommend you watch the YouTube video about the helical myocardial band entitled 'Fransisco [*sic*] Torrent-Guasp's New Science of the Helical Heart' (Truthbubbles, n.d.).

Having gained a familiarity with the basic heart development to day 35, we can now go to the treatment table for a practical session.

Exercise on the development of the heart

https://youtu.be/6Xt6n1yepoM

In the above two sections, we have looked at the development of the eye and that of the heart, as examples of how you could work with any aspect of embryological development. Now we will progress with using our fourth dimensional osteopathy to look at the birth process.

DELIVERY ON TIME: MEMBRANOUS BIRTH MEMORY

Birth is probably one of the most traumatic events our physiology will experience. Luckily (though maybe it's not luck but mammalian evolution), our physiology is designed to accommodate these forces to an amazing level by not having the sutures of the skull fully formed at the time of birth.

As stated in Chapter 14 on treating babies and children, I will not go into the birth process in great detail, as that needs to be covered by a paediatric training course. However, for those of you who do already work with babies and children, you will find these next two sections fascinating.

For the previous nine months before birth, assuming the child was not born prematurely, the embryo and developing foetus is surrounded by

a highly fluid environment. Energetically, if the parents are happy with regard to the forthcoming child, they both will be sending their love towards the child in the womb. During the latter stages of the pregnancy, the baby is getting much larger and there it is less space for it to move around and so it is more cramped within the uterus. Consequently, the fasciae and membranes will be relatively stiffer than when there was more space, but a baby is much more flexible than later in life, so this is just a marginal difference.

Birth starts

It has been revealed in a study by Condon and his team that the foetal lungs secrete a hormonal stimulus which passes to the maternal uterus and stimulates the onset of contractions. This hormone is secreted when the foetal lungs are ready and have sufficient surfactant present to survive life in air outside the womb:

> In conclusion, our studies provide important evidence that augmented production of SP-A by the maturing foetal lung at term provides a key hormonal stimulus for the cascade of inflammatory signalling pathways within the maternal uterus that culminate in the enhanced myometrial contractility leading to parturition. This hormonal signal, transmitted to the uterus by foetal AF macrophages reveals that the foetal lungs are sufficiently developed to withstand the critical transition from an aqueous to an aerobic environment. (Condon *et al.* 2004)

In a 'normal' birth the baby's occiput is described as lying to the left aspect of the mother's pelvis. This position is guided by the shape of the mother's pelvis and the spiral nature of the uterine muscles. There is always a reciprocal tension between the pelvic shape and the baby's head position, as the baby's head always attempts to lie in the widest diameter of the maternal pelvis. Hence in the upper pelvis this widest aspect is lateral and in the lower pelvis it is greatest in the anterior/posterior (A/P) direction. Consequently, the baby's head has to rotate to accommodate the changing pelvis shape. The so-called normal birth is where the baby's head moves in the best manner to fit in with these shape changes.

First and second stages of labour

During the first stage of labour, the baby's occiput lies towards the left side of the upper maternal pelvis. As contractions proceed the baby then has to rotate its head, as it descends into the lower aspect of the maternal pelvis, where the widest diameter is A/P. The occiput is leading the birth journey, so that this rotation of the baby's head results in the baby's occiput lying at the anterior aspect of the mother's pelvis, face towards the lower sacrum.

The mother's pelvic floor and uterine cervix then have to soften and dilate to open up the birth canal for the baby's head, the cervix needing to widen to 10 cm. The uterine contractions pulling the cervix wider and larger, plus the pressure of the baby's head against pelvic floor, will open the pelvic floor and the vaginal exit.

These changes result in the extending of the baby's neck and the occiput presenting first. In her article for mothers on a normal birth (with excellent diagrams of the second stage, which I recommend viewing), Arora describes the second stage of labour as: 'This is the active stage. During this time, the baby is pushed out of the uterus and into the world through the vaginal canal' (Arora 2018).

You will see from reading and viewing images of the second stage that these movements by the baby demand quite strong rotational and extension motions of the head and neck, whilst being under strong downwards compression by the maternal uterus. Such forces demand much accommodation by the plates of the foetal skull, and consequently the bones of the cranial base and vault move in their relationship to each other during this process. Having only soft skin and membrane at the vault fontanelles during the time of birth allows these accommodating skull motions to occur.

Exercise on birth process and the meninges

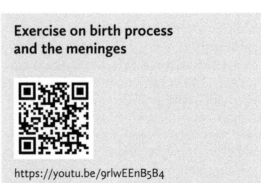

https://youtu.be/9rlwEEnB5B4

BIRTH AND THE CENTRAL NERVOUS SYSTEM

A number of years ago, after using the timeline approach with birth and the meninges for some time, I realised that the central nervous system (CNS) must undergo a series of changes during birth also, but differently from the meninges. For example, the onset of birth and the first uterine contraction will be reacted to differently by the CNS, as the calm, peaceful, warm state of the uterine environment would have been drastically changed with that first uterine contraction.

Around that same time, I was invited to have an experience of Holotropic Breathing, a technique developed by Stanislav Grof, MD PhD, and Christina Grof, PhD. They developed Holotropic Breathing to reduce the mental shock of the birth process and how it played out in later adult life. An award-winning book on the topic was published in 1992: *The Holotropic Mind: The Three Levels of Human Consciousness and How They Shape Our Lives* (Grof and Bennett 1992).

For anyone who has not heard of Holotropic Breathing or not experienced this, it is a technique where you have to hyperventilate, under carefully controlled conditions and with helpers to check you are OK, for two hours. The person leading my Holotropic experience had me lying on a foam mattress, whilst I listened to varying types of music. This, according to the Grofs, helps the psyche to unravel and process some of the mental birth traumas. This was then followed by my having to draw what I felt with crayons, in whatever way it came up, and then discuss my drawing with the group present. The whole session lasted about two and a half hours.

A few weeks later I realised that as osteopaths we could achieve the same result in 20 minutes or so, not two and a half hours, by going through the timeline approach to birth, but this time having our practitioner awareness on the CNS not the membranes.

The onset of contractions

The sudden start of contractions, even when stimulated by the chemical output of the foetal lungs which signals they are ready to receive air, will have been a considerable shock to the foetal CNS. That warm, comforting uterine environment suddenly becomes threatening, with a squeezing that does not go away and is then shortly followed by another, and only seems to get worse. Even though these first early contractions are not as powerful as later ones, they are still a big change for the state of the CNS compared with moments previously.

The Grofs call the stage before the start of contractions: 'A time of peace and joy of a healthy womb' and describe the start of contractions for the CNS of the baby as: 'An unbearable feeling of being stuck in Hell with no way of escaping' (Grof and Bennett 1992). I am not sure if I find this description a little excessive, but that sense of 'What on earth is happening? I don't like it, I can't escape, what's happening to me?' does come across in these words.

The big squeeze

As the contractions continue unabated and get stronger, and as the baby descends further into the pelvis, it meets what I call 'the big squeeze' as the baby's head enters the true birth canal. This is the point where the baby's head undergoes maximum shape change and moulding as it gets severely squeezed.

When the brain undergoes very severe shock for any reason beyond its tolerance level, it goes into a protective shutdown as the input stimulus is beyond what it can cope with. We call this shutdown fainting or being knocked out, or just not knowing what happened to us for a period of time. From clinical experience working with the CNS and birth, a baby's brain does something similar and shuts down with deep shock during this big squeeze phase. The mother's pelvis is having to open wider, and the baby's head is changing shape, as its head is forcing that shape change of the mother's pelvis.

The Grofs describe this stage as the: 'Death versus Rebirth Struggle. Second clinical stage of childbirth; intense struggle for survival.' Again, they use highly graphic words, but they are correct. If the baby does not cope and manage this big squeeze, it can die.

Having passed through this stage, the head emerges, presenting itself to the world. This is when the body fluids of the baby are then squeezed back up into the head, as the torso is still under contractile pressure, but the head is now just under atmospheric pressure. This then allows the shape of the baby's head to restore as much as possible. This again will be a huge change for the brain tissue, as it undergoes another massive shape change. This is then followed by the delivery of the rest of the body and being wrapped in the mother's arms and closeness to the mother's breast. The Grofs describe this last stage as the: 'Death versus Rebirth Experience. The child is born. Intense ecstatic feelings of liberation and love. A new world begins.'

As we know, the CNS is involved with our psyche. If the CNS does not get an opportunity to resolve any of its birth shocks, then these stresses can and do play out as life patterns. For example, if the CNS went into shock with the onset of contractions but had not since that time released the stresses and shock, then the person could have difficulty moving on in their life, and need to stay somewhere safe and secure, perhaps not taking chances, even if such opportunities may open and progress their life.

As an adult, if the CNS has not yet released the shock and distress of the big squeeze, then the individual may repeatedly have feelings that life is on top of them, and that there is only deep tension that will not go away – a feeling of being unable to cope with everything that is happening to them. If the CNS did not release the stress and shock of the head reverting towards a more

normal shape, and the concept of now being outside and separate from the mother, the adult person can be left with a sense of not being able to stand on their own two feet, and needing continual support much of the time. These psychological scenarios may seem familiar as you may have seen these character types in other people you have met.

The Grofs found that their Holotropic Breathing method released these psychological issues and behavioural patterns in the adult. Since I have been teaching this osteopathic timeline approach in Europe for quite a number of years, I have had students who, after attending this course, have come on my other courses, a few months or even years later. Quite a few of the students have privately said to me when meeting them again that their life has been very different since the timeline course and that their mental negativity has significantly reduced. The Grofs' theory appears to be verified, and as osteopaths we can do this in 20–30 minutes, not two and a half hours!

Exercise on birth and the CNS

Please note: *I strongly recommend* that you do *not* practise this session on birth and the CNS, if you have just done the timeline approach to birth and the membranes. It would be too much for your friend/family member's physiology as they are both very powerful methods of working. I suggest you do the birth and meninges session first, and then this birth and CNS session several days later.

https://youtu.be/hGxem8ijmpo

POST BIRTH: A PHYSICALLY TRAUMATIC TIME

Once the baby is born, the child starts growing up and becomes more adventurous. This may lead to accidents and injuries. The traumatic forces within the physiology will enter many tissues and organs. These will include the musculoskeletal system tissues: bone, periosteum, fascia, muscle, joints, ligaments. However, the same traumatic forces will also penetrate into the blood vessels, organs and all aspects of the nervous system. We know from our existing palpatory skills that such tissues become compressed and denser and feel heavier. We know that the fluctuation of the cerebrospinal fluid becomes poorer. Around these areas the blood vessels seem to constrict and the whole musculoskeletal system tightens. At the same time the digestive system frequently shuts down due to the sympathetic response.

If we are able to treat the time of the event as if it happened very recently, it becomes easier to release the physical shock and gain a deeper rebalancing of the various tissues and organs. As a consequence, a greater level of health and potency can be expressed within the tissues.

Exercise on a physically traumatic time

In the next practical you will be selecting to palpate an area where your friend/family member has experienced an accident, injury, or fall at some time in the past. This may be either the recent or more distant past, it does not matter. Please make sure they do NOT inform you *when* the event happened, only to *which area of their body*. In this practical we will be using timelines to diagnose as close as possible when the event happened, and then treat the event as if it happened recently.

https://youtu.be/mr1xLBnsfGQ

I will discuss working with timelines to help emotional shock and stresses in the next chapter, as it will be more appropriate at that point.

I hope you will take your time to enjoy working through these various timeline approaches a few times, before progressing to the next chapter. Using timelines can be quite revolutionary in how you diagnose and help your patients.

REFERENCES

Arora, M., 2018. Normal delivery – signs, benefits, process and tips. Available from: https://parenting.firstcry.com/articles/pregnancy-tips-for-normal-delivery/?ref=intelink.

Britannica.com, 2012. Mesoderm. Encyclopaedia Britannica. Available from: https://www.britannica.com/science/mesoderm.

Britannica.com, 2018. Space-time. Encyclopaedia Britannica. Available from: https://www.britannica.com/science/space-time.

Britannica.com, 2019a. Ectoderm. Encyclopaedia Britannica. Available from: https://www.britannica.com/science/ectoderm.

Britannica.com, 2019b. Endoderm. Encyclopaedia Britannica. Available from: https://www.britannica.com/science/endoderm.

Carroll, S., 2010. What is time? One physicist hunts for the ultimate theory. Wired. Available from: https://www.wired.com/2010/02/what-is-time/

Condon, J.C., Jeyasuria, P., Faust, J.M., & Mendelson, C.R., 2004. Surfactant protein secreted by the maturing mouse fetal lung acts as a hormone that signals the initiation of parturition. *Proceedings of the National Academy of Sciences of the United States of America.* 101(14): 4978–4983. Available from: https://doi.org/10.1073/pnas.0401124101.

Grof, S., with Bennett, H.Z., 1992. *The Holotropic Mind: The Three Levels of Human Consciousness and How They Shape Our Lives.* San Francisco: HarperCollins.

Jarvis, G.E., 2016. Estimating limits for natural human embryo mortality. *F1000Research.* 5: 2083. Available from: https://doi.org/10.12688/f1000research.9479.1.

Kallen, A., 2022. Here's how long it takes sperm to reach the egg after sex. Flo Health. Available from: https://flo.health/getting-pregnant/trying-to-conceive/fertility/how-long-does-it-take-sperm-to-reach-egg#:~:text=Usually%2C%20the%20sperm%20reaches%20the,for%20up%20to%20five%20days.

Kocica, M., Corno, A., Lackovic, V., & Kanjuh, V., 2007. The helical ventricular myocardial band of Torrent-Guasp. *Seminars in Thoracic and Cardiovascular Surgery. Pediatric Cardiac Surgery Annual.* 52–60. Doi: 10.1053/j.pcsu.2007.01.006.

Leeds University, 2013. Human heart development slower than other mammals. Available from: https://www.leeds.ac.uk/news-health/news/article/3368/human-heart-development-slower-than-other-mammals.

MIT Technology Review, 2009. Space physicists calculate number of universes in the multiverse. Available from: https://www.technologyreview.com/2009/10/15/123729/physicists-calculate-number-of-universes-in-the-multiverse/

Nazario, B., 2020. Conception: from egg to embryo slideshow. Available from: https://www.webmd.com/baby/ss/slideshow-conception#:~:text=The%20fertilized%20egg%20starts%20growing,attaches%20to%20the%20fallopian%20tube.

Tan, C.M.J., & Lewandowski, A.J., 2020. The transitional heart: from early embryonic and foetal development to neonatal life. *Fetal Diagn Ther.* 47: 373–386. Available from: https://www.karger.com/Article/Fulltext/501906#.

Truthbubbles, n.d. Fransisco [sic] Torrent-Guasp's New Science of The Helical Heart. YouTube. Available from: https://www.youtube.com/watch?v=N6ORMHi9rcU.

Wertheim, M., 2018. Radical dimensions. Available from: https://aeon.co/essays/how-many-dimensions-are-there-and-what-do-they-do-to-reality.

CHAPTER 16

The Inner Relationship of Mind, Body and Emotions

WHERE IS 'THE MIND'?

As any practitioner who has been in clinical practice for a while will know, it is impossible to separate the mind from the body. Perhaps the terms 'psycho-physiology' or 'mind-body' are more correct. Much thought has gone into the question: where is the mind? Communication pathologist and neuroscientist Caroline Leaf expresses this conundrum as follows:

> The mind uses the brain, and the brain responds to the mind. The mind also changes the brain. People choose their actions – their brains do not force them to do anything. Yes, there would be no conscious experience without the brain, but experience cannot be reduced to the brain's actions. The mind is energy, and it generates energy through thinking, feeling, and choosing. It is our aliveness, without which, the physical brain and body would be useless. That means *we* are our mind, and mind-in-action is how we generate energy in the brain. (Leaf 2021)

As has been mentioned in the chapters covering differing aspects of the anatomy, emotional feelings are felt in the body, not in the brain. Whenever we feel particularly strong sensations, they frequently go to specific areas. Nobody from any culture in the world has ever put their hand on their forehead and said: 'Oh he/she loves me!'

They always feel it in the heart, and will put their hand to their heart to connect to that feeling.

We also have what we call 'gut feelings'. Such colloquial terminology was probably created way back in the history of our language, as such feelings are part of being a human. Having a gut feeling about something can be both in the form of a positive intuitive insight, an inspiration, and also in the form of a negative warning feeling about something.

Again, we all undergo such experiences at varying times of our life. Most people do not talk about such experiences as they may think the listener would view them as being foolish, or not being logical, which for many people is an absolute cardinal sin in Western society. Should we trust these heart-felt emotions and our gut feelings?

Rebecca D. Heaslip from Leadership Insight quotes Richard Branson, an internationally well-known and highly successful individual, speaking on this topic:

> I do a lot by gut feeling and a lot by personal experience. I mean if I had relied on account- ants to make decisions, I most certainly would never have gone into the airline business. I most certainly would not have gone into the space business, and I most certainly would not have

gone into most of the businesses that I'm in. (Heaslip 2012)

As an osteopath, I find that when working with patients I agree with Branson on both levels, that of doing a lot by both gut feeling and personal experience. By this I mean that I use both intellect and experience along with intuitive insight, as has been described in Chapter 3 in the diagnosis section.

However, in this context, what is a gut feeling, or intuition? On one level our intuition is our brain processing information at a level below our conscious thinking. It then sends signals via the brain stem vagal nuclei and vagus nerve to both the heart and the gut tube. Such signals may then create part of what we experience in those organs. However, both the heart and the gut send afferent signals to the brain via the vagus nerve, and the heart sends more afferent signals to the brain than efferent signals going the other way.

HEART MEMORY AND HEART TRANSPLANT PATIENTS

As the afferent signals from the heart are greater than the efferent signals, this demonstrates quite clearly that the heart needs to communicate with the brain about aspects of its information.

> ...the heart sends more information to the brain than the brain sends to the heart. More recent research shows that the neural interactions between the heart and brain are more complex than previously thought. In addition, the intrinsic cardiac nervous system has both short-term and long-term memory functions and can operate independently of central neuronal command. (Heart Math Institute 2001)

A study done in 1976 on the effects of love emotions and heart disease came up with some intriguing results:

> Without loving companionship, human beings are more vulnerable to cardiovascular and other illness. Research supporting this conclusion comes from many directions. An early Israeli study of 10,000 married men with heart disease found that one simple questionnaire item had a dramatic moderating effect, even in the presence of high cholesterol, EKG abnormalities, and high anxiety (Medalie and Gouldbourt,

1976). Among those men who said 'Yes' to the question, 'Does your wife show you her love?' only 52% developed angina. Among the group who said 'No' to the same question, 93% developed angina! (Saybrook University 2009)

The above quote further verifies that we feel love, or a lack of it, in our heart not our brain. The subjects who did not feel love being expressed in their marriage developed angina, not symptoms from reduced brain blood flow.

There have been a number of heart transplant recipients who have gained information, feeling and sometimes lifestyle changes based on aspects of the heart donor's personality or lifestyle. I shall not go into specific case histories here, but I do strongly recommend that you look at the work of Paul Pearsall and his colleagues. In their 2005 article, they give ten really fascinating case studies where the donor affected the recipient in some very clear manner: 'According to this study of patients who have received transplanted organs, particularly hearts, it is not uncommon for memories, behaviours, preferences and habits associated with the donor to be transferred to the recipient' (Pearsall *et al.* 2005).

Such cases as described above do demonstrate that the heart does contain memory within its own tissues. However, these heart memory cases as described should not negatively influence anyone's decision about whether to undergo such an operation. Heart replacement surgery may give many more years of life to the recipient.

THE 'DIGESTIVE BRAIN'

It is increasingly acknowledged that our digestive health is strongly influenced by mental states such as stress and anxiety. The coeliac plexus receives signals from both the vagus as well as the greater and lesser splanchnic sympathetic nerves. This plexus, as discussed in Chapter 9, supplies the stomach, liver, gall bladder, spleen, kidney and small intestine. Consequently, the sympathetic fight or flight impulses can tighten up and restrict the blood flow to these organs along with that of the gut tube. Therefore, it can easily cause stress/anxiety-based gut issues.

Stress-based gut issues become more clearly expressed in people without any known gut pathological state, a functional condition. According to Harvard University:

> In addition, many people with functional GI disorders perceive pain more acutely than other people do because their brains are more responsive to pain signals from the GI tract. Stress can make the existing pain seem even worse.
>
> Based on these observations, you might expect that at least some patients with functional GI conditions might improve with therapy to reduce stress or treat anxiety or depression. Multiple studies have found that psychologically based approaches lead to greater improvement in digestive symptoms compared with only conventional medical treatment. (Harvard Health Publishing 2021)

This statement by Harvard University that psychological based approaches lead to improvement in digestive symptoms is highly relevant to us as osteopaths. Our treatments, particularly if we are working at the level of the involuntary mechanism, definitely have a calming and restorative nature on the CNS and autonomic nervous systems, particularly if you consciously choose to work on these systems.

In modern society, many people suffer from too much happening in their lives, too much of importance to concentrate on, too many demands. We have all experienced this from time to time. As long as it is just a phase in our life which has a definite end point that is within the foreseeable future, then the negative effect on our nervous system and emotional system will probably be minor. However, there are many people who spend much of their life in such circumstances. The consequences start with anxiety type symptoms, which, if left unassisted, become stronger and more frequent until eventually the person feels exhausted and sinks into depressive states. As has been mentioned in Chapter 12 on the brain, such states can be palpated as anxiety feeling buzzy and depressive states feeling like the battery has run out of charge.

Different parts of the body express emotions of differing types. Anxiety, apprehension, fear, lack of love, worry, aspects involving negative intimacy, etc. can create tensions in differing locations. Nummenmaa and his team did some research into where we feel a variety of emotions in our body. They grouped these into two groups, basic and non-basic. The basic were: anger, fear, disgust, happiness, sadness and surprise. The non-basic were: anxiety, love, depression, contempt, pride, shame and envy. Their conclusions were:

> We conclude that emotional feelings are associated with discrete, yet partially overlapping maps of bodily sensations, which could be at the

core of the emotional experience. These results thus support models assuming that somatosensation, and embodiment, play critical roles in emotional processing. Unravelling the subjective bodily sensations associated with human emotions may help us to better understand mood disorders such as depression and anxiety, which are accompanied by altered emotional processing, ANS activity, and somatosensation. (Nummenmaa *et al.* 2014)

I recommend reading the above article by Nummenmaa *et al.*, and especially looking at the Figure 2 image (see web page in the references). This image displays the areas of the body which have high or low levels of activity for each emotion, and is worth viewing as these scientific findings relate to clinical findings by osteopaths.

DIFFERING ORGANS AND DIFFERING EMOTIONS

In East Asian medicine, differing organs are considered to be associated with different emotions. Lee and his team looked at these organs and emotions from a scientific perspective. Their conclusions were:

> The visualisation of emotions on a human body template created for the present study revealed that specific patterns existed between the visceral system and corresponding emotions such that anger corresponded with the liver, happiness with the heart, thoughtfulness with the heart and spleen, sadness with the heart and lungs, fear with the kidneys, heart, liver, and gallbladder, anxiety with the heart and lungs, and surprise with the heart and gallbladder. Furthermore, the present findings showed that the heart had significant associations with most of the emotions listed, other than anger and fear. (Lee *et al.* 2017)

The diaphragm and our emotions

As has been said in Chapter 9, the diaphragm in our patients is rarely found in a good state. Being the functional midpoint between the cranial base and sacrum has much to do with this diaphragm state, but we must acknowledge that emotions have a profound influence also. In the English language we have an idiom: 'butterflies in my stomach', this being said after experiencing or anticipating an action which created/creates nervous anxiety which is felt in the upper abdomen. Examples may be: when you are about to go on a first date with someone, if you were about to parachute out of an aeroplane, or before exams as a student.

In these examples, a sense of anxiety was created, even if the actual experience resulting from the event was highly positive. The source of that upper abdominal anxiety can be from the coeliac plexus of nerves becoming more active, and/or the influence of the diaphragm tightening up, commonly both. Breathing exercises, which have been used for thousands of years in yogic philosophy (known as pranayama), can be used to reduce emotional tensions. The breathing exercises work via the lungs to help the vagus and parasympathetic nervous system to counterbalance the sudden sympathetic activity, but the breathing exercises also have a direct mechanical effect of relaxing the diaphragm muscle itself.

I give my patients the following exercise, which is very effective at making the lower ribs work with our breathing. In many people the diaphragm gets locked up as do the lower ribs. Ask the person to place their hands on the respective sides of the lower aspects of the costal margin, so that their middle fingers just touch each other in the midline over the upper abdomen. Then ask them to breathe normally, but as they do so, to focus on their fingertips moving laterally away from each other during the inhalation phase. This action stimulates the 'bucket handle' type motion of the lower ribs, an action which frequently becomes lost as the stress levels in the breathing pattern increase.

EXERCISES

Here are three exercises which you will find of particular value when wishing to assist your patient who has stress and/or emotional tensions:

1. The small head within the big head.
2. Sympathetic and parasympathetic balancing.
3. Head, heart and gut balancing.

Each of these three approaches is quite different and you may find each has benefit for differing types of patients. It is very important to appreciate that as osteopaths, when proceeding with such approaches, we do not need to know, nor should we enquire as to, the cause of the emotional/stress issues of the patient. That is none of our business!

Exercise 1: The small head within the big head

This is the approach which comes from working with timelines (see Chapter 15), but as will become clear, is more appropriate to be included here.

About 30 years ago when palpating the head, I experienced a finding which was quite fascinating. I had my hands on the lateral aspects of the skull and after a while of just feeling the involuntary mechanism, I felt as if my hands were being drawn in, and settled to an energetic place, which felt as if I was holding a much smaller head, smaller than that of the patient's adult size. Initially I dismissed this experience, but when I experienced it the following week on another patient, I realised this was not coincidence, nor imagination, but a palpatory reality. I realised that what I was feeling was a child-sized head, even though the patient was an adult. The quality of this small head was tight, but not the type of tightness associated with mechanical trauma. There was no directional force vector, just an 'implosion' type quality, as if the head membranes and central nervous system were tightening up from within, not from without. Such a palpatory quality is of the type associated with mental tension/distress.

I realised that this needed further investigation and I then carried out a timeline assessment to discover the age of this 'small head' within the 'big head'. As I did so, I found the age at which this head energetically became 'stuck' and hence left this imprint of tension and created a small head at that same age as indicated by the timeline, when a negative event happened in childhood. I then proceeded to reduce these emotional shocks which were creating the small head sensation, and as I did so, this small inner head grew in size back towards the adult sized head. This process had very profound positive benefits to the patient, without my needing to know the nature of the problem.

Exercise on the small head within the big head

https://youtu.be/K6hRTUHSXow

Exercise 2: Sympathetic and parasympathetic balancing

This approach involves the practitioner attuning their awareness to the two aspects of the autonomic nervous system initially individually, then afterwards both simultaneously. The role of the practitioner is to help these two systems have a better interrelationship with each other. In doing so the physiology can find the best autonomic state to be in at any particular time. As has been stated above, frequently they are out of balance with one or both being hyperactive.

Exercise on sympathetic and parasympathetic balancing: Vagus and adrenals

https://youtu.be/nGgYXUw26oc

Exercise 3: Head, heart and gut balancing

I developed this approach about four years ago, after hearing a talk on the latest advanced methods of coaching and psychological approaches to helping clients. The speaker discussed how we have head thinking, heart emotion and gut feelings, and how some people have a lack of one or two of these three components.

You may have come across people who are 'all in their head'. Everything they do is purely based on much intellectualisation, little or no emotion or feeling. It is as if staying in the head they feel safer, not connecting to emotions or feelings. Likewise, you may have seen people who are lacking in 'common sense' or rationalisation, being more impulsive. Such people have a tendency to live by their emotions or gut feelings the whole time.

The healthy reality is that we need to access and use all three aspects of ourselves. If one or two aspects are neglected or shut away, then we become out of balance. If the legs on a three-legged stool are equal in length, then the stool is stable and comfortable to sit on. If one or two legs are shorter, then it becomes very uncomfortable to sit on. Similarly, life becomes less comfortable if one or two of these three aspects are significantly diminished.

The speaker, having described this balancing approach, then went on to say that six one-hour sessions could make a very big change to the client. A few days after hearing this presentation, I realised that as osteopaths we could make the same level of change in one or two sessions of just 20 minutes!

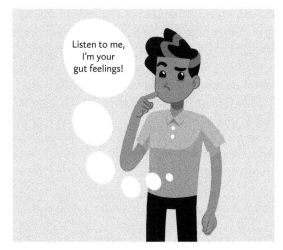

Listen to me, I'm your gut feelings!

Figure 16.1 Types of thoughts, feelings and emotions felt in the head, heart and gut.

Exercise on the head, heart and gut

https://youtu.be/2EyIqbGsE2A

REFERENCES

Harvard Health Publishing, 2021. The gut-brain connection. Available from: https://www.health.harvard.edu/diseases-and-conditions/the-gut-brain-connection.

Heart Math Institute, 2001. Heart-brain communication. Available from: https://www.heartmath.org/research/science-of-the-heart/heart-brain-communication/

Heaslip, R., 2012. Trust your brain...trust your heart... TRUST YOUR GUT! Available from: https://leadership-insightblog.com/2012/07/25/trust-your-braintrust-your-hearttrust-your-gut/

Leaf, C., 2021. How are the mind & the brain different? A neuroscientist explains. Available from: https://www.mindbodygreen.com/articles/difference-between-mind-and-brain-neuroscientist/

Lee, Y.S., Ryu, Y., Jung, W.M., *et al.*, 2017. Understanding mind-body interaction from the perspective of East Asian Medicine. *Evidence-Based Complementary and Alternative Medicine*. 7618419. Available from: https://doi.org/10.1155/2017/7618419.

Nummenmaa, L., Glerean, E., Hari, R., & Hietanen, J.K., 2014. Bodily maps of emotions. *Proceedings of the National Academy of Sciences of the United States of America*. 111(2): 646–651. Available from: https://doi.org/10.1073/pnas.1321664111.

Pearsall, P., Schwartz, G., & Russek, L., 2005. Organ transplants and cellular memories. Available from: https://www.paulpearsall.com/info/press/3.html.

Saybrook University, 2009. Emotion is at the heart of the heart. Available from: https://www.saybrook.edu/blog/2009/03/09/emotion-heart-heart.

CHAPTER 17

The Inner Relationship of Inter-Tissue Relationships

In this chapter I will explore relationships between tissues and structures within the body. Some of the connections will have a logical anatomical relationship, however some appear to have a functional relationship even though there is no obvious anatomical relationship present. When working at the functional relationship, it can help unlock tensions and strains which otherwise may be difficult to fully resolve.

When working with the practical sessions, you as the practitioner will need to be able to have what is known as 'divided awareness' when palpating. Divided awareness is having your awareness fully on more than one tissue at the same time. This is not easy until you become more adept and experienced at working with the involuntary mechanism, hence my decision to place this chapter here. We all have, however, experienced divided awareness in other aspects of our lives.

When someone first learns to drive a car, they are totally focussed on a set number of things: other road users, pedestrians, their steering and indicators, the gears (if not an automatic gearbox), the rear-view mirror, the car speed and the correct use of their feet on the pedals. These are all in addition to knowing where they are going and road signs/instructions along the way. To the beginner, that is a lot to think about, and the brain has no space for any other information nor activity. However, after a few weeks of regular driving, the person can also listen to the car radio whilst on their journey, whilst still carrying out all the necessary driving skill requirements. So, if you do find that divided awareness when palpating is a little tricky, just be patient, you will develop these skills, in the same way that the driver learns to listen to the radio whilst driving.

Let us now look at a variety of interrelated body tissues. Having read this chapter, you may discover some interrelationships within the body of your own that I have not mentioned, so this certainly is not intended to be a definitive list.

Each of the sections below has its own practical exercise. The exercises do require you as the practitioner to be deeply centred before undertaking the practical. It is only by being deeply centred that your palpation and divided awareness skills will be sufficient to palpate the qualities occurring between the tissues described.

THE ETHMOID, XIPHOID AND COCCYX, MIDLINE FINE TUNERS!

Although it is a delicate bone, the ethmoid is pre-formed in cartilage and is therefore described as a cranial base bone, along with the other base bones such as the sphenoid, occiput and temporal bones. We must remember that the sphenoid, occiput and temporal bones are bones which are both vault and base bones, so actually the ethmoid is the only pure cranial base bone. As we know, the sphenobasilar symphysis (SBS) is a highly significant midline suture. It adapts to the various mechanical forces acting upon it as a bony fulcrum working in harmony with the Sutherland Fulcrum, which is the fulcrum of the meninges. As cranial practitioners, we are fully aware that although this suture at the SBS does ossify, it nevertheless still maintains its plasticity in how it functions and modifies to respond to mechanical forces.

The xiphoid is a little bone which articulates with the sternum at its inferior end. The manubrium articulates with the sternum, and like the SBS, this junction fuses though should still retain some springiness, some plasticity and flexibility. Likewise, even after fusing to the sternum, the xiphoid still retains plasticity at its sternal attachment. The xiphoid has important diaphragmatic muscular origins. The sternum is a bony fulcrum for the rib cage and is therefore important to consider when looking at thoracic mechanics.

The coccyx articulates at the inferior part of the sacrum. It is delicate but also has important muscular attachments. I once had a patient who had their coccyx removed surgically. Naturally this created complications for the pelvic floor tissues and organs as they lost their posterior coccygeal attachment. The coccyx is also the point of attachment of the pia mater, which on this patient did feel rather strange having lost its final attachment. However, with this patient, I also found that the sacrum itself felt unstable in a manner I had never felt before. This was an independent sensation from the pia and pelvic floor disturbances. It was as if the sacral bone had lost some of its innate stability.

These three bones, the ethmoid, xiphoid and coccyx, are three midline small bones, each being immediately adjacent to a significant midline bone. Each of these three ossify very much later compared with other bones of the body, in the early 20s. Could the ethmoid, xiphoid and coccyx be fine tuners for the function of their adjacent structures: ethmoid to the SBS, xiphoid to the manubrium and sternum, and the coccyx to the sacrum? If so, then it would give the ethmoid, xiphoid and coccyx a functional relationship with each other.

I looked further into this with patients where I needed to treat the ethmoid, xiphoid or coccyx and found that by looking at the functional relationships between them there were frequently issues which needed treating in all three fine tuners, and that they all benefitted by treating the other two.

So, if you have a patient where the ethmoid, xiphoid or coccyx is not functioning as well as you consider necessary, do look at their other 'fine tuning friends' and their interrelationships.

Exercise on the ethmoid, xiphoid and coccyx

https://youtu.be/ZYcxoefhUts

THE SKIN AND CENTRAL NERVOUS SYSTEM

As discussed in Chapter 4 on the topic of embryology, the skin and the nervous system both arise from ectodermal tissues, forming the layer next to the amniotic sac, and being the closest of the three germ layers to the side of implantation into the mother's uterine wall.

There are some skin conditions which include stress or tensions as a direct aetiological factor, which significantly aggravate the skin tissue. These include eczema, rosacea, lupus and psoriasis. When teaching a course to osteopathic students on the tissue relationships within the body, the feedback from students was that purely working on the skin, before working on the skin – CNS relationship, was highly soothing to the nervous system. This indicates that the functional relationship is a two-way process.

Probably like me, you do not get patients coming into your practice where their primary complaint is a skin condition, such as those mentioned above. However, this does not stop you from helping such conditions, whilst you also work on their region of primary concern. If you

can assist or reduce the skin irritation/itchiness, as well as their main symptoms, they will be very grateful.

Exercise on the ectodermal relationships between the skin and the brain

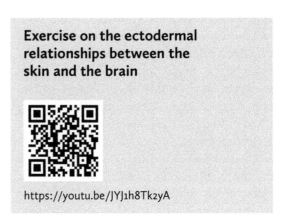

https://youtu.be/JYJ1h8Tk2yA

LUNGS AND THE POSTURE

I am grateful to a good friend and colleague Nicholas Gossett, who inspired me to look into the relationship between the lungs and the posture.

In very simple embryological terms, the lungs grow out of the ventral aspect of the foregut as a lung bud around the fourth week of intrauterine life. The heart by this time is making progress in being formed and the liver is forming immediately under the septum transversum, which becomes our future diaphragm muscle. The heart and the liver move away from each other as the embryo lengthens and extends from its flexed posture, and the lungs then grow into the space created by this process. In some people, and it can appear more commonly expressed in teenagers, the lungs do not energetically fully open out into the thoracic space available, resulting in an inward retreating on the bronchial tree, back towards the initial lung bud at the posterior aspect of the thorax. If the lungs keep this energetically restricted state, it pulls on the shoulder

girdle and also creates an increased flexion of the thoracic spine, creating a poor posture.

Now, we must also accept that in teenagers there is a variety of physiological, hormonal and psychological changes occurring all at once, making life tricky for both them, and probably their parents, by possibly creating a further psychological family feedback loop. However, we should still bear in mind that 'stuck lungs' can and sometimes do significantly add to teenage postural stresses.

Exercise on the lungs and posture

https://youtu.be/2qefoTLB1ik

MENINGES AND THE EYES

As we saw in Chapter 15 when looking at the embryology of the eye, the eye develops initially from brain tissue which later develops into the retina and optic nerve. However, we also have the sclera and choroid layers and a pigment epithelium, the latter being a fine layer lying between the choroid and the retina layer.

This arrangement had my 'little grey cells' thinking and making comparisons of the eye layers with the arrangement of the meninges around the brain. The outer sclera, as we know, is the white outer protective layer of the eye. Iqbal describes the outline anatomical aspects of the outer sclera as: 'Covering the posterior 5/6 of the eyeball, having a varying thickness between 1 mm at the posterior aspect of the eye, 0.3 mm where the ocular muscles insert, 0.6 mm at the "eye equator" and 0.8 mm at the corneoscleral junction' (Iqbal 2022).

The sclera is composed of strong white collagen fibres which are laid down in a variety of directions. Recent findings indicate that the sclera, which was once considered an inert tissue due to its being highly resistant to infection, tumours and foreign materials, is now being seen in a different light: 'Evidence now demonstrates that although the sclera has low baseline metabolic requirements, it constantly remodels throughout life to maintain its functions' (Dawson et al. 2011).

When I read how this highly strong collagenous tissue surrounding and protecting an organ, which is formed from brain tissue, remodels throughout life to maintain its functions, I started to become fascinated about the similarities between the sclera and dura mater. Both tissues have as their main function to protect the delicate and vital organ within, sight being our primary sense. Both are highly collagenous with the fibres laid down in a variety of directions. Both are the outer layer of the three non-bony layers outside of brain tissue, the retina

effectively being brain tissue. Like the sclera, the dura does not have a high metabolism.

Both the dura and sclera lie adjacent to bony protections, that of the orbit for the sclera, and the cranial base and vault for the dural meningeal layer. As stated by Dawson et al. (2011), the sclera constantly remodels to maintain its function. The dura, as we know well, modifies itself throughout life in order to work as a fulcrum to adjust to mechanical shocks and traumas, at the Sutherland Fulcrum. Embryologically, both are formed primarily by the neural crest cells and to a lesser extent, the paraxial mesoderm. Here we have two tissues with a high level of similarities.

I then considered the next layer inside the sclera, the choroid of the eye. Like the arachnoid mater in comparison with the dura, it is much more delicate and thinner than the sclera: 'The average subfoveal choroid thickness was 330 ± 65 μm (range, 189–538 μm), and was influenced significantly by age ($P = 0.04$)' (Read et al. 2013). Putting these measurements into millimetres to compare with those of the sclera quoted above gives an average figure of 0.33 mm, making the choroid thinner. Likewise, the arachnoid mater is much more delicate and thinner than its outer neighbour the dura.

The choroid is a highly vascular layer which lies between the sclera and the pigment epithelium. It furnishes the blood supply to the retina via the pigment epithelium in a similar way that the blood vessels in the subarachnoid space supply the outer aspects of the brain via the much more delicate pia mater.

The retinal pigment epithelium is the next layer within after the choroid and is the intimate covering of the functional aspect of the retina of the eye. Similarly, the pia mater is intimate and inseparable from the brain tissue immediately underneath it.

Between the retina and choroid layers lies the retinal pigment layer (RPE). The cells of the RPE layer are very securely joined, creating a barrier between the layers either side. Its function is to protect the retina and help to maintain the health of its physiology, and also to allow the photoreceptors to register the light entering the retina (UCL Institute of Ophthalmology 2022).

Again, I began to consider the similarities between the layers of the eye, the sclera through to the retina, with the layers of the skull, dura mater through to the brain tissue. Knowing that the retina is effectively modified brain tissue further increased my curiosity as to this possible relationship. When looking at the eye tissues of patients, I have since found it also very useful clinically to look at the interrelationships of the eye layers with the layers of the meninges and the grey cells of the brain tissue, as in doing so there appears to be a better tissue resolution when treating.

Exercise on the meninges, eyes and the brain

https://youtu.be/AgbxFBOP_og

THE PERICARDIUM AND THE MENINGES

In Chapter 10 we looked briefly at the heart and the pericardium. Here we will focus on the functional and anatomical similarities of the heart and pericardium to the meninges, and then proceed to a practical exercise where you may experience the palpatory similarities. The pericardium consists of three layers which protect the heart. The meninges are the three protective layers of the brain. The heart is fundamental to our circulation and highly significant to our emotions; the brain is fundamental to most body functions and develops our thinking.

As discussed in Chapter 10, the fibrous pericardium is the outermost of the three layers of the pericardium and consists of strong collagenous fibres. This is continuous with the tendon of the diaphragm tissue. Like the dural covering of the brain, it is the strongest of the three layers of the pericardium. The dura mater has significant similarities with the fibrous pericardium in terms of tissue composition and function, both being highly collagenous. The main role of both of these layers is to give strong but flexible protection to the organ within.

The second layer of the pericardium is the parietal layer. This is a more delicate layer just within the fibrous layer and is immediately adjacent to the fluid-containing pericardial cavity. In the same way, the arachnoid mater is immediately adjacent to the dura mater and lies adjoining the fluid-filled subarachnoid space.

The innermost of the three layers of the pericardium, the visceral layer, lies on the inner surface of the pericardial cavity and is effectively the 'skin' of the muscular myocardium, though not composed of myocardium tissue. In the same manner, the innermost of the three layers of the meninges, the pia mater, is on the inner surface of the subarachnoid space and is the effective 'skin' of the brain tissue though not the brain. Blood vessels pass through the visceral layer of the pericardium to supply the myocardium, and equally blood vessels pass through the pia mater to supply the brain tissue.

Could these similarities be a coincidence, or could there be a functional relationship occurring between the pericardium and the meninges? I had to find out. I started palpating friends and family members to see if there was a similar palpatory quality between these structures, and much to my amazement, there did seem to be so: the dura mater relating to the fibrous pericardium, the arachnoid mater to the parietal pericardium, and the visceral layer to the pia mater.

I then started looking at my patients and palpated both the meninges and the pericardium to see if there were any clinical findings to corroborate my theory that these layers were functionally related. Again, to my surprise I did find with some frequency that when a patient had a specific tension or disturbance of one or more layers of the meninges, the same layer (or layers) had a tension or disturbance to the pericardium.

I must point out that these pericardial findings were subtle and I feel most likely would not have been detected medically.

Exercise on the meninges and pericardium

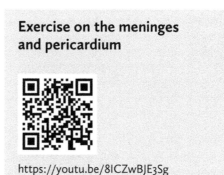

https://youtu.be/8ICZwBJE3Sg

INTERRELATIONSHIPS OF THE SYMPATHETIC NERVOUS SYSTEM (SNS)

As has been discussed in previous chapters, the sympathetic nervous system prepares our physiology for high demand, e.g., to escape from danger, or take part in sports and physically demanding hobbies. The SNS also comes into action during times of emotional distress, where the brain and emotions perceive an event as dangerous, without the need for physical activity to escape the danger, being solely an emotionally stressful event.

The main systems of the body involved in this process are the central and autonomic nervous systems, respiratory/cardiovascular systems, digestive system and liver, the kidneys and bladder, the skin, and the musculoskeletal system. Let us look at the interrelationship of some of these organs. In the practical session, I will lead you through a few examples and then you will have the skill to explore more types of such interrelationships yourself.

When the sympathetic system becomes more active, lung activity increases to ensure more oxygen is entering the circulation to meet the needs of increased body metabolism from changes to other body tissues and organs. As mentioned in Chapter 16, emotional stress (a common factor) can cause tightness in the diaphragm muscle and thus affect the lungs and their relationship to the sympathetic system.

Now, we are going to do an exercise where we put one hand on the lungs and the other hand on a variety of differing tissues and organs to get a sense of whether we can detect any sense of communication between the two, both being sympathetic partners when activated by the SNS. Having used the lungs as the communication reference point, we could follow this process with another area for the referencing hand contact.

I have found this process very beneficial when working with a patient where there is clearly an overactive SNS associated with ongoing stress/emotional issues. It has helped to diagnose and then treat situations where the interrelationship is not occurring or not beneficial to the physiology.

Exercise on the palpating sympathetic nervous system

https://youtu.be/ZptNaSSSWLY

In this chapter I have hoped to open your awareness to the possibility of tissue and organ links which you may never have previously considered, and that it has stimulated your thoughts to sometimes be outside the known physiological box. This could never be a complete list of tissue and organ interrelationships to explore at the treatment table, and so I do trust that you will look further into other possible interrelationships.

You may consider that some of these interrelationships are of no particular therapeutic benefit. However, you may find that a new patient arrives on your doorstep, where looking in this manner is just what is required for their specific physiology. In my career, I have certainly found that the more I look at interrelationships within the physiology, whether within the same system or between systems, the better my patients seem to respond.

REFERENCES

Dawson, D., Ubels, J.L., & Edelhauser, H., 2011. Cornea and sclera. In: Levin, L.A., Nilsson, S.F.E., Ver Hoeve, J., *et al.*, eds. *Adler's Physiology of the Eye*. 11th edition. Elsevier, pp. 71–130. Available from: https://www.researchgate.net/publication/281572472_Cornea_and_Sclera.

Iqbal, A., 2022. Anatomy and physiology of cornea and sclera. Available from: https://www.academia.edu/27920412/ANATOMY_AND_PHYSIOLOGY_OF_CORNEA_AND_SCLERA.

Read, S.A., Collins, M.J., Vincent, S.J., & Alonso-Caneiro, D., 2013. Choroidal thickness in childhood. *Investigative Ophthalmology & Visual Science*. 54(5): 3586–3593. Available from: https://iovs.arvojournals.org/article.aspx?articleid=2189684#:~:text=The%20average%20thickness%20from%200.5,the%20per.

UCL Institute of Ophthalmology, 2022. The retina and retinal pigment epithelium (RPE). Available from: https://www.ucl.ac.uk/ioo/research/research-labs-and-groups/carr-lab/bestrophinopathies-resource-pages/eye/retina-and-retinal.

CHAPTER 18

Working at the Intracellular Level Along with Tissue and Cellular Consciousness

In this chapter I will describe the main organelles in a standard human cell and then explore some of these in practical sessions at the treatment table. I will then proceed to discuss what I describe as 'cellular consciousness', as a palpatory experience.

CELLULAR ANATOMY

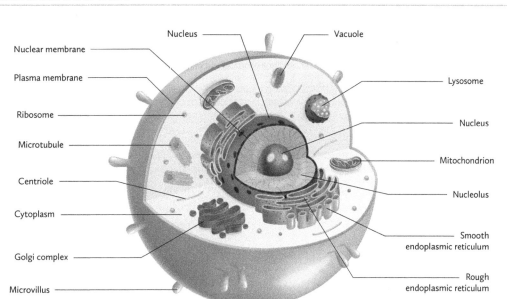

Figure 18.1 A typical cell and its organelles. Note: Some cell types are highly specialised and different to this image, e.g., mature red blood cells have no nucleus. Muscle cells and nerve cells are also highly specialised and also differ.

In Chapter 6 we looked at the fascia and the extracellular matrix which lies between the cells of the body, it being called a matrix because it is much more than just a fluid medium. In the same manner that we can take our awareness from the fascia (or any other tissue) to the matrix between the cells, so we can take our awareness to the cell membrane and even inside the cell wall. We have to remember that we palpate with our awareness, our third hand. Our third hand is very clever as it can operate at the microscopic level just as easily as at the gross level, *if* we can visualise that level in our awareness. Consequently, we need to have a sense of the anatomy at that cellular level. To make life easier, I shall be describing a generalised cell, not a specialised cell such as a neuron or a muscle cell, though these too could be explored on your own if you so wish after having read this chapter and undertaken study of the anatomy of those particular cells.

The cell membrane

We start with the cell membrane. It is better to call it a membrane rather than the cell wall as it is extremely thin and not a rigid structure as in the plant kingdom. As an indication: 'Plasma membranes range from 5 to 10 nm in thickness. For comparison, human red blood cells, visible via light microscopy, are approximately 8 μm wide, or approximately 1,000 times wider than a plasma membrane' (LibreTexts Biology 2019).

To help us get a greater grip on how thin the cell membrane is, we need to comprehend the size of one nanometre. The mathematical term 'nano' means one billionth so therefore one nanometre equals one billionth of a metre, or one millionth of a millimetre. Such an incredibly small distance is difficulty to imagine and visualise! To give you an example for comparison, a human hair is approximately eighty thousand to one hundred thousand nanometres thick.

So, if the human cell membrane is just 5–10 nanometres in thickness, that makes it 10,000–20,000 times thinner than this sheet of paper that you are now reading from! However, the cell membrane is not just amazing for its small size, it is an incredible structure in its own right, because it controls what enters and leaves the cell and how the cell responds to its environment.

Bruce Lipton, a well-known American cell biologist, in his bestselling book *Biology of Belief*, considers the cell membrane to be the brain of the cell, stating: 'I believe that when you understand how the chemical and physical structure of the cell's membrane works, you'll start calling it, as I do, the magical membrane... I refer to it in my lectures as the magical mem-Brain' (Lipton 2008).

The cell membrane is a phospholipid structure, with the fatty lipid molecules in the centre and the water-based phosphate molecules on the outer and inner aspects. The fatty layer effectively creates an insulator preventing electrically charged molecules, the water-based molecules, passing through the membrane. The vast majority of cell nutrients are charged, water-based molecules, and need a special mechanism to enter the cell. Likewise, the cell needs a mechanism for dispersing its waste products. This is achieved by the cell allowing specific molecules to pass through this insulating fatty layer via special molecules called channel proteins.

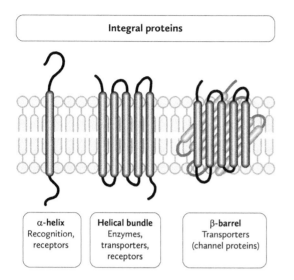

Integral proteins

α-helix	Helical bundle	β-barrel
Recognition, receptors	Enzymes, transporters, receptors	Transporters (channel proteins)

Figure 18.2 Integral proteins traversing the cell membrane.

These channel proteins have an outer lipid-based amino acid and an inner water-based amino acid. This water-based inner amino acid allows the water-based nutrients and waste products to pass though the fatty central aspect of the membrane. According to Lipton, these channel proteins in some states are wound up like a coiled ball, but when activated by specific molecules, the channel proteins unwind into a tube allowing those specific molecules to enter the cell, unlocking the gateway to pass through the membrane.

There are also integral membrane proteins (IMPs), which play a key role in cell function. There are two basic types of IMPs, receptor proteins and effector proteins. Lipton in his chapter on the Magical Membrane further describes the receptor proteins as 'the cell's sense organs' which 'respond to specific environmental signals' (Lipton 2008). These receptor proteins are influenced by electrical signals from the environmental molecules resulting in a shape change which then allows its signals to be read by the cell. Lipton also states: 'Receptor antennae can also read vibrational energy fields such as light, sound, and radio frequencies' (Lipton 2008).

The effector proteins are how the cell responds to the stimuli from its environment. We know that the nucleus and the DNA are a vital part of any cell. However, Lipton describes how the genes within the DNA strands do not control their responsiveness or actions, rather it is these effector proteins or their by-products which form an active sleeve which then surrounds the DNA strands:

> In contrast to conventional wisdom, genes do not control their own activity. Instead, it is the membrane's effector proteins operating in response to environmental signals picked up by the membrane's receptors, which control the 'reading' of genes so that worn-out proteins can be replaced, or new proteins can be created. (Lipton 2008)

Whether you do or don't agree with Lipton's description of the cell membrane as the 'cell mem-Brain', it cannot be denied that it is much more than just a container for the cell contents. Being able to respond to sound, light and radio frequencies in addition to molecular stimuli, along with the consequent interaction with the DNA, does imply that it plays a profound role in cellular health and function.

Cytoplasm/cytosol

Having entered the cell membrane, we are now in the environment of the cytoplasm or cytosol. This is the gel-like fluid between the cell membrane and the nucleus, the nucleus having its own nucleoplasm. The cytoplasm has a different biochemistry to the extracellular matrix.

Within the cell, the aqueous aspect, which contains water, organic molecules and dissolved ions, is the cytosol, of which the highest proportion (approximately 70 per cent) is made up of water molecules. Within these water molecules are ions of potassium, sodium chloride, bicarbonate, amino acids, magnesium and calcium. There are, however, differences between the cytosol and the extracellular matrix on the other side of the cell wall, as the levels of potassium are much higher within the cell. The cell wall plays an active role in maintaining these differences (Biology Online 2021).

The cytosol is the medium in which all of the cell organelles and the cell cytoskeleton are located and interact with each other. As stated above, the cytosol contains approximately 70 per cent water molecules. Tatomir goes further in making us realise just how much we are made up of water in her description of intracellular fluid (cytosol):

> The definition of intracellular fluid refers to the fluid found inside of the cell. Intracellular fluid represents around 40% of total human body weight and is comprised of water, dissolved electrolytes, and proteins.
>
> There are several important differences between intracellular fluid versus extracellular fluid. For example, intracellular fluid represents 40% of human body weight, while extracellular fluid constitutes 20% of body weight. While intracellular fluid is only found on the inside of cells, a majority of extracellular fluid is found in all of the spaces of the body located outside of the cells, while a small percent is located within the blood plasma. (Tatomir 2022)

The cytosol contains electrolytes, the key one being potassium. This has a positive charge and is involved in the opening and closing of the transport channel proteins, as described above. The intracellular fluid/cytosol also contains magnesium, sodium, chloride and bicarbonate ions. The differences between the fluids either side of the cell membrane are that the extracellular matrix contains a higher concentration of sodium and calcium whereas the intracellular cytosol contains higher levels of potassium and magnesium ions.

As we will see in our next practical session, these differences of the fluid quality either side of the membrane can be experienced on palpation. We will do this exercise on the cytoplasm in conjunction with the organelles. Before we move on to discuss the organelles, we need to mention the ribosomes.

Ribosomes

These are very tiny structures within the cell which are free floating or attached to the endoplasmic reticulum and have no surrounding membrane. Ribosomes are present in all living cells. They are made up of RNA molecules and proteins which synthesise new proteins. They do this by converting the gene code into amino acids which they then build into more complex proteins.

The cell organelles

The cell organelles are structures within the cell that have their own membrane or envelope. In this section I will be outlining the main organelles within a so-called typical cell, not a specialised cell such as muscle or nerve.

Endoplasmic reticulum (ER)

The ER is a highly significant structure within the cell. It is a very large organelle: 'In animal cells, the ER usually constitutes more than half of the membranous content of the cell' (Rogers 2020). The ER is considered to be larger than the nucleus. Also, like the ribosomes, the ER is always present within the cell, whereas the nucleus is not always present, as can be seen in mature red blood cells. The ER has open connections to the nucleus membrane, but also extends out as far as the cell membrane.

The ER, having commenced at the nuclear envelope, opens out into a series of tubular cisterns and interconnected sheets. The tubular cisternae sacs create a 3D network whereas the sheets are membrane-enclosed and extend across the cell cytoplasm. The smooth ER tubular cisterns, which are found closer to the cell membrane, synthesise lipids and steroids and also store the main enzymes and any manufactured by-products already produced from these enzymes. The rough ER contains ribosomes, which gives it a rough texture, and is just involved in the synthesis of proteins.

In *simple* terms this important structure is mainly responsible for:

> ...the transportation of proteins and other carbohydrates to another organelle, which includes lysosomes, Golgi apparatus, plasma membrane, etc. They provide the increased surface area for cellular reactions. They help in the formation of the nuclear membrane during cell division. They play a vital role in the formation of the (cellular) skeletal framework. They play a vital role in the synthesis of proteins, lipids, glycogen and other steroids like cholesterol, progesterone, testosterone, etc. (A Level Biology 2022)

Nucleus

The nucleus has an estimated diameter of 5–20 microns (5–20 x 0.001 mm), giving it a diameter approximately one to two thousand times greater than the thickness of the cell membrane. Containing the DNA, its main role is to regulate gene expression and the information required to synthesise proteins. Within the nucleus lies the nucleoplasm, which is of a similar nature to the cytosol on the other side of the nuclear envelope. The nuclear envelope surrounding the nucleus contains pores which allow large proteins, such as RNA, to pass in and out of the nucleus.

Muscle, liver and bone cells are unusual in that they often have more than one nucleus, being known as a multinucleate cell or syncytium. By contrast the erythrocytes in the blood lose their nucleus after maturation.

Mitochondria

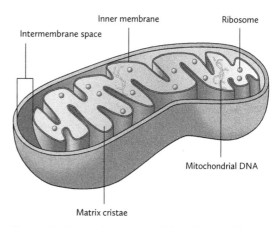

Figure 18.3 Internal structure of the mitochondrion.

It is generally agreed that the mitochondria originally started as independent free-living micro-organisms, as they contain their own DNA. These early organisms then either infected larger singe cell organisms or were engulfed by them and the two created a mutually beneficial symbiotic relationship. The larger partner gave a better and safer environment for the mitochondria and in return, the mitochondria gave a greatly increased energy. This relationship then became a permanent arrangement, and the mitochondria became organelles inside the larger cells.

This evolutionary giant step forwards which then led to multicellular organisms starting to appear is considered to have happened very early: 'Mitochondria arose through a fateful endosymbiosis more than 1.45 billion years ago' (Martin 2010). The mitochondria are effectively the power plants of the cell as they generate energy by converting glucose into adenosine triphosphate (ATP), a highly energy-rich molecule. Being independent cells within the human cell, the mitochondria have an inner and outer membrane, their own DNA, ribosomes and matrix (cytoplasm).

Golgi body/apparatus

The Golgi body (GB) or Golgi apparatus consists of membranes which are either tubules or small sacs, also referred to as vesicles. Within the cell, the GB is located close to both the nucleus and the endoplasmic reticulum (ER) so that it can easily receive protein metabolites from the ER. As these proteins emerge from the ER, they then enter the GB for additional chemical changes and processing. Carbohydrates may be added to the proteins and these glycoproteins then get taken to the rest of the cell, being transported via other vesicles.

Another function of the GB is to create new cell vesicles out of its own membrane. These new vesicles are then filled with the newly produced chemicals from within the GB, which then pass through the cytoplasm to the cell membrane.

Vesicles

There is a variety of different types of vesicles within the cell. Lysosomes are vesicles which contain digestive enzymes which break down larger molecules into smaller ones. Consequently, their function is to break down substances within the cell by a phagocytic action, which may be a danger to the cell.

Vacuoles

These vesicles, like the lysosomes, also have a protective function for the cell, by isolating dangerous substances in addition to containing cell waste products. The vacuoles' role also includes the removal of invading bacteria by their digestive processes. In addition, vacuoles have an important responsibility for maintaining cell chemistry by balancing the cell pH, as well as helping to maintain cell internal pressure to the required physiological level.

Transport vesicles

These are vesicles which basically transport proteins and other molecules from one destination to another within the cell or even across the cell membrane and out of the cell.

Secretory vesicles

These vesicles, as the name implies, secrete material which the cell wants to be removed from within the cell. These may be harmful or toxic substances, or they may be substances which are beneficial and even required by other cells in different areas of the body. There are some specialised secretory vesicles such as the synaptic vesicles which release neurotransmitters, which have been stored within the cell but are released when appropriate. Other specialised secretory vesicles are those within the endocrine system which secrete their stored hormones when stimulated to do so.

For this next practical you will need to be very highly centred. I strongly recommend doing this when not tired or fatigued, and in a calm state of mind.

Exercise on a journey inside the cell

https://youtu.be/nAw1gQ64sl8

CELLULAR CONSCIOUSNESS

What do I mean by the term cellular consciousness? When we think, feel, or intuit as a person, this could be described as functions of our consciousness, this being our consciousness as an individual. Earlier I mentioned how the cell membrane has receptors, some of which can detect and respond to electrical impulses, light waves, sound waves and radio waves. Is detecting information and responding to it a level of consciousness?

The definition of consciousness by Oxford Languages (the source of the Google online dictionary) is: 'The state of being aware of and responsive to one's surroundings.' The Merriam-Webster online dictionary gives two definitions: 'a: The quality or state of being aware especially of something within oneself. b: The state or fact of being conscious of an external object, state, or fact.' Quite clearly from all three of these definitions, there is a 'cellular consciousness'.

There have been times when treating a patient with a chronic condition that I have been aware of two aspects to the patient's symptoms. Firstly, there is the complaint, where the patient describes where they feel the aches, pains and discomforts, altered function, in specific aspects of their physiology. Here is a common example: 'My right leg is now painful with some pins and needles in the toes, but I also feel the sharp pains in my back which have been there for six months now.' Such a statement is an expression of the person's consciousness stating their symptoms.

However, on a number of occasions when working on a patient at a subtle or deep inner level, I have become aware of another symptomatic expression. This is different from the patient's expression, and is how the cells in a localised area have been feeling within themselves, having to put up with the ongoing discomfort caused by the condition. This seems to be an expression of the cells being unhappy to live in the midst of the highly disturbed tissue state, pressure, or compression, to live with poor circulation, to live within the poor physiology.

This is not the expression of the person's symptoms, the individual consciousness, but more the expression of a cellular consciousness, expressing how they are fed up, angry and/or irritable at having to live like that. It is almost as if the cells are communicating their own cry for help which is expressed differently from that of the patient. This tissue consciousness conveys itself to me, the practitioner, in the first person; for example: 'I am feeling fed up being here, as other areas are not doing their job', or 'I'm really angry at having to live inside this (tissue state) all the time.' This is very different to the patient saying: 'the pain is at this place', or 'it hurts there'.

When a person says: 'My right leg is now painful with some pins and needles in the toes, but I also feel the sharp pains in my back which have been there for six months now', the patient's consciousness is expressing their symptom picture of a low back pain, with pain in the right leg and pins and needles in the foot. However, the cellular consciousness in the lower spine may express itself as: 'I'm totally fed up with living in a compressed and restricted manner, it's just been too long now, I feel like giving up!'

Such cellular consciousness or 'cellular emotions' can be significantly different from the patient's emotions, which may feel quite OK. When such cellular consciousness expressions come to my awareness, it is not that I have been thinking on that level, expecting to feel them, nor predetermining my thoughts, nor is this just a guess. In Chapter 3 I discussed how sometimes we can get an insight at the intuitive level, not intellect; getting a sense of this cellular consciousness happens at this more profound 'inner level'. The understanding just seems to come to the practitioner's awareness.

I must point out that such experiences do not occur with all of my patients, and perhaps that may be due to there being times where I am not in the required highly receptive state to experience them. Like you the reader, I am not perfect! Equally, even when I am 'tuned in' to my patient's tissues when highly centred and aware, the cellular consciousness may not be expressing negativity at that time. As I have said above, cellular consciousness tends to be expressed with more chronic and severe physiological disturbances. However, if and when it does appear to you, do accept and acknowledge these expressions.

What to do if this cellular consciousness presents itself to your awareness? Remember that in Chapter 3 we looked at how A.T. Still probably worked at a level of a deep universal compassion for his patients. I think that this cellular consciousness expression is the cells calling for understanding and compassion for what they, the cells not the person, have to experience living in the midst of the cellular turmoil. We can acknowledge this cellular consciousness and mentally offer compassionate understanding for how the cells are having to live under those circumstances, and, in the case of chronic conditions, for months or years.

When you as a practitioner do this, it is as if the cells ease their distress and soften, and give you the impression that they are informing you: 'Thank goodness, someone finally understands my having to exist like this.' As I have said, this is an expression from a cellular level, not your patient saying out loud: 'Ah, I'm glad you understand my condition.'

Some of you may already have had therapeutic experiences which relate to this concept of cellular consciousness, and the cell expressing itself to your awareness directly without the words being spoken by the patient. Do not forget that the patient may be totally unaware of such cellular expressions; he or she just wants the pain gone, their medications reduced, etc.

If I get a sense of the cellular consciousness being expressed, generally I do not tell the patient what I experienced. The cells had probably been attempting to communicate their distress to their owner for quite some time *before* the onset of symptoms, unless it was caused by a sudden physical trauma. However, the patient did not listen to, or ignored this cellular consciousness messaging, hence the development of symptoms.

Exercise on cellular consciousness

https://youtu.be/yxhRdwD4Wow

I hope you have found this chapter inspiring, as it takes you further on your inner journey into the physiology. Hopefully in doing so, it has thereby further stretched your concept of the scope of osteopathy and enhanced how you can treat your patients. With regard to working at the cell membrane and intracellular level, you may come across patients where working at such a level is appropriate. Systemic conditions, being those which are influencing the whole physiology and hence every cell of the body, might be an area for such considerations.

REFERENCES

A Level Biology, 2022. Endoplasmic reticulum – structure and function. Available from: https://alevelbiology.co.uk/notes/endoplasmic-reticulum-structure-and-function/

Biology Online, 2021. Cytosol. Available from: https://www.biologyonline.com/dictionary/cytosol.

LibreTexts Biology, 2019. Membranes. Available from: https://bio.libretexts.org/Courses/University_of_California_Davis/BIS_2A%3A_Introductory_Biology_(Easlon)/Readings/15.1%3A_Membranes#:~:text=Plasma%20membranes%20range%20from%205,wider%20than%20a%20plasma%20membrane.

Lipton, B., 2008. *The Biology of Belief*. 5th edition. Carlsbad, CA: Hay House Inc.

Martin, W., 2010. The origin of mitochondria. Scitable. Available from: https://www.nature.com/scitable/topicpage/the-origin-of-mitochondria-14232356/

National Nanotechnology Initiative, n.d. Size of the nanoscale. Available from: https://www.nano.gov/nanotech-101/what/nano-size.

Rogers, K., 2020. Endoplasmic reticulum. Encyclopaedia Britannica. Available from: https://www.britannica.com/science/endoplasmic-reticulum.

Tatomir, J., 2022. Location & composition of intracellular fluid. Available from: https://study.com/learn/lesson/intracellular-fluid-location-examples-composition.html#:~:text=Also%20referred%20to%20as%20cytoplasm,%2C%20dissolved%20electrolytes%2C%20and%20proteins.

CHAPTER 19

Experiences of Refined Perception

SUTHERLAND'S TERMINOLOGY

William Sutherland spoke about 'liquid light' in a number of lectures between 1949 and 1950, which were then transcribed by Dr Anne Wales in the chapter 'The Tour of the Minnow' within the book *Teachings in the Science of Osteopathy* (Sutherland and Wales 1990). In an earlier publication, *Contributions of Thought* (Sutherland 1967), a series of transcripts of Sutherland's lectures, Anne Wales took notes from seven different lectures which Sutherland gave about the tour of the minnow and presented them in one version, therefore it is more comprehensive than the version in *Teachings in the Science of Osteopathy*.

OBSERVATION BY DR WALES OF DR SUTHERLAND TREATING A PATIENT

For many years I have been intrigued by Sutherland's use of the term 'liquid light' in his later teachings. I feel certain that he 'saw' or perceived, the liquid light often when he was treating. Dr Wales once personally told me, whilst being my table tutor, that sometimes a 'golden glow' would slowly develop over Sutherland's patients when he treated them (Wales 1980). Sutherland also used terms such as 'fluid within a fluid' and 'Breath of Life':

> It is like the beam that goes out from the Lighthouse: It lights up the ocean but does not touch it. Sometimes I call it a 'fluid within a fluid', or the 'liquid light'; something that you turn on in this dark room and the darkness disappears. Where does it go? It is something that is invisible; the 'Potency', the 'Breath of Life' or Dr Still's 'highest known element.'

> The Intelligence in the power of the Tide. We refer to the potent fluctuation of this Tide and to something that is intelligent, something invisible. We are referring to the Breath of Life in that Tide. (Sutherland 1967)

The Cambridge Dictionary definition of potency is strength, influence, or effectiveness (Cambridge Dictionary 2022). Dr Sutherland chose his words carefully to describe such experiences.

> Do you know anything about sheet lightning? You see its manifestation all through the clouds, but it doesn't touch the clouds. I want you to see this invisible 'liquid light' or the 'Breath of Life', as sheet lightning and a transmutation; the sheet lightning all through the nerves, not touching the copper tube. (Sutherland and Wales 1990)

Dr Wales had earlier transcribed Sutherland's analogy of a nerve fibre as an insulated copper wire, hence his saying 'not touching the copper tube'.

In the same presentation, Sutherland said: 'In this picture there is also a transmutation from the cerebrospinal fluid, that "highest known element" formed in the "copper tube"' (Sutherland and Wales 1990).

In all these Sutherland quotes and others, he chose to use such terms as 'Potency' 'highest known element', 'liquid light', 'Breath of Life', 'liquid within a liquid'. These are certainly not throwaway phrases!

SUTHERLAND CHOSE HIS WORDS CAREFULLY

Before becoming an osteopath, William Sutherland worked in the newspaper industry for 12 years. During this time, he would have been taught how to use words carefully and to put their precise meaning to purpose. Consequently, when giving his lectures, he would have chosen his words professionally and with conscious intent. These words and phrases are all powerful, which in my mind relate to the spiritual nature of the human being, not the mental or physical levels.

Many people from cultures all over the world talk of our having a mind, body and spirit, with reference to these being fundamental components of us all, as human beings. Perhaps this is why Dr Wales, when transcribing Sutherland's words, chose at times to write some of these extraordinary terms with first letter capitalisation, to take their significance to a higher level for the reader. It is also intriguing that many cultures talk of the highest levels of spiritual growth as enlightenment or to become enlightened. Such a description indicates that the individual expresses an inner light to their consciousness, and perhaps why some people have described seeing a glowing 'light' around such individuals' physiology.

The prefix 'en' in English means: 'To cause (a person or thing) to be in the place, condition, or state of the stem' (Dictionary.com 2022), the stem being the end part of the word. Therefore, the word enlightened literally means 'to cause or place a person to be in the state of light'. By this definition, Dr Wales's first-hand observation of a golden glow developing around patients as Sutherland treated them literally describes a process of becoming enlightened, although probably only temporarily.

So, are we describing here the interchange point between physical, mental and spiritual within the physiology of the patient, and within the perception of the practitioner? I personally think so. However, we still need to be down to earth when discussing such phenomena. Therefore, let us look at the current science, and see if there could be any scientific verification for such occurrences.

SCIENCE AND PHYSIOLOGICAL PHOTOLUMINESCENCE

Could light be generated with the human physiology? Light as we are aware, travels faster than anything else we know. Light also illuminates matter around it. Could the physiology express `en-light-en-ment'? It is now being considered by some researchers that it is light which is the communication medium within our nervous system. 'This form of communication involves light; that neurons, indeed all living cells, can generate light and may use this to send messages to each other' (Moro *et al.* 2022). If as Moro implies, that all living cells produce light, then this may explain why under the treatment process Anne Wales and other observers perceived light emanating from the body of people when Sutherland was treating them.

Friz Popp, a biophysicist who was responsible for creating the term `biophotons' was fascinated by the concept of bio luminescence and undertook research into this concept:

`The phenomenon of ultraweak photon emission from living systems was further investigated in order to elucidate the physical properties of this radiation and its possible source. We obtained evidence that the light has a high degree of coherence because of (1) its photon count statistics, (2) its spectral distribution, (3) its decay behaviour after exposure to light illumination, and (4) its transparency through optically thick materials. (Popp et al 1984)

Popp found that light is a major controlling factor of the biological organism. Looking at more recent studies, Burgos and his team found that:

> Ultraweak Photo Emissions (UPE) are correlated only with intracellular signalling metabolic intermediates. These findings strongly support the notion that UPE is linked to intracellular metabolism. Another explanation for the results of our analysis of extracellular metabolites is that the time course of respiratory burst (measured up to 9,000 seconds) was too short for studying the flow of metabolites from the cytoplasm to the extracellular medium.
>
> In summary, we report a strong correlation between ultraweak photon emission intensity, nicotinamide adenine dinucleotide phosphate (NADPH) oxidase activity and intracellular metabolism. (Burgos et al. 2017)

NADPH in its reduced form is a chemical which has been found to be essential in the physiology, creating the vital forces which enable many of the chemical reactions occurring in the body:

Reduced nicotinamide adenine dinucleotide phosphate (NADPH) is an essential electron donor in all organisms. It provides the reducing power that drives numerous anabolic reactions, including those responsible for the biosynthesis of all major cell components and many products in biotechnology. (Spaans et al. 2015)

This finding and conclusion of Burgos, that a strong correlation occurs between ultraweak photon emission intensity and intracellular metabolism, is highly intriguing when we consider what would have been happening when Sutherland's students witnessed a light emission developing over his patients when treating them. This would imply that Sutherland, either consciously or not, was working at an intracellular level with his patients.

Miyamoto and his team wrote about ultraweak photon emission and studied the electronically excited states which are active in such physiological expressions:

> The chemistry behind the phenomenon of ultraweak photon emission has been the subject of considerable interest for decades. Great progress has been made on the understanding of the chemical generation of electronically excited states that are involved in these processes. Proposed mechanisms implicated the production of excited carbonyl species and singlet molecular oxygen in the mechanism of generation of chemiluminescence in biological systems. (Miyamoto et al. 2014)

When the experience of liquid light was described by Sutherland and Rollin Becker, this was at times of high potency expression within the patient. So, when reading Sutherland's and Becker's accounts, albeit in non-scientific terminology, they have a high correlation to these scientific descriptions.

Similarly, the 'chemical generation of electronically excited states', as described above by Miyamoto, again is fascinating for us as practitioners. For anyone who has experienced what we as practitioners call potency (and I am sure many of you have), the term 'electronically excited states' fits in perfectly with our palpatory experience. However, the palpatory experience of potency is not just a random excited state, nor is it a chaotic excited state, but a feeling of high 'coherence' of an 'electronically excited state' within the physiology, whilst deep therapeutic change occurs. Therefore, the combination of this phenomenon of 'ultraweak photon emission' alongside the 'electronically excited state', to my mind is a highly accurate description of the experiences had by practitioners who have experienced liquid light when treating patients (see practitioner experiences below).

Mae-Wen Ho has carried out much scientific work and written the book *The Rainbow and the Worm* on bioluminescence. I was fortunate enough to join her over lunch for a discussion when she came to speak at one of the Sutherland Cranial College of Osteopathy conferences in the UK. In one of her papers on bioluminescence, she states that:

> The organism is a dynamic liquid crystalline continuum with coherent motions on every scale. Evidence is presented that biological (interfascial) water, aligned and moving coherently with the macromolecular matrix, is integral to the liquid crystallinity of the organism;

and that the liquid crystalline continuum facilitates rapid intercommunication throughout the body, enabling it to function as a perfectly coherent whole.

> They give brilliant dynamic liquid crystal displays in colours of the rainbow. The colours depend on the coherent alignment of molecular dipoles in liquid crystal mesophases. (Ho *et al.* 2006)

Thus, from the above research papers, it can be seen that the body can and does emit light. Also, the physiology when expressing a liquid crystalline state emits, according to Ho, not only light but a 'rainbow' of colours. This adds further intrigue to this light phenomenon which some practitioners experience, as some practitioners have told me that when working they experience different colours in the physiology in different anatomical locations (see practitioner experiences below).

Ho did this research on a worm, not a highly complex organism like a human with a highly complex neural physiology, and with perhaps the potential to have a much greater and more powerful coherence, light coherence not being the same as light intensity. For an example of light coherence think of laser light compared with the light from a light bulb. They have totally different qualities and can be therefore put to very differing uses.

THE MITOCHONDRION

Let us consider an aspect of the physiology which we looked at in Chapter 18, the mitochondrion. The mitochondrion is the energy provider for cellular function, resulting in ATP formation. In the practical exercise for Chapter 18 one of the aspects we looked at was the mitochondrion. At the time of writing, I have taught this exercise to about 250 people during some of the courses I teach, taking the student to the mitochondrion within the cell. I make sure I do not inform the students what they may or may not experience during the practical, to ensure I do not influence what they feel.

After the practical, I ask for their experiences. Approximately 80 per cent or more of the students then report feeling a sense of bright (often white) light when taking their awareness to the mitochondrion, which was not there before they took their awareness to that structure. Having a high number of students expressing similar types of experiences when taking their awareness during the practical to the mitochondrion is way beyond coincidence, especially as none of the students had pre-expectations and with many saying that they thought they would not feel anything at all, before the practical started.

Could it be that when we are working at a coherent level of our practitioner awareness, at the same time feeling high levels of potency within the patient at the treatment table (such as described in many of the experiences listed below), the mitochondrion becomes more coherent and emits all light frequencies at the same time, and so emits bright white light? Could this be the 'liquid light' as described by Sutherland and Becker? Perhaps.

There has been much research undertaken on the benefits of meditation and brain wave coherence. For example, a 2016 paper by Tomljenović and colleagues showed:

> Changes in EEG patterns after meditation practice were found mostly in the theta band. An interaction effect was found on the left hemisphere ($p<0.10$). Theta power decreased on the left, but not on the right hemisphere. Increased theta coherence was found overall and in the central, temporal and occipital areas ($p<0.10$). Decrease in alpha power was found on channels T3 ($p<0.10$), O1 ($p<0.05$) and O2 ($p<0.10$). An interaction effect was found in the delta frequency band ($p<0.06$), too. A trend for power decreasing was found on the left, and a trend for power increasing on the right hemisphere. (Tomljenović *et al.* 2016)

Interestingly, the process of meditation allows the day-to-day consciousness of the individual to become significantly more settled and the person becomes more still within themselves, which has been demonstrated to result in a greater coherence of the physiology. When we work as practitioners, we prepare ourselves by centring, to allow our awareness to become more still and settled, in order to work to the best of our ability. Probably this too creates an increased coherence of the practitioner's consciousness, the feeling of being still and centred and clear-thinking within oneself. Perhaps over a period of years and gaining a repeated experience of being centred and still within one's own consciousness, and centred within one's physiology, will progress the development of experiencing refined consciousness and perception whilst working.

REFINED PERCEPTION

As practitioners we should not shy away from the potential of having such experiences when we treat our patients, nor dismiss such experiences of others. I call such experiences as those, 'refined perception'. Let us discuss this topic further as such experiences happen to very many cranial practitioners over a period of years (not weeks or months), and explore how it could occur.

When we first start cranial palpation, we must shift our palpation from efferent (what am I doing, feeling) to afferent sensing (how my is hand being moved by another's body tissues), in order to feel the flexion and extension of the involuntary mechanism (IVM). This is a major shift in our osteopathic palpation and perception and once gained, like riding a bicycle, is never lost (though it can go 'foggy' if not used regularly). Through regular practice we refine our perception to feel more delicate anatomical tissues. We learn how to feel the IVM in membranes, not just bone tissues, and we progress to feeling the cerebrospinal fluids and body fluids. We may then progress, perhaps on our second or third training course, to feeling the brain as a tissue and so on.

By practising the exercises in this this book, you will find yourself having explored and gained afferent feedback of more and more refined tissues and fluids, e.g., the endosteum of the bone (Chapter 5), the extracellular fluid (Chapter 6), the arachnoid and pia (Chapter 7), the pericardium (Chapter 10), the eye (Chapter 11), anatomical areas within the brain (Chapter 12), and even going inside the cell wall (Chapter 18).

As our perception refines, so we gradually open our awareness to ever finer levels of the physiology. We are doing this through the sense of touch. However, all of our senses can also become refined. We have a phrase in the English language (and this is probably true for other languages): 'That does not smell right!', referring to a situation or something someone said, not a real unpleasant nasal smell. You cannot quite explain why, but you get the insight that something is not right, that things don't add up. However, maybe we are smelling it!

> Humans can smell fear and disgust, and emotions are contagious, according to a new study. The findings, published in the *Journal of Psychological Science*, suggest that humans communicate via smell just like other animals:
>
> 'These findings are contrary to the commonly accepted assumption that human communication runs exclusively via language or visual channels,' write Gün Semin and colleagues from Utrecht University in the Netherlands. (Ghose 2012)

Dogs can be trained to tell when someone with epilepsy is about to have a seizure. Dogs can also detect when a diabetic person needs to take their medication. I once treated a patient (a home visit) whose dog, a springer spaniel, would sit next to me when treating his owner. The dog would nudge my elbow and whimper when I shifted just my mental awareness (no body movement)

1 cm from 'near' to 'in' the key area of severe pain in her body!

When we are in fear we sweat more and secrete different chemicals from our skin. Dogs (and probably other animals) can smell or sense pain, fear and changes in electrical activity. Animals in the African savannah will suddenly behave very differently when one spots a top predator. Those that were not within seeing distance can then react very quickly, partly by sound but also by smelling fear on the wind.

As osteopaths, we develop a very highly refined perception of touch. Is it that our nerve endings in our fingers become more sensitive? Is it that our nerve fibres from our upper extremities get better at sending the signals? I doubt it. I consider it most likely that it is our brain sensory input to our conscious awareness that changes over time.

The thalamus in the brain has now been demonstrated to be the region which filters what gets sent to the conscious mind: 'The thalamic reticular nucleus (TRN), the major source of thalamic inhibition, regulates thalamocortical interactions that are critical for sensory processing, attention and cognition' (Li *et al.* 2020).

There is also the possibility that the individual sensory nuclei in addition to the thalamus, e.g., the visual and sensory cortices, also get refined as our osteopathic experience increases. Therefore, I would like to postulate that these central nervous system refinements, probably along with others not yet understood, open our osteopathic perceptions to subtle sensory information such as light fields, smells and tactile experiences that we could not previously experience.

We all know that some people have narrow vision and only see what they want to see and not the big picture; they lack peripheral vision. This term can be referring to a psychological narrow vision but can also refer to the purely visual experience, the person not noticing people or things away from their main focal area. As practitioners, not only are we refining our tactile/afferent sensing abilities, but we are also becoming more adept at working with our peripheral vision in addition to our focal vision.

When palpating the physiology of our patients, we let our awareness settle on the health, the stillness within the patient, in addition to the areas of ill health or mechanical disturbance. In order to palpate the stillness within our patients, we too, as practitioners have to allow our own awareness to settle to a more still and refined level. In my considered opinion, I think that perhaps it is this experience of allowing our own awareness to settle to increasing levels of still-ness within ourselves which results in a minute level of expansion of our consciousness to occur. I consider this to be the process of how such experiences, over years and years of repetition, culminate in the practitioner gaining refined perception whilst working, as the awareness develops the neural circuitry to then perceive such levels of the human physiology.

When I spoke to many practitioners about their experiences of refined perception whilst treating, they too agreed on this being the mech-anism of how such experiences seem to develop with increasing years of being a practitioner. Not everyone finds their sensory refinement is the same (see the refined perception feedback examples below). Some people see liquid light but in different ways and manners from others. Some practitioners get a shift in their palpatory perception at times when working as if they somehow feel a level which they describe as being 'beyond anatomy' after having felt highly specific anatomical detail. Some people say they see colours in the physiology. We are all unique and so our refined perception also expresses our individuality. A number of practitioners said they do not see liquid light, but then said they do perceive areas of 'darkness' within some patients' physiology (this being nothing to do with the patient's skin colour). This, to my mind, meant they were seeing the lack of light within tissues in those areas.

Many practitioners have said that they some-times get such experiences and other times not. Feelings of fatigue and tiredness are expressions of dulled awareness and so are likely to limit such experiences. However, palpation is a two-way process, as we are palpating the living physiol-ogy of our patients. Maybe, the phenomenon of refined perception depends on both the state of the practitioner and that of the patient's physiol-ogy, during any specific treatment session.

FURTHER THOUGHTS ON DIVIDED AWARENESS

As was discussed and utilised in Chapter 17, we use divided awareness at times when working. In such circumstances you have one part of your attention on one aspect of the physiology and another part of your awareness on another region or aspect. Or, you may have your attention on the whole physiology at the same time as a part, giving each equal levels of your attention. These skills usually develop gradually over a period of time, by culturing and training the mind to work in a special manner. This training and culturing of the brain will (like learning any other skill) develop new neural pathways as this higher ability grows. Divided awareness is not the same as refined perception. However, its usage by a practitioner tends to occur and be used more as their cranial career progresses. Perhaps the developing ability to use differing parts of awareness consciously at the same time adds to the coherence and the ability to experience aspects of refined perception.

As has been implied above, the descriptions and words chosen by Still, Sutherland and Becker such as liquid light, highest known element, sea around us, fluid within a fluid, etc., are all descriptors pertaining to that part of us which is spirit, not mind or body. Some very experienced practitioners from the UK that I talked to about their experiences (see below) said that to use or talk about the terms spirit or spiritual was considered an absolute 'no-no' and likely to send the profession back many years, to the dark ages. However, they then continued to encourage me to talk about this, saying it was high time that these spiritual aspects were discussed openly, within the profession.

Interestingly, Kok Weng Lim, a UK practitioner and friend, told me about a 2010 Cranial Academy Conference he attended in the USA, which was entitled 'SPIRIT and MATTER: Osteopathic Reflections on Function, Fluid and Fascia', directed by Dr Paul Lee. So quite clearly using the term spirit has been able to be discussed at national conference level for many years now, in the USA. This conference information (thank you to Kok Weng Lim) gave me vindication that including this chapter in the book was appropriate.

I would like to finish this chapter with a quote from Peter Armitage, who wrote a paper entitled 'Experiencing stillness'. Peter kindly gave me a copy of this paper in order that I can quote from it:

> Where can we find the help to progress? In Stillness itself. If we have left even a little room for ignorance, for 'not-knowing-yet', it allows space in our mind where the Potency, which I consider as the agent of Stillness, can emerge and make knowledge available to us. If we are convinced that we already know, there is no such space.
>
> We look from the heart of our stillness into the heart of stillness in our patient.
>
> When I was willing to let go of the need to locate, to pin down, to define, to compare (which generally made me anxious anyway) I found awareness of a different order altogether: of Stillness which is deep peace, perfect and unchanging; of Health entire, untouched, unharmed, invulnerable. Full of Love, it has the quality of transcendence, of being independent of any physical structure whatever, beyond space and time and distinct from the universe. (Armitage 2018)

THE EXPERIENCES OF OSTEOPATHS

As the author, I did not want to write only about my own experiences of liquid light during treatment, and so I contacted a number of very highly experienced practitioners and fellow teachers of Sutherland's approach. The responses below have been transcribed exactly as spoken to me by the practitioner. I wished to get experiences from osteopaths all over the world, not just the UK; the practitioners who kindly gave their experiences are from Australia, Finland, Germany, Italy, New Zealand, Switzerland, the UK and the USA.

I have quoted their experiences but have kept them anonymous, the reason being that I would not wish the reader to give higher importance to one person's experience than another just because they were a famous teacher, and the other not. Some responses were just a few sentences and others were a longer conversation and therefore a longer quote. Some people replied, humbly saying that their experience was not significant or not what I was seeking, and then sent me a beautiful expression of what they experience.

I hope you find these experiences of fellow osteopaths interesting, and maybe some of them are similar to your own. Do always remember that whatever you experience during a treatment session, it is your genuine, and thus an important, experience. As long as the experience came without your ego taking supremacy at that moment,

I suggest you acknowledge that it happened and trust the information or the inspiration, which may have occurred as a consequence. Perhaps you may wish to keep a diary of your osteopathic experiences of refined perception.

These are just experiences from practitioners; they are not trying to score points for the best experience.

Practitioner experiences of refined perception

'When doing a CV4 I get a sense of potency down the midline. The vector looks as if liquid light and an electrical current within that water lights up, like moonlight arising and illuminating the shape of the water. Sometimes I see colours in areas of the patient's body, sometimes as darkness, etc. Relaxing our attention away from intellectual thought, our senses expand to see, hear, feel, smell, things not normally available to our awareness or perception.'

'Sometimes you seem to know when a treatment is finished when the quality of the air in the room and the light in the room changes. The air seems to sparkle or get a different tint, more like silvery gold and there seems to be more energy. I feel more awake as well. Lymphatics sometimes show up as light when treated.'

'The time I have really had that overriding feeling of liquid light is when I have been treating a very subdued baby who has had a birth hypoxia or similar, that has rendered the CNS impotent and the whole involuntary mechanism is hankered and tethered down. When I have approached the third ventricle and it has lit up, there is always a feeling of liquid light, the baby usually has this other-worldly smile and the mother recognises an awakening of her child. It is a truly magical moment. It also seems that development then takes off better even if it is hampered by limitations of brain damage.'

'I am able to experience liquid light at times.'

'I'm simply in awe when liquid light happens to come into my perception. It gives me a soothing feeling of "what appeared to be complicated actually is simple" and "everything is all right".'

'Sometimes when I am treating, I feel like my vision is a bit fuzzy or the room seems a bit dim. Then suddenly it feels like the sun has come out and everything seems brighter and clearer. At first I thought that the sun had literally come out from behind the cloud, but then I sensed that there had been a shift in the patient and I hypothesised that I had somehow replicated this within myself. It's perhaps like the shift in tissues after a CV4 but I haven't necessarily (or at least not intentionally) performed a classic CV4.'

'Since I started to study the senses in the child, I start to imagine each of them in their own physiology. I tried to feel their function as well their anatomy. For example, the vision activation due to the light passing through the eyes and deeper in the brain and the nervous system. So, I tried to do the same with the liquid fluids, blood and lymph. If I look to the entire vascular system, some sparkling can appear from far away and light up the full body. The feeling I have is a general increase of the light, potency, temperature and vitality of the entire body. I can't separate the feelings.

The first time I saw the light was in Africa more than 15 years ago working with people near to death. In some cases, I felt the light moving away from them before the death.

In some situations after a surgery, I felt the vitality and light coming in. Children born sick have low potency and thin light in the eyes. Healthy children have brighter light, in the eyes and the liquid.'

'I do not perceive as light but do get a sense of

refined touch, like a refined sight, touch, smell, etc. when treating my patients.'

'Every day there are at least three new expressions of Light. The Liquid Light is a sweet, warm, honey-like substance. The newborn expresses a constant transparent filtered golden/orange light that extends outwards and feels like grace. If neutral is well established in a person, then Light occurs as a central fire in the third ventricle and spreads downwards through the central canal.'

'A 63-year-old patient had issues when she was a newborn baby. As I was working on her birth issues, light filled the room and her tissues, as if light was working through her whole body.'

'White floating as if coming from somewhere within the patient, could be light, like a small typhoon that comes to the patient, very "alive". Sometimes it's like a fog over the patient that turns to rain of either silver or golden colour.'

'I remember an early experience, back in the 1980s, some months after doing my first Osteopathy in the Cranial Field course. I do not recollect any mention of the term liquid light on the course, and my palpatory skills were basic! I was seated at the head, aiming to release the occiput and condylar parts, using the principle of Balanced Ligamentous Tension, with added fluid drive from foot dorsiflexion. I remember a shaft of light, travelling up the spinal cord from the sacrum, or possibly the coccyx, in a slight spiral, at speed, to the condylar parts, connecting the two. There are other occasions since, when I have the sense that something has "happened"; and I sometimes see colours in a person's energy field, but I have never repeated that early experience.'

'I experience a huge door with liquid bright light, it feels like the ocean itself, the potency of the ocean in the body, beyond the fluid filling the room. When the change in perception happens, it will be going on not just in the body. It is like a doorway from the body to wholeness.

Wisdom comes to me and Light spreads (when working with fluids, lateral fluctuation) through the body and through the room. If you change your perception, of course you can see more clearly where the fluid wants to go, the Master Mechanic. Perception shifts to perceive what is needed in the treatment at that moment.'

'This was an extreme experience when on an osteopathic course, looking at the heart and head electromagnetic fields at the same time. It was like an explosion of light above the patient and myself, the practitioner. It was like a firework all over the place, then her body started to expand, and the Long Tide came up and it was really powerful, very beautiful. At the time this occurred it was the end of the course, I felt very connected, a very special feeling within myself. I felt very centred, less of my own body pains in my own spine. It was easy to get into this "different space", not thinking, just "being there".

Since...especially when working on vascular system, I get a perception of light flares. Sometimes I get perception of light in the tissues. Now I start working with this light, going into a more deeply centred, meditative state and then I feel my own body expanding, and I let happen what has to happen for that person. You can feel the light, the expansion, the cellular expansion, not on structure any more, as if the body does not exist any more.'

'I get experiences of peace and calm, being breathed in the body of a child, her body not being separate from the rest of the universe (when treating a child with teething issues).

Another experience can happen when I ask myself, "Can I see some light? Can I see a flame or a sense of 'ignition'?" Tied in with a sense of ignition styles in the 3rd or 4th ventricle.

Also fire or flame when treating patients, a sense of where fire or heat, where the Tide is working.

This is the same phenomenon as Liquid Light but different perception of it. It was like a glimpse of a fish under the water, a sliver of something, fish/whale, like a movement of quicksilver. A sense of knowing, "That was the treatment." It was having senses of quicksilver or the sun rising up, everything being filled with light. Like a room of being warmth, light and heat.'

'Some "knockout moments" with potency especially with neonates and when working on 23-week-old premature babies. Somewhere I feel a spark which is often in the central nervous system. It's like a spot in that darkness. I then identify the disparity in the expression and acknowledge it. I let the baby feel and acknowledge it. Then letting the baby feel where it wasn't and then soft potency creeps through. Sometimes it just gets bigger and outside the body. It's as if the body says I like that feeling and I want it everywhere. I wasn't doing anything, no fluid drives no CV4, just acknowledging, and something will happen. This was my biggest experience of shift of potency.

When I'm working, I am focussed but at the same time slightly disengaged. Quite a lot of the time I'm working at a level which I call "not anatomy" but still clear and sharp, not sleepy or "zoned out". It's like being defocussed, like looking at a 3D picture. I'm empathising with tissues or "beyond that", beyond normal physiology. It's like feeling something "way beyond" palpation, like being on another dimension.

Definitely have had experiences of "a bit dark" in a part of the body.

Whilst working on an 18-month-old child, whilst working "four hands" with a colleague, I was on the sacrum and suddenly I got hit by tingling occurring all over his body. Then there was a massive electrical charge, my hair stood up and I felt an immense surge of warmth of unconditional love. The whole body filled with incredible sensation of heat and love, tears came to my eyes.'

'When treating I feel lots of different levels. I can be aware of ligaments, fluids, etc., i.e., anatomy based, also emotions of different qualities. It's not just focussing on what you see, but sometimes liquid, light or like sky behind the clouds.

I don't see pictures but I do sense things. Sometimes I feel that as a light or something comes into balance. It's a different quality of energy, very relaxing, like an inner sunbathing compared to a storm. It makes me feel loved or blessed, as if you are not on your own. It's very warm and comforting. If I don't get over focussed there is something that is allowing change or allowing movement. Or allowing flow. When I can think about it, it feels very restful.

Sometimes it is about perception. I can be focussed on a point of balance with the tissues or I can focus on what allows that movement. Sometimes, it feels like there is a quality within that which you could call "finer", a finer frequency. I don't feel it all the time, sometimes I just feel "the sludge" of inertia, despair or whatever.

Over the years through work on myself, my attention has freed itself, allowing me to go into a different state of consciousness, and so be aware of different things, like a freeing of my attention, so there is less interference. It's as if my subtle senses are now free.

I do see areas that are dark, but also black, syrupy "gloop" like tar, sometimes sticky.

Occasionally I have experiences of the room becoming much brighter, and sometimes I also get experiences of "stillness enveloping the room" when working on courses. I sometimes experience something similar with a client and then something appears, an energy appears. A silence comes and descends, and when it has finished its work, it disappears.

Had one patient who felt "all this light coming in", that I didn't feel but she did.

Something happens and you feel more humble and safer. Then something internally relaxes and there is a change in your own state. Patients sometimes at these moments fall asleep or feel light within, etc., an experience that is not their normal.'

'I had this experience when newly qualified and working with a very experienced practitioner, our working "four hands": I felt extraordinary clouds of light, like the Aurora Borealis occurring, like clouds of light going through the tissues.

I'm aware when there is no light, it's like a grey cardboard box, no light, nothing there. Experiencing a lack of light. I suppose in my treatment, I'm quite visual, so I work with that sense of light. It's like the "tour of the minnow", there is like a spotlight that I follow. It's as if something is becoming illuminated and then that's what I work with.

Yes, the sun coming out from behind the clouds type of experience, that's an experience I am familiar with.

Occasionally, I experience a kind of "choppy light" not integrated or coherent light, it can then feel like a wet or dry choppy sea, or feeling like very dry crackling when standing under a dry electricity pylon when it is crackling.

I do experience changes within me. It happens as a transformational light in my system and another level of perception happens. This is nonlinear. We each need to go through our own process of purification.

When such experiences occur, I know it's true. I get an experience, then I know the truth of it. It's as if I'm on the edge of consciousness. When working, it seems important to illuminate the perception without defining it in any way because everyone's experience is so different.'

'When I treat there seems to be a different understanding compared to ordinary life. Things become clear about things I'm trying to understand.

Within me, I get a sense of a fluid uplift that defies gravity, and it has a quality of light golden glow.

I get a feeling of that quality of light, that glow and beauty. It is the difference between that form of clay and the living, it gives me sense of the life quality. When I take my body and remove the "clay" and what remains is the life-ness like a golden sunlight. A non-material light. I don't see it with my eyes, but I feel it with an inner eye. A quality of stillness and knowing.

When I am treating patients, it is as if some part of me is defocussed along with being focussed at the same time. It's like another level of consciousness comes across us as practitioners at a certain level when in treatment. A prayerful space. We are tuning into that level of what Sutherland describes as the Master Mechanic.

If you look at the tiny spaces, it's like you go through the looking glass. You then perceive many clues to opening your awareness. Then to that space between the cells, possibly subatomic particles? That space between is what is nourishing creation. That's what makes us not a lump of clay!

To me it has a lot to do with the consciousness of the heart. And the opening of the heart, I feel like my awareness is in my heart more than my brain, and the opening of the heart, the awareness that I'm here, I'm me and the patient, they're them, and they have got everything they need within their system. Somehow in the acknowledgement of my separate nature and their separate nature, there becomes paradoxically a sense of union.

When I ask the tissues how they would like to be held, I find the body takes me, moves my hands, and takes me to match the compression, "this is the way I am" and makes it happen. I'm then matching in my hands, my heart and my awareness.'

'Sometimes I see colours in my mind's eye, not my physical eyes. I do get experiences of a Shift Point during treatment, to a state of Being. When this happens, I can go there but can't invite yourself there. I have to allow it to happen.

I once had an experience on working on sacrum prone, the whole thing just "came alive".

I do get feelings that something from the horizon washes through me, enabling me to be able to perceive "something" from outside that washes through us, and sustains us.'

'When teaching as a practical tutor, I can see, feel, interact without touching. I find that a sense of "feeling the whole room" also happens from the same state. Sometimes it is as if I'm on a potency experience journey. There are points where I become more afferent, and no longer "in the way of these things happening".'

'When teaching, I get experiences of being in the room, knowing where the mechanism is not functioning properly, without looking nor touching.

Sometimes I see liquid light in the spinal column and throughout. I do not see colours except for sometimes "golden light" and sometimes "blackness" in or around the patient.

These types of experiences happen when I'm in a state of stillness, but do not happen if I'm not so healthy.

Sometimes I feel an energetic shift within the patient, as if that change in energy goes through myself.

I feel as if I'm working at a spiritual or quantum-mechanical level rather than the level of mechanical "linear" anatomy.'

'I perceive on different levels of perception. I always have to be very "in my body", very grounded and anatomy focussed. It is like when you are not "at home" then the "mail cannot be read". Then when I have a deep level of the anatomy it is as if the anatomy lets go and I then start to get these perceptions as if beyond the anatomy. Sometimes the body lights up. Sometimes it is as if a light shines in a particular place, particular direction. I call it a breadcrumb of a light trail, showing me where the potency will be treating. When the treatment has finished in that location, the light moves to somewhere else. This continues until the treatment has finished.

It is as if we are "given" this information, we do not "go and find it".

At such times I feel more than just me, no separation between me and everything else.'

'I find myself entering a state of calm solemnity, a peaceful state within as if that is my starting point. I get an experience of what I call a non-compressible substance which moves within me, like a fluid. I call it love, or the vital principal or a divine presence. This within me then connects to the same level within the patient. I find it very important to acknowledge the anatomy at a deep detailed level first to get a clear intellectual understanding of the diagnosis. Somehow this makes these deeper levels of awareness happen more easily.'

'I attain a phase where I perceive a change in the room, the patient, the tissues, and myself. I can perceive this on one, two, three or all four levels at the same time. I don't know what makes me perceive it, it just comes to me. This is either a conscious perception or unconscious, whether I can be aware of it or not.

When I experience a change in the patient's tissues it is in my consciousness not my hands, and then I experience a change in the luminosity in the patient. I get a sense that it is more than "just me" working in the patient, as at such times, liquid light arrives which mixes and disperses within the patient. It's like seeing coffee in a glass jug and then seeing milk being poured into the coffee and seeing the milk mix, but one liquid has far more energy than the other.

Sometimes I get a sense of immediate light appearing within the patient, like a light switch being turned on. Patients can sometimes feel this dramatic event, saying, "I felt that."

Such experiences are as if my individual consciousness identifies with me, the room and the patient. In those moments, the interaction of consciousness and physical form of the world synchronise and change. I just wait, whilst very awake in my head and body, but my thoughts become quiescent and "the other" level of consciousness can take over.'

'I do find I can experience a level where I can augment potency as a deliberate procedure. To do that I have to be in the right place: the sea around us, the long tide, the space around the patient and around me. At the end point some patients see colours but I never see light nor colour, though I do see darkness. I feel at the end that the patient is "plugged into" the biosphere, more transparent, some of their form dissolves. I often feel the autonomics more than the Tide. I frequently get to a state where my mind shifts to a different state allowing myself to be "taken somewhere" and I'm not in charge.'

'I get experiences of liquid light when the treatment goes systemic, a sense of global engagement. It's like an effervescent sensation in the tissues, a luminosity. There becomes a sense of homogeneity, the fractionisation dissolves. If the de-fractionisation occurs locally, it creates a local activation of the fluids, and the liquid light occurs there.

Within myself I feel a sense of relationship to the natural world, a heightened state of awareness, like the Sea Around Us is constantly perceivable.'

'I get to a point of "beyond anatomy" which changes the state of what I am identifying, a realm of unity, truth, peace, harmony, oneness, a state of God. Just to say, I don't mind using that word!

I feel that potency is an emissary of stillness.

To stay with the stillness and I will be shown what has to be done.

I feel that the terms: "liquid light", "fluid within a fluid", "transmutation", "breath of life", "something that is invisible", "sea around us", are all signposts that Sutherland and Becker were giving us, for our professional journey. They did not hold back on using such very specific spiritual phrases, because they were used for our signposting benefit.

It was my experience in the early years of practice that the consistent use of the fulcrum, which represents a functioning point of stillness, along with the "heart-to-heart" concept would often take me during treatments to what I described as a "region beyond anatomy". All the anatomical-physiological detail I had carefully marshalled and struggled to contain would vanish, in favour of boundless space.'

'I feel a softening of my eyes, and then a sense of stillness, in or above, my sternum that opens out, and I'm no longer directing something. It's a sense of expanding, of opening and the smaller becoming bigger. I'm not the one doing it. I'm the one that is not doing anything. During this time my palms tingle and I feel a body warmth. I absolutely get this feeling that the anatomy disappears, and that I'm holding the field not a temporal bone, for example. I'm not holding it, I'm just in it. A sense of potential, full of something.

I get a very common feeling of being at one with my patients as if there is no difference, the same, and at one with nature and my surroundings, a sense of "unity". If I hear a dog barking when in this state, I wonder why I am barking!'

'I was treating a teenage girl who had just had a severe impact to her tarsus from someone who accidently trod fully on her bare foot, whilst he was wearing heavy boots. Whilst waiting for the ambulance to arrive, I held her foot. After a while I had a sense of violet light coming from the foot. A short while later, I then felt a dramatic flash of white light from the foot and felt a dramatic tissue quality change. The girl then said she felt a sudden change and now no pain. Then the ambulance arrived to take her to the hospital and after a wait, she had an X-ray taken. When she returned to the event where I was attending, she said the hospital could not see any evidence of a fracture.

When I see gold light it seems to happen when there is a change happening within the heart and when I feel a change in the ovaries, I see magenta light.'

'Sometimes I see a sense of golden light develop over the whole patient during a treatment. Commonly I see or feel "dark areas" in my patients. Most patients after my having made an accurate, fine-level tissue diagnosis, the anatomy that I have been very conscious of just disappears and I feel that I am working at a level "beyond anatomy" as if more at the quantum mechanical level. During such times I feel very clear and aware within myself, and a sense of oneness or unity with the patient and my surroundings.'

Contributors are listed in alphabetical order below (not by quote order, which are presented in order of when I spoke to the person):

Peter Armitage, Clare Ballard, Luca Bregant, Karen Carol, Matthew Carratu, Giles Cleghorn, Christine Conroy, David Douglas-Mort, Richard Feeley, Maxwell Fraval, Nicholas Gossett, Philip Hartnol, Shawna Higgins, Jim Jealous, Sandra Kaspar, Robert Paul Lee, Kok Weng Lim, Guglielmo Lo Giudice, Maire Maine, Anne Mamok, Connie Mansuetto, Timothy Marris (author), Simone Odermatt, Hilary Percival, Mark Rosen, Dorothy Smith, Daniella Steoffin, Pekka Taipale, Susan Turner, Joyce Vetterlein, Mark Wilson.

REFERENCES

Armitage, P., 2018. Experiencing stillness. Draft. Expanded and reprinted as Armitage, P., 2019. *Experiencing stillness. Sutherland Cranial College of Osteopathy Magazine.* 41(Summer): 20–21.

Burgos, R.C.R., Schoeman, J.C., Winden, L.J.V., *et al.*, 2017. Ultra-weak photon emission as a dynamic tool for monitoring oxidative stress metabolism. *Scientific Reports.* 7(1): 1229. Available from: https://doi.org/10.1038/s41598-017-01229-x.

Cambridge Dictionary, 2022. Potency. Available from: https://dictionary.cambridge.org/dictionary/english/potency.

Dictionary.com, 2022. En. https://www.dictionary.com/browse/en.

Ghose, T., 2012. Humans can smell fear – and it's contagious. NBC News. Available from: https://www.nbcnews.com/health/body-odd/humans-can-smell-fear-its-contagious-flna1c6927562.

Ho, M.W., *et al.*, 2006. The liquid crystalline organism and biological water. In: Pollack, G.H., Cameron, I.L., & Wheatley, D.N., eds. *Water and the Cell.* Dordrecht: Springer. Available from: https://doi.org/10.1007/1-4020-4927-7_10.

Li, Y., Lopez-Huerta, V.G., Adiconis, X., *et al.*, 2020. Distinct subnetworks of the thalamic reticular nucleus. *Nature.* 583: 819–824. Available from: https://doi.org/10.1038/s41586-020-2504-5.

Miyamoto, S., Martinez, G.R., Medeiros, M.H.G., & Di Mascio, P., 2014. Singlet molecular oxygen generated by biological hydroperoxides. *Journal of Photochemistry and Photobiology B: Biology.* 139: 24–33. Available from: https://doi.org/10.1016/j.jphotobiol.2014.03.028.

Moro, C., Liebert, A., Hamilton, C., *et al.*, 2022. The code of light: do neurons generate light to communicate and repair? *Neural Regeneration Research.* 17(6): 1251–1252. Available from: https://doi.org/10.4103/1673-5374.327332.

Popp, F A et al. "Biophoton emission. New evidence for coherence and DNA as source." *Cell biophysics* vol. 6,1 (1984) [Online]. [2 May 2023] Extract available from https://pubmed.ncbi.nlm.nih.gov/6204761.

Spaans, S.K., Weusthuis, R.A., van der Oost, J., & Kengen, S.W., 2015. NADPH-generating systems in bacteria and archaea. *Frontiers in Microbiology.* 6: 742. Available from: https://doi.org/10.3389/fmicb.2015.00742.

Sutherland, W.G., 1967. Tour of the minnow. In: Wales, A.L., ed. *Contributions of Thought: Collected Writings of William Garner Sutherland 1914–1954.* Kansas City, MO: Sutherland Cranial Teaching Foundation, p. 243.

Sutherland, W.G., & Wales, A.L., eds., 1990. *Teachings in the Science of Osteopathy.* Portland, OR: Rudra Press, pp. 227–232.

Tomljenović, H., Begić, D., & Maštrović, Z., 2016. Changes in trait brainwave power and coherence, state and trait anxiety after three-month transcendental meditation (TM) practice. *Psychiatria Danubina.* 28(1): 63–72. Available from: https://pubmed.ncbi.nlm.nih.gov/26938824/

Wales, A., 1980. Conversation with Timothy Marris during Sutherland Cranial Teaching Foundation Training course, London. 20 September.

CHAPTER 20

Conclusion

YOUR INNER JOURNEY AND DEEPENING CENTRING

I hope you have enjoyed your inner osteopathic journey as you read and participated in the practical exercises of this book, and in your own inner journey of becoming more profoundly centred when palpating and treating the physiology.

This inner process of deepening your centring ability and experience is key to allowing your palpation to become more profound, and consequently your diagnoses to be more profound and accurate. As a result, your skill in easing patients' symptoms will increase, and you will also be able to address much more profound aspects underlying their symptoms. It is the reduction of underlying issues which helps prevent patients' symptoms returning. It is the resolution of underlying mechanical tensions within the physiology which makes osteopathy stand apart from other branches of medicine.

REVIEW AND SUMMARY

In Part 1, you were shown the best way to use this book: that of reading each chapter in turn and not jumping ahead to what you thought would be the most interesting chapters. If you followed this guidance, then you will have gained far more than if you did skip chapters. We then looked at your inner perception and the osteopathic toolbox; this focussed on how to centre ourselves and what we keep in the toolbox and take to any treatment table. Part 1 concluded with a discussion of diagnosis and palpation of fluids, to prepare ourselves for Part 2.

In Part 2, having discussed ourselves as the practitioner, we moved on to exploring our patients' tissues through chapters on bone, fascia and cells, cerebrospinal fluid and meninges, limbs and spine, abdomen and pelvis, thorax, cranial nerves, brain, and hormonal systems. Hopefully these chapters and the associated exercises will have deepened your experience of each of these topics when treating your patients.

In Part 3, we progressed further to look at the body in new ways at deeper, inner levels. I introduced the topic of working with babies and children as this is a very rewarding field for osteopaths. If you have not yet undertaken a course on paediatric osteopathy, I strongly recommend such a course. We also looked at the fourth dimension and how to use this in our osteopathic work. The enormous subject of mind and emotions had to have a chapter to itself, and Part 3 was the correct placement for such a powerful topic.

The inter-tissue relationships chapter may have opened your eyes and palpation to new possibilities for a deeper inner understanding of our patients. The progression inside the cell to explore cellular consciousness again may be a new experience for you, but hopefully it will open your awareness to new diagnostic possibilities. I felt compelled to finish this book by discussing refined perception from a scientific perspective, instead of dismissing the topic altogether. Having discussed such experiences with colleagues, I now feel validated in including this topic.

To summarise, this book has been about your journey as a practitioner to experience new levels of the physiology. At the same time, hopefully, you will have experienced deeper and more profound levels of yourself, from becoming more centred, both as a person and as a practitioner. If so, then it will have allowed you to assess and diagnose more profoundly and to treat areas which perhaps are new to you. It has hopefully made you realise that there is much more to osteopathy than just treating muscles and joints (if that is how you worked before), and that the scope for osteopathy to help your patients is far greater than you previously considered.

As has been mentioned earlier in the book, we do need to work in harmony and alongside our medical colleagues, as often conventional medical treatment is very important too, for the wellbeing of our patients. However, we as osteopaths can assist and help the physiology alongside such medical treatments. If in contact with the patient's general practitioner, do keep your diagnoses simple and at a level which they can accept, coming from an osteopathic practitioner. Remember, most medical practitioners think that osteopaths only work on the musculoskeletal system. Consequently, do not give our medical colleagues diagnoses at the levels sometimes explained in this book: give your findings and diagnoses based on their comprehension, not that of an advanced-level osteopath.

So, having completed the book, what should you do next? First of all, continue with your regular centring, if you had not been doing so previously. Second, let what you have gained from reading this book and practising the exercises change the way you work: my aim for this book is not to intellectualise physiology, but to present a living palpatory experience that you can take to your clinical setting, with patients. Third, be open to working on new levels within your patient's physiology. This will result in a more profound diagnosis and treatment plan, and thereby help your patients to a higher degree.

I would love to hear of your experiences, thoughts, or learnings from reading this book and participating in the practical sessions. My email is: tim.marris@osteopathashford.com.

With attending courses, working with similarly trained colleagues, and self-study, I learned more deeply about the roles of the circulatory (arterial, venous and lymphatic) systems. Through this learning, I gained an understanding of how as osteopaths we can directly influence these vessels and how to improve the blood flow and drainage from their target tissues. I was not able in this book to go into the depth required on these topics, and I warmly recommend the reader to attend a course on the 'Rule of the Artery' or 'The Circulation', if you get the opportunity.

I would like to leave you with these final words: you never finish learning about the physiology, never finish progressing in your palpation skills, and never finish deepening your inner stillness when working on patients, or in your life as a whole.

Subject Index

Author Index